HAIR AND SCALP DISORDERS

Edited by **Zekayi Kutlubay**
and **Server Serdaroglu**

Hair and Scalp Disorders
http://dx.doi.org/10.5772/63002
Edited by Zekayi Kutlubay and Server Serdaroglu

Contributors

Safvet Örs, Anastasia Nesterova, Anton Yuryev, Selda Pelin Kartal, Ayse Serap Karadag, Emin Ozlu, Murat Küçüktaş, Arzu Kilic, Melike Kibar, Serap Gunes Bilgili, Goknur Ozaydin Yavuz, Ibrahim Halil Yavuz, Shin-Ichi Osada, Ekaterina Vorotelyak, Ekaterina Kalabusheva, Vasily Terskikh, Elina Chermnykh, Khitam Al-Refu, Burhan Engin, Eduard Vsevolodov, Hilal Gokalp, Tugba Kevser Uzuncakmak, Filiz Cebeci, Melek Aslan Kayıran, Burak Tekin, Gurkan Yardimci, Filiz Canpolat, Bilgen Erdoğan, Zekayi Kutlubay

Published by InTech

Janeza Trdine 9, 51000 Rijeka, Croatia

Publishing Process Manager Romina Skomersic
Technical Editor SPi Global
Cover InTech Design team

First published April, 2017
Printed in Croatia
Legal deposit, Croatia: National and University Library in Zagreb

Additional hard copies can be obtained from orders@intechopen.com

Hair and Scalp Disorders, Edited by Zekayi Kutlubay and Server Serdaroglu
p. cm.
Print ISBN 978-953-51-3097-0
Online ISBN 978-953-51-3098-7

For EU product safety concerns:
IN TECH d.o.o., Prolaz Marije Krucifikse Kozulić 3, 51000 Rijeka, Croatia,
info@intechopen.com or visit our website at intechopen.com.

Meet the editors

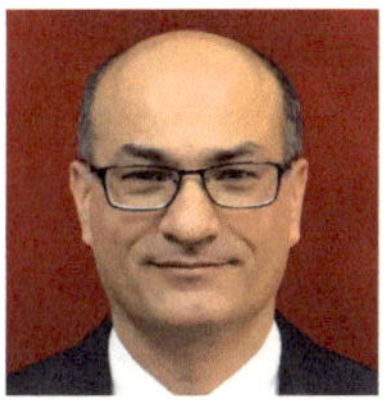

Zekayi Kutlubay, MD, is a chief physician of Istanbul University Cerrahpasa Medical Faculty Hospital. He is also an associate professor in the Department of Dermatology at Istanbul University Cerrahpasa Medical Faculty in Turkey. He has coauthored over 40 publications and supervised several master, doctoral, and postdoctoral students. His actual research interests are focused on psoriasis, pediatric dermatology, autoimmune bullous diseases, urticaria and allergic diseases, Behçet's disease, vasculitis, lasers, cosmetic dermatology, facial rejuvenation, hair diseases, mesotherapy, botulinum toxin, and fillers.

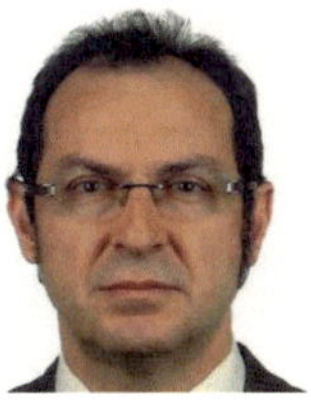

Server Serdaroglu, MD, is the head of the Department of Dermatology at Istanbul University Cerrahpasa Medical Faculty. He is also a professor in the Department of Dermatology at Istanbul University Cerrahpasa Medical Faculty in Turkey. He has coauthored over 30 publications and supervised several master, doctoral, and postdoctoral students. His actual research interests are focused on psoriasis, hair diseases, pediatric dermatology, autoimmune bullous diseases, urticaria and allergic diseases, lasers, and cosmetic dermatology.

Contents

Preface

This textbook contains the latest advances and scientific knowledge from the leading experts in hair biology, hair disorders, and clinical trichology.

During the past 40 years, the interest in hair loss and disorders has significantly increased. In addition, recent advances in molecular biology have evolved our understanding of hair biology. One of the main goals in publishing this book is to increase our knowledge about hair pathology, new treatment options, and modalities.

This book is organized into ten sections. Each section deals with hair biology, hair genetics, hair diagnostics, hair loss types, pathogenesis, treatment options, and restoration techniques. This book also emphasizes on various genetic and nongenetic alopecia types, differential diagnosis, and the measurement of hair loss. One chapter of the book is devoted to natural products for hair care and treatment. Besides, a comprehensive chapter on psychocutaneous disorders of the hair and scalp is presented within this textbook.

We hope that the current book will provide interesting knowledge and different useful methods for recognizing and improving hair loss problems. We believe that this textbook will serve as a comprehensive guide to many physicians dealing with hair disorders in their clinical practice. It will hopefully be a valuable resource for dermatologists, educators, other physicians, and medical students.

We offer our special thanks to Ms. Romina Skomersic, Publishing Process Manager, for her invaluable help in this book project.

We are thankful to our wives and our children for their understanding regarding missed family time.

Assoc. Prof. Dr. Zekayi Kutlubay, MD
Associate Professor of Dermatology
Department of Dermatology
Istanbul University Cerrahpasa Medical Faculty
Turkey

Prof. Dr. Server Serdaroglu, MD
Professor of Dermatology
Department of Dermatology
Istanbul University Cerrahpasa Medical Faculty
Turkey

Section 1

Introduction

Chapter 1

Introductory Chapter: Hair Loss

Zekayi Kutlubay and Server Serdaroglu

Additional information is available at the end of the chapter

http://dx.doi.org/10.5772/66984

1. Introduction

Hair loss (alopecia) is a prevalent dermatological course and it has an impact on both females and males of all ages. For centuries, hair has been the most important sign for the females. Healthy hair is an essential factor for physical well-being and females can show their charm, beauty and personal power with healthy hair. That is why hair loss can cause psychological problems for women rather than for men.

The term alopecia comes from the Greek *alopex*, 'fox', originally referring to mange in foxes, and can be associated with a wide variety of conditions such as genetic, autoimmune, infectious and environmental. Many people face this dermatological condition. The appearance of hair loss can diversify according to what causes this disease. The whole body and scalp can be affected abruptly and gradually. Temporary and permanent hair loss can occur. Sometimes, it is not necessary to apply any treatment to grow hair again, but sometimes, it is an obligation to treat hair loss. Sometimes, hair will not re-grow.

Hair is one of the characteristic features of mammals. Hair is an essential speciality for protecting humans from environmental factors, producing sebum and pheromones and apocrine sweat. It affects someone's role in sexual and social relationships. Hair acts a major role for thermoregulation and it is a resource for stem cells [1].

Hair is a derivate of the epidermis. Hair has two different parts: one of them is the hair shaft and the other is the follicle. The generation of hair depends on the follicle. Cortex, cuticle cells and a medulla for some types of hairs are the parts of the hair shaft. Hair follicle is an essential part for hair growth and it grows continuously. The continuous growth and rest sequence is named hair cycle. The span of hair growth depends on many endocrine, neural stimuli and vascular stimuli. Various factors such as age, localization of the hair and nutritional habits have an impact on the nature of hair.

Nearly there are 5 million hair follicles in humans, and scalp has 100,000 of them. Mainly terminal hairs are on scalp, eyelashes and eyebrows, whereas vellus hairs cover the rest of the body [2]. Hair is formed in two different parts: follicle is located under the skin and it is the living part and the other one is the hair shaft, above the skin surface, and it is fully keratinized non-living part. Hair development is a continuous cyclic process. Hair growth cycle consists of growth (anagen), regression (catagen), rest (telogen) and shedding (exogen); mature follicles go through all of these process. The location of the hair, hormonal balance, personal nutrition and age can affect the duration of the phases [3, 4].

Especially feminine appearance, attractiveness, personal image and sexuality can be affected according to the healthy hair. Hair is an important point for a healthy look, social image and communication. All individuals complain about hair loss without thinking about age and gender but hair loss can have more dramatical effects on females than on males, because hair loss can change the life quality and social communication. That is why dermatological clinics take much interest in hair loss problems.

Hair loss can be due to a wide variety of causes such as scarring and non-scarring diseases.

Alopecia areata (AA), which is an inflammatory disease, causes non-scarring patchy hair loss of the scalp and whole body; it occurs depending on genetic and autoimmune basis [5]. The lifetime coincidence of this chronic disease is 2.1%. This inflammatory disease begins with circular hair loss with sudden sharp borders [6]. The etiology of this disease can be genetic, infectious, immunological, environmental or psychological even though the etiopathogenesis is not known. Some genes such as TRAF1/C5 locus can be a reason for genetic disposition [7]. Some autoimmune disorders, such as Hashimoto's thyroiditis or vitiligo, which are related to diseases of T-cell, can accompany hair loss problems. Some studies point out that the risk of alopecia areata can be increased by the history of atopy [8]. In the pathogenesis of the disease, cytokines such as IFN-gamma, interleukins and TNF-alpha are important factors. The patients with normal appearing underlying skin are presented with asymptomatic and patchy hair loss. The beginning point of this disease is generally scalp hair, and then it can spread to eyebrows, eyelashes and total body. If a patient has a limited involvement, it can re-grow spontaneously. But some patients have a chronic and recurrent course, with many attacks over years.

Physicians think that the treatment of alopecia can be so challenging. Variable treatments with different effects can be applied to the patients. These treatments consist of systemic, intralesional or topical corticosteroids, systemic or local phototherapy, cyclosporine-A, acupuncture, interferon-α, anthralin, topical immunotherapy agents, topical minoxidil and photodynamic therapy [9–11]. Although the stem cells of hair follicles spread into the scalp typically in order to re-grow hair, there are no useful and existing treatments to recover alopecia areata. It is a chronic disease and the consequences can be disruptive for psychological and physical appearance. The impressiveness of treatments decreases due to the spontaneous relapses and remissions and these courses can be unpredictable. This application has been shown as allergic contact dermatitis; topical sensitizers have a major role to begin a delayed-type (type IV) hypersensitivity reaction by acting as haptens. To make a complete antigen, these sensitizers help to bind to an endogenous protein. There are some applications to aim topical sensitization such as dinitrochlorobenzene, SADBE and DPCP [11].

The quality of life is also affected by AA; in most studies, AA is the sort of alopecia, and psychological and social factors have an impact on this disease. The incidence of lifetime major depressive symptoms and anxiety disorders in AA patients was estimated as 39% in one study [12]. Besides, antisocial personality disorder and post-traumatic stress disorder were observed at a high rate in those patients. In AA patients, antisocial personality and post-traumatic disorders were found at a high rate.

Androgenetic alopecia occurs commonly in males and it is a male-type hair loss. This disease is known as the most common form of hair loss; it is progressed by alopecia areata, tinea capitis, telogen effluvium and scarring alopecia [13]. The most essential point of this course is genetic and hormonal reasons. It has been found that middle-aged white men are generally exposed to this disease. This problem affects mostly 30% of white men at the age of 30, 50% at the age of 50 and 80% at the age of 70 [14]. Androgenetic alopecia begins with gradual thin hair in the temporal area and then it follows reshaping of the anterior part of the hairline. According to Norwood-Hamilton classification, it ends with baldness. Androgenetic alopecia is also observed in women, but the thinning of hair happens in different areas. In women, this disease does not commence on marked baldness; it is found especially on the crown. The progression is mostly seen according to the Ludwig scale [13]. Medications approved by the Food and Drug Administration (FDA) to treat male-pattern hair loss include minoxidil and finasteride. By using these medications, hair loss may be reversed or slowed in early phases.

Scarring alopecias or **cicatricial alopecias** are a group of rare inflammatory hair loss diseases; hair follicles are devastating permanently in these diseases. The most common symptom of this disease is the loss of apparent follicular ostia in a scarring area. The most important histopathological characterization of this disease is the replacement of the hair follicle structure made from fibrous tissue. Cicatricial alopecias have various types such as primary cicatricial alopecia, secondary cicatricial alopecia and hereditary cicatricial alopecia. The reason for primary cicatricial alopecia is the destructive inflammation of the hair follicle which is referred to different etiologies and it is generally autoimmune processes.

It is essential to examine the whole scalp and skin biopsies for finding the main reason for cicatricial alopecia are necessary. There are three main groups for primary cicatricial alopecia: lymphocytic, neutrophilic and mixed. It is classified according to the types of inflammatory cells examined histologically where hair follicles are affected. It could be so difficult to differentiate the primary cicatricial alopecia types because of the various forms of this disease and it ends with complete hair loss. The most visible symptom of this disease is the active inflammation. In this condition, the most substantial aim for treatment is to stop or slow down the development of this disease. For the patients with lymphocytic primary cicatricial alopecia, topical and intralesional corticosteroids and antimalarials can be applied and in persistent conditions, systemic immunosuppressive agents can be tried. The applications of antibiotics and retinoids are the most essential medications to treat neutrophilic cicatricial alopecia.

Telogen effluvium is characterized by diffuse loss of telogen hair. Telogen effluvium is a non-inflammatory disease. The main reason for this disease is still unknown, but it is most frequent reason for hair loss. In a normal scalp, 90–95% of the hair follicles are in the anagen phase, and 5–10% are in the telogen phase. It is normal to lose 100 hairs in a day. In telogen effluvium disease, the ratio or the number of hair follicles increases. According to various follicular cycles, five types of functional telogen effluvium have been found. The types include the immediate anagen release, delayed anagen release, immediate telogen release, delayed telogen release and short anagen phase. The pathological causes of this disease are exogenous factors, inflammatory diseases, some drugs and connective tissue disorders such as systemic lupus erythematous, stress, organ dysfunctions, endocrine disorders, syphilis and nutritional causes.

This disease can be seen as acute and chronic and it is classified according to its duration. If the duration of disease is shorter than 6 months, it is known as acute telogen effluvium; if the hair loss is longer than 6 months, it is accepted as chronic telogen effluvium. The hair loss can be apparent 2 or 3 months later in acute telogen effluvium disease. The aetiologic factors or events of telogen effluvium may not be detected in 33% of the patients. Some tests can be applied to patients such as the hair-pull test and the result of this test is positive. In addition to that, inflammation is not found in telogen effluvium. In the trichogram test, the telogen hair ratio reaches above 25% in telogen effluvium. A fine evaluation is to be done to understand the real cause and the most substantial factors: to treat telogen effluvium is to find the natural process of telogen effluvium. If the triggering factor of this disease can be found and stopped, hair loss will generally decrease within 3–6 months [15, 16].

Trichotillomania was observed several years ago, but there have been little data about treatment and its etiology. It can be described as an impulse control disorder and it is identified by chronic hair pulling. Trichotillomania (hair-pulling disorder) is a type of tractional alopecia. In every types of hair loss, this disease has also affected the quality of life and relations in a negative way. When we look at the history of the disease, it was identified in *DSM-III-R* (*Diagnostic and Statistical Manual of Mental Disorders*, Third Edition) in 1987; in that study, continual hair pulling was described as a psychiatric disorder. Hair pulling is not known as rational behaviour in medical condition (e.g., dermatological problems) and it is a psychiatric disorder. The repeated attitude cannot be stopped and finally it causes hair loss. The reason for this disease can also be subjective nuisance and deterioration in social life. The patients not only pull the hair from the scalp but they also pull the hair from other body areas such as the eyebrows, beard, eyelashes, arms, groin and moustache.

The symptoms of trichotillomania resemble the obsessive-compulsive spectrum, so this disease is mainly included among psychiatric diseases [17]. Trichotillomania usually begins in early ages and become chronic with gradual events. It can also be seen in adolescence at the beginning of 12 years. The adults can also face this disease at old ages. Trichotillomania can be confused with AA in older patients in the first phase of the disease because it appeared mostly in females [18, 19]. When we observe more than a third of paediatric patients with trichotillomania, there have been many psychiatric disorders such as attention deficit-hyperactivity disorder, anxiety disorder, obsessive-compulsive disorder and depression. But unfortunately, the studies show that 40% of the trichotillomania patients could not be diagnosed and 58% patients never received correct medications [20].

Trichophagy is a kind of disease which is described as putting the hair into the mouth. Trichophagy can cause serious diseases such as vomiting, ileus and weight loss. Hair swallowing has been shown in 5–18% of these patients [19, 21].

2. Diagnosis

It has been understood that there have been many reasons for hair loss. Dermatologists always apply different methods for finding the main evidence of the disease. The dermatologist also will carefully look at patient's scalp and hair. For instance, they have to pull their patients' hair to get the true results, and it is named as 'pull test'. Pulling hair test can be helpful to describe the process of hair loss. And dermatologists should sometimes observe the whole body to understand the ratio of hair loss. To make sure about the evidence, they also use blood tests. By using blood tests, they can find other reasons for hair loss such as iron deficiency, anaemia, thyroid disease or vitamin deficiencies. The dermatologists can also apply punch biopsy to detect histopathological reasons. All of the applications should be done to find out some clues in your scalp [22].

Although medical treatment is a useful method for patients and physicians, the results of treatment could be unsuccessful. Instead of other techniques, hair transplantation should be used for androgenetic alopecia. Hair transplantation method is essential not only for androgenetic alopecia but also good for other kinds of hair loss. The other kinds of problems include cicatricial alopecias, congenital alopecias, post-burn sequelae and alopecia areata [23]. Lately, hair transplantation has been common for treating hair loss. 'Follicular unit transplantation' and 'Follicular unit extraction' are the main types of this method. In follicular unit transplantation, occipital region is the main area for taking skin patches; they can be separated manually to grafts and put to the recipient area. 'Follicular unit extraction' is the other method in order to treat hair loss. In this method, 1-mm diameter micrografts are taken from the donor area and they are transferred to predrilled holes. This technique is less painful and more comfortable for patients because it does not cause a linear scar. The essential disadvantage of this treatment is that patients should spend much more time for extracting grafts. Due to the 'punched–out' sites, donor transferring into the area can be limited [24, 25].

3. Psychosocial effects

Alopecia occurs not only for physical reasons but also because of psychological problems. They have a major role in this serious condition. It has a significant psychological impact on the quality of life.

The incidence of alopecia always increases because of the psychological problems. Patients with alopecia are exposed to mental disorders such as post-traumatic stress disorder, social phobia, depression, anxiety and suicidal thoughts. Psychological/psychiatric disorders have been detected at rates up to 60% in dermatology patients treated as inpatients [26].

Mental disorders are observed to be a higher risk among women with scarring alopecia. Hair loss can be an important reason for psychological/psychiatric problems such as embarrassment, depression, anxiety about their appearance, low self-esteem, anger, less social and sexual activity and even suicidal thoughts. Because of the connection between alopecia and mental disorders, dermatologists and psychologists/psychiatrists have to find the main reasons for the hair loss together [27, 28].

The aim of this chapter is to review the latest developments in the understanding of hair loss and its treatment. The contents cover the molecular and cell biological aspects of hair follicles through to the pathogenesis of alopecia, its treatment with topical and systemic agents, and new treatment options such as hair transplantation, mesotherapy and platelet-rich plasmas (PRPs).

Author details

Zekayi Kutlubay* and Server Serdaroglu

*Address all correspondence to: zekayikutlubay@hotmail.com

Department of Dermatology, Cerrahpasa Medical Faculty, Istanbul University, Istanbul, Turkey

References

[1] Buffoli B, Rinaldi F, Labanca M et al. The human hair: from anatomy to physiology. Int J Dermatol 2014;53:331–341.

[2] Krause K, Foitzik K. Biology of hair follicle: the basics. Semin Cutan Med Surg 2006;25:2–10.

[3] Wolfram LJ. Human hair: A unique physicochemical composite. J Am Acad Dermatol 2003;48:S106–114.

[4] Stenn KS, Paus R. Controls of hair follicle cycling. Physiol Rev 2001;81:449–494.

[5] Ito T, Aoshima M, Ito N, Uchiyama I, Sakamoto K, Kawamura T et al. Combination therapy with oral PUVA and corticosteroid for recalcitrant alopecia areata. Arch Dermatol Res 2009;301:373–380.

[6] Mirzoyev SA, Schrum AG, Davis MD, Torgerson RR. Lifetime incidence risk of alopecia areata estimated at 2.1% by Rochester Epidemiology Project, 1990–2009. J Invest Dermatol 2014;134:1141–1142. DOI: 10.1038/jid.2013.464.

[7] Rallis E, Nasiopoulou A, Kouskoukis C, Roussaki-Schulze A, Koumantaki E, Karpouzis A et al. Oral administration of cyclosporin A in patients with severe alopecia areata. Int J Tissue React 2005;27:107–110.

[8] Smith JR, Akin RS, Wells MJ. Alopecia areata treated with efalizumab: a case with significant hair re-growth after long-term therapy. J Drugs Dermatol 2009;8:758–760.

[9] Strober BE, Siu K, Alexis AF, Kim G, Washenik K, Sinha A et al. Etanercept does not effectively treat moderate to severe alopecia areata: an open-label study. J Am Acad Dermatol 2005;52:1082–1084.

[10] D'Ovidio R. Alopecia areata: news of diagnosis, pathogenesis, and treatment. Ital J Dermatol Venereol 2014;149:25–45.

[11] Holzer AM, Kaplan LL, Lewis WR. Haptens as drugs: contact allergens are powerful topical immunomodulators. J Drugs Dermatol 2006;5;410–416.

[12] Colon EA, Popkin MK, Callies AL, Dessert NJ, Hordinsky MK. Lifetime prevalence of psychiatric disorders in patients with alopecia areata. Compr Psychiatry 1991;32:245–251. DOI: 10.1016/0010-440X(91)90045-E.

[13] Elston CA, Elston DM. Hair Disorders: Finding the Root of the Problem. May 24, 2016; Accessed August 20, 2016. Available at http://reference.medscape.com/features/slideshow/hair-disorders#page=2.

[14] Ellis JA, Sinclair R, Harrap SB. Androgenetic alopecia: pathogenesis and potential for therapy. Expert Rev Mol Med 2002;4:1–11. DOI: 10.1017/S1462399402005112.

[15] Shapiro J. Clinical practice. Hair loss in women. N Engl J Med 2007; 18;357(16):1620–1630. DOI: 10.1056/NEJMcp072110.

[16] Harrison S, Sinclair R. Telogen effluvium. Clin Exp Dermatol 2002;27(5):389–395. PMID: 12190639.

[17] Van Ameringen M, Patterson B, Simpson W. DSM-5 obsessive-compulsive and related disorders: clinical implications of new criteria. Depress Anxiety. 2014;31:487–493. DOI: 10.1002/da.22259.

[18] Papadopoulos AJ, Janniger CK, Chodynicki MP, Schwartz RA. Trichotillomania. Int J Dermatol 2003;42:330–334. DOI: 10.1046/j.1365-4362.2003.01147.x.

[19] Fettahoğlu EÇ. Hair loss related to primary psychiatric disorders. TURKDERM 2014;48:52–55. DOI: 10.4274/turkderm.48.s12.

[20] Cohen LJ, Stein DJ, Simeon D, Spadaccini E, Rosen J, Aronowitz B, et al. Clinical profile, comorbidity, and treatment history in 123 hair pullers: a survey study. J Clin Psychiatry 1995;56:319–326. PMID: 7615485.

[21] Tolin DF, Franklin ME, Diefenbach GJ, Anderson E, Meunier SA. Pediatric trichotillomania: descriptive psychopathology and an open trial of cognitive behavioral therapy. Cogn Behav Ther 2007;36:129–144. DOI: 10.1080/16506070701223230.

[22] Spano F, Donovan JC. Alopecia areata: Part 1: pathogenesis, diagnosis, and prognosis. Can Fam Phys 2015; 61:751–755.

[23] Ors S, Ozkose S, Ors S. Follicular unit extraction hair transplantation with micromotor: eight years experience. Aesthetic Plast Surg 2015;39(4):589–596.

[24] Kutlubay Z, Kucuktas M, Engin B. Hair transplantation in the cicatricial alopecias. Hair Ther Transplant 2013; 3:109. doi:10.4172/2167-0951.1000109.

[25] Harris JA. Follicular unit extraction (FUE). In: Avram MR, Rogers NE (eds), Hair Transplantation, Cambridge Medicine, Cambridge, 2010; 23–34.

[26] Gupta MA, Gupta AK. Psychiatric and psychological co-morbidity in patients with dermatologic disorders: epidemiology and management. Am J Clin Dermatol 2003;4:833–842. PMID: 14640776.

[27] Yazıcı E, Erol A. Psychiatric approach to alopecia. Turkiye Klinikleri J Cosm Dermatol-Special Topics 2015;8:73–78.

[28] Aghaei S, Saki N, Daneshmand E, Kardeh B. Prevalence of psychological disorders in patients with alopecia areata in comparison with normal subjects. ISRN Dermatol 2014;2014:304370. DOI: http://dx.doi.org/10.1155/2014/304370.

Section 2

Hair Biology

Chapter 2

Anatomy and Physiology of Hair

Bilgen Erdoğan

Additional information is available at the end of the chapter

http://dx.doi.org/10.5772/67269

Abstract

Hair is one of the characteristic features of mammals and has various functions such as protection against external factors; producing sebum, apocrine sweat and pheromones; impact on social and sexual interactions; thermoregulation and being a resource for stem cells. Hair is a derivative of the epidermis and consists of two distinct parts: the follicle and the hair shaft. The follicle is the essential unit for the generation of hair. The hair shaft consists of a cortex and cuticle cells, and a medulla for some types of hairs. Hair follicle has a continuous growth and rest sequence named hair cycle. The duration of growth and rest cycles is coordinated by many endocrine, vascular and neural stimuli and depends not only on localization of the hair but also on various factors, like age and nutritional habits. Distinctive anatomy and physiology of hair follicle are presented in this chapter. Extensive knowledge on anatomical and physiological aspects of hair can contribute to understand and heal different hair disorders.

Keywords: hair, follicle, anatomy, physiology, shaft

1. Introduction

The hair follicle is one of the characteristic features of mammals serves as a unique miniorgan (**Figure 1**). In humans, hair has various functions such as protection against external factors, sebum, apocrine sweat and pheromones production and thermoregulation. The hair also plays important roles for the individual's social and sexual interaction [1, 2].

The hair follicle serves as a reservoir for epithelial and melanocyte stem cells and it is capable of being one of the few immune privileged sites of human body. Hair follicle development is related to the interactions between epithelial and mesenchymal cells. Many genes play substantial role in this interaction and also in hair follicle cycling [3–5].

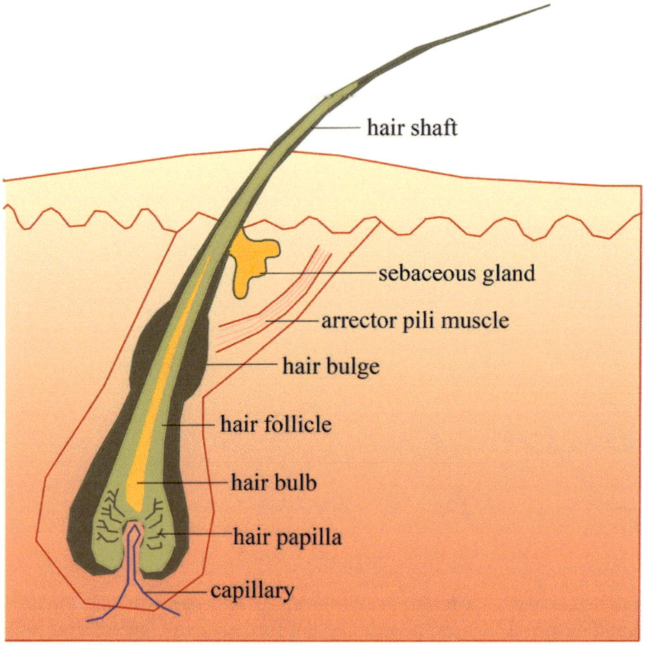

Figure 1. Diagram of an anagen follicle.

The aim of this chapter is to enhance the knowledge of the complex anatomy and physiology of the hair in a simple manner (**Table 1**) [2, 5].

Anagen	Growth stage of hair follicle cycle
Catagen	Regression and involution stage of hair follicle cycle
Telogen	Resting stage of hair follicle cycle
Exogen	Active hair shaft shedding stage of hair follicle cycle
Kenogen	Telogen follicle without club hair form
Club hair	Fully keratinized, dead hair formed at telogen stage
Lanugo hair	Fine hairs on the fetus body; shed in utero or within the first weeks after birth
Vellus hair	Non-pigmented, and generally non-medullated; short hairs
Terminal hairs	Large and pigmented hairs
Hair matrix	Consists of rapidly proliferating keratinocytes that move upwards to produce the hair shaft
Follicular dermal papilla (DP)	Onion-shaped portion of hair bulb surrounded by hair matrix cells, consists of mesenchymally derived tissues
Hair bulb	Lowermost portion of the hair follicle, includes the follicular dermal papilla and the hair matrix
Isthmus	The lower portion of the upper part of hair follicle between the opening of the sebaceous gland and the insertion of arrector pili muscle

Infundibulum	Uppermost portion of the hair follicle extending from the opening of the sebaceous gland to the surface of the skin
Bulge	Segment of the outer root sheath located at insertion of arrector pili muscle
Inner root sheath (IRS)	Guides the hair shaft and helps to take a shape; coats the hair shaft up to the isthmus level
Outer root sheath (ORS)	Extends along from the hair bulb to the infundibulum and epidermis serves as a reservoir of stem cells
Connective tissue sheath (CTS)	Significant mesenchymal follicular layer that adheres to the basement membrane of the hair follicle and interacts with the follicular dermal papilla

*Data from Refs. [2, 5].

Table 1. Glossary of terms for hair anatomy and physiology.

2. Hair and follicle morphology

In utero, type and distribution of each hair follicle over the entire body are determined. The genes that are expressed before the signs of hair follicle formation constitute the precise spacing and distribution of the follicles. The protein products of these genes are presented during the different phases of hair cycle, indicating that they are so important for the normal development and distribution of follicles as well as for the ongoing growth process [4, 5].

The initial "message" for the development of all types of skin appendages is from the dermal mesenchyme (stage 0) and hair follicle development begins with the accumulation of epithelial cells to form epithelial placode after the initial mesenchymal signals (stage 1). Thereafter, the epithelial placode expands and generates the primary hair germ (stage 2). The second signal arises from epithelial placode and constitutes a cluster of adjacent mesenchymal cells which later develops the dermal papilla (DP). The ultimate signal from this primitive dermal papilla to the epithelial placode cells indicates a rapid proliferation and differentiation. This consecutive signaling process finally leads to the production of the mature follicle.

In the second stage of development, hair germ elongates into a cord of epithelial cells and forms the hair peg (stages 3 and 4). It is surrounded by mesenchymal cells that eventually transformed to the fibrous sheath. Derived from the epithelial cells of the hair peg, hair matrix cells form the hair shaft and inner root sheath (IRS). Outer root sheath (ORS) generates two bulges along the side of the hair follicle, the proximal bulge serves as a reservoir for epithelial stem cells and the distal bulge evolves to sebaceous glands. During the development of bullous peg (stages 5–8), the hair bulb and the main cell layers of the mature hair follicle are also formed [2–4, 6].

Several molecular pathways, growth factors, proteins and genes play substantial roles for the development of the hair follicle. Canonical (β-catenin dependent) WNT (wingless-type integration site) signals are candidates for the initial dermal message, and it is believed that they precede other activators and regulators of appendage development. β-Catenin is the downstream mediator of WTN signaling. Activation of this β-catenin pathway seems to be essential for the epithelial ability of the hair follicle production [7].

Ectodysplasin (EDA) and its receptor (EDAR) are another important pathways involved in the placode stage of hair morphogenesis. The mouse EDAR mRNA is expressed in the epithelium before placode formation, and then becomes restricted to placodes, whereas the EDA mRNA is still expressed even after placode formation [3, 6, 8]. In the placode stage, activated WNT and EDAR control the localized accumulation of sonic hedgehog (SHH), which is essential for the downgrowth of the hair germ [2]. In contrast to EDA and EDAR, members of the bone morphogenic protein (BMP) family of secreted signaling molecules seem to be inhibitors of placode formation. The antagonist named Noggin neutralizes BMP activity via regulation of lymphoid enhancer factor 1 (LEF1) expression [4]. EDAR is necessary for placode development in primary hair follicles but not for induction of secondary hair follicles, which utilize signaling pathways that involve Noggin and SRY-box 18 (SOX18) expression within the dermal papilla [9, 10].

In summary, the formation of placodes in response to the first dermal signal involves activation of EDA/EDAR signaling in the epithelium, followed by epithelial WNT signaling, and subsequent activation of BMP signaling. The actions of EDA/EDAR and WNT promote placode formation, whereas BMP signaling represses placode fate in adjacent skin [6].

Human hair follicle morphogenesis occurs only once. Lanugo, vellus and terminal hairs follow the same basic architectural principles. The first "coat" that is formed is fine, long, variably pigmented lanugo hair, which is shed in an anterior to posterior wave during last trimester of gestation. A second coat of fine, shorter, unpigmented lanugo hair then grows in all areas except the scalp and is shed 3–4 months after birth. After these first two cycles, hair starts to grow in an asynchronous "mosaic" pattern rather than in waves [2].

3. Hair anatomy

3.1. Classification of the hair

Nearly whole body surface is coated with the hairs except a few areas like palms, soles and mucosal regions of lips and external genitalia. Most of these are tiny, colorless vellus hairs. The ones located in several areas like scalp, eyebrows and eyelashes are thicker, longer and pigmented and are called terminal hairs. Humans have approximately 5 million hair follicles and 100,000 of them are located on the scalp [11] (**Table 2**) [2].

Basically terminal hairs are found on scalp, eyebrows and eyelashes at birth while the rest of the body is covered with vellus hairs. In puberty, some vellus hairs (i.e. beard, trunk, axilla and genital area) by the influence of androgens differentiate to terminal hairs, which are long (>2 cm), thick (>60 μm), pigmented and medullated. The bulb of the terminal hairs is located in the subcutaneous fat; however, the bulb of vellus hairs is in the reticular dermis. Vellus hairs are thin (<30 μm), short (<2 mm) and mostly nonmedullated.

The hair is classified into three main ethnic subgroups (Asian, African and European). However in a recent study, this classification is expanded to eight main subgroups by considering three parameters: curve diameter, curl index and number of waves [12].

http://dx.doi.org/10.5772/67269

Total count	Almost 5,000,000
Scalp hair count	80,000–150,000
Hair cycle ratios of scalp hair	Anagen: 85–90%
	Catagen: 1%
	Telogen: 10–15%
Duration of hair cycle phase	Anagen: 2–6 years
	Catagen: 2–3 weeks
	Telogen: 3 months
Physiologic hair shedding rate (scalp)	~100–200/day
Hair shaft production rate (scalp)	~0.35 mm/day, 1 cm/month
Hair shaft diameter and length	Vellus: 0.06 mm; 1–2 mm
	Terminal: >0.06 mm; 1–50 cm
Hair patterns	Scalp hair
	Pubic and axillary hair
	Phalangeal hair
Hair shaft pigmentation	Dark hair: predominance of eumelanin
	Blond/red hair: predominance of pheomelanin

*Data from Ref. [2].

Table 2. Basic data of human hair follicles.

Structural features of the hair follicle have to be considered during the classification process. Hair shaft diameters, hair follicle density and follicular infundibulum volume are some of them. Hair shaft diameters represent little variations and hairs are found to be thicker in androgen dependent areas. Hair follicle density is much more condense in the forehead and follicular infundibular volume is also bigger. It is important just because of the large follicular infundibular volume that is associated with more follicular reservoir ability [1, 13].

3.2. Structure of the hair

Hair is consisted of two distinct structures: follicle—the living part located under the skin and hair shaft—fully keratinized nonliving part above the skin surface. The arrector pili muscle, takes place between the hair bulge area and dermoepidermal junction. Above the insertion of the arrector pili muscle, sebaceous glands and, in some certain regions, apocrine glands are opened into the follicle.

Hair shaft is consisted of three layers: cuticle, cortex and in certain cases medulla. Flat and square-shaped cuticle cells are adhered tightly to the cortex cells proximally. Peripheric movements of cuticle cells make the direction of the distal free edge upward and cause extensive overlapping. These imbrications are crucial. By interlocking with the cuticle cells of inner root sheath, they contribute to the follicular anchorage of the growing hair. These imbricated surfaces also facilitate removal of dirt and desquamated cells from the scalp. Cuticle has also important protective properties and barrier functions against physical and chemical insults [14–16].

During the migration of the cells from the hair bulb to compose the cortex, the shapes of them become more fusiform. These cells coalesce tightly and are placed parallel to the axis of the shaft. Axial keratin filaments (microfibrils) that are formed from multiple hard α-keratin intermediate filaments (α-KIF) molecules, packs each cortex cells. Several microfibrils come together to form larger units called macrofibril which represents almost 50% of the cortex material. The cortex comprises the bulk of the shaft and also contains melanin [2, 15, 16]

Medulla is located in the center of the hair shaft preferably presented in coarser fibers. The hair medulla contains structural proteins that are markedly different from other hair keratins and eosinophilic granules that are filled by an amino acid, citrulline and eventually form internal coatings within the membranes of mature cells [14, 16, 17].

The follicle is the essential growth structure of the hair and basically has two distinct parts: upper part consisting of infundibulum and isthmus whereas the lower part comprising of hair bulb and suprabulbar region. The upper follicle remains constant, while the lower part has continuous cycles of regeneration [1, 2, 16, 18].

The infundibulum, the uppermost portion of the hair follicle extending from the opening of the sebaceous gland to the surface of the skin, is a funnel-shaped structure filled with sebum, the product of the sebaceous glands. The upper part named acroinfundibulum, the keratinization of epithelium turns into the "epidermal mode", with formation of stratum granulosum and stratum corneum like a similar manner to epidermis [1, 14, 16].

The isthmus is the lower portion of the upper part of hair follicle between the opening of the sebaceous gland and the insertion of arrector pili muscle. At the isthmus level, epithelium keratinization begins with the lack of granular layer named "trichilemmal keratinization" [14, 16]. Only few differentiated corneocytes remain and the invagination of the epidermis in this area must be considered as highly permeable for topically applied compounds [19]. Hair follicle stem cells are thought to reside in the bulge area on the isthmus close to the insertion of the arrector muscle [20]. Lineage studies have proven that bulge cells are multipotent and that their progeny generate the new lower anagen hair follicle [21]. One of the most distinguishing features of stem cells is their slow-cycling nature, presumably to conserve their proliferative potential and to minimize DNA errors that could occur during replication. They migrate in a downward direction. On entering the hair bulb matrix, they proliferate and undergo terminal differentiation to form the hair shaft and inner root sheath. They also migrate distally to form sebaceous glands and to proliferate in response to wounding [16, 20, 22].

The suprabulbar region of the follicle, below the isthmus and above the hair bulb, is comprised of three layers from outermost to innermost: outer root sheath, inner root sheath and hair shaft (**Figure 2**).

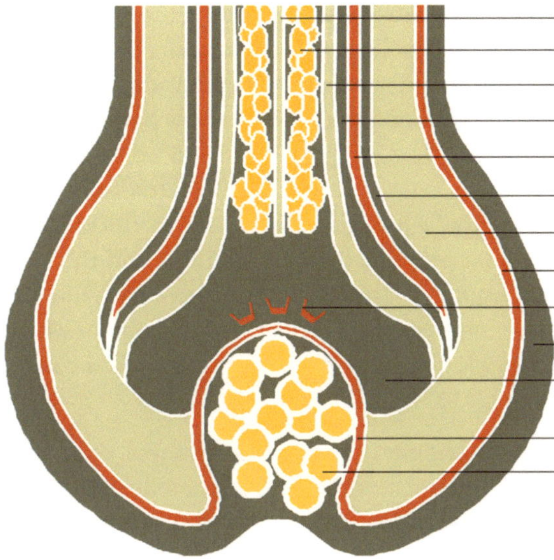

Figure 2. Diagram of proximal hair follicle.

Outer root sheath (ORS) extends from the epidermis at the infundibulum and continues to the hair bulb and its cells change considerably throughout the follicle. In the infundibulum, it resembles epidermis, whereas in the isthmus level, ORS cells begin to keratinize in a trichilemmal mode. Keratinocytes in the ORS form the bulge area at the base of the isthmus. At the lower tip of the hair bulb it consists of a single layer of cuboidal cells, becoming multilayered in the region of the upper hair bulb. In some follicles, there is a distinct single cell layer interposed between the outer and inner root sheaths, known as the companion layer [23]. Companion layer cells show numerous intercellular connections to the inner root sheath and are thought to migrated distally along with the inner root sheath to the isthmus region and to form the plane of slippage between the inner and outer root sheaths [1, 3, 14, 16]. The ORS of the hair follicle also contains melanocytes, Langerhans cells and Merkel cells. These cells take place in certain functions of the follicle such as acting as a sensory organ and serving as an immunologic sentinel for the skin [5].

Inner root sheath (IRS) contains three layers: Henle's layer, Huxley layer and cuticle layer. The innermost layer is the cuticle of IRS whose cells interlock with those of the hair cuticle. This connection, anchoring the hair shaft to the hair follicle, is so tight. The inner root sheath hardens before the presumptive hair within it, and so it is thought to control the definitive shape of the hair shaft. Each of the three layers of IRS undergoes abrupt keratinization. This occurs at different levels in each layer; however, the patterns of change are similar. Keratinization first appears in Henle's layer, the outermost. Huxley layer is keratinized above the Henle's layer at the region known as Adamson's fringe. The IRS coats and supports the hair shaft up to the isthmus level where the IRS disintegrates [3, 14, 16].

The expanded onion-shaped portion of the lower hair follicle, including the hair matrix and the follicular papilla is known as the hair bulb which is the active reproductive portion of the hair follicle. The hair bulb encloses folicular dermal papilla, mucopolysaccharide-rich strome, nerve fiber and capillary loop. The matrix cells are localized to the lowermost portion of the follicle and surround all sides of the follicular papilla. The hair shaft and IRS are derived from the matrix cells. The IRS is derived from the lower and laterally located matrix cells, whereas the hair shaft is originated from upper and centrally located cells. In addition to producing the main structural components of hair, they also produce the hair keratins, and their associated proteins (KAPs) [24]. Melanocytes reside among matrix stem cells to produce the pigment of the hair. During their differentiation phase, matrix cells phagocytose melanin or pheomelanin from the dendritic elongations of melanocytes. The hair assumes its color via the amount and the type of the phagocytized major pigment [1, 3, 16, 25].

Follicular papilla, which is derived from a condensation of mesenchymal cells at the early stages of follicular embryogenesis, is one of the most important players during the induction and maintenance of the follicular epithelial differentiation. It is responsible for determining the follicle type. The volume and secretory activity of follicular papilla and also the number of matrix stem cells determine the size of the anagen hair bulb, the duration of anagen phase and the diameter of the hair shaft [11, 26, 27]. Moreover the follicular papilla is an essential source of growth factors [1, 3, 16, 28].

3.3. Molecular structure

Keratin proteins can be divided into two major families: the type I (acidic) keratins and the type II (basic-neutral) keratins. About 54 functional keratin genes (28 type I and 26 type II keratins) have been identified to date. There are 11 type I hair keratins, designated K31–K40, and 6 type II hair keratins, designated K81–K86, and the remainder are epithelial keratins [24].

The keratin-associated proteins (KAP), is a large group of proteins which constitutes the matrix of the keratin. The matrix proteins are separated to three major subgroups according to their amino acid compositions [29]. Different hair and epithelial keratins are expressed in the various concentric layers of the hair follicle, with hair keratins found primarily in the cortex and hair cuticle [1, 2].

3.4. Hair follicle innervation and vascularization

Nerves related to the hair follicle are identical to the dermal nerve network including sensory afferents and autonomic sympathetic nerves. Smaller nerve fibers form a circular layer around the bulge area of terminal follicles and the bulb area of vellus follicles. There are several types of nerve endings associated with the hair follicle: free nerve endings, lanceolate nerve endings, Merkel cells and pilo-Ruffini corpuscles. Each nerve ending responds to distinct stimulus. Free nerve endings transmit pain, lanceolate nerve endings detect acceleration, Merkel cells responsible of pressure sensation and pilo-Ruffini corpuscles detect tension. Perifollicular nerves related neuromediator and neuropeptides,

http://dx.doi.org/10.5772/67269

that is, substance P, calcitonin gene-related peptide influence follicular keratinocytes and hair follicle cycling [1, 3, 16].

Cutaneous vascularization is provided by arterioles, which are concentrated at the lower portion of the hair follicle and compose vascular network. During the hair cycle phases, there are some alterations in the density of perifollicular vascularization due to the upregulation of vascular endothelial growth factor expression [1].

3.5. Immunology of hair follicle

The immunology of hair is very amazing and complicated. The hair follicle represents an immune privileged (IP) site, which is defined basically as a location in the body where foreign tissue grafts can survive for longer periods of time without immune rejection. This specialized immune environment of IP is required to prevent destructive immune reactions in critical regions. Other immune privileged sites include the anterior chamber of the eye, testis, brain and placenta. Hair follicle IP has a unique characteristic of recurring in a cyclic pattern.

Until recently, the IP of the hair follicle is considered to be restricted to the matrix region during the anagen phase. However, evidence has accumulated that the IP of the hair follicle extends to the bulge region and is present at this site during the entire hair cycle. Since the bulge represents the hair follicle stem cell niche, sustained IP in this region may be essential for the survival of the follicle.

Hair follicle IP occurs during anagen [30]. Thus hair follicle IP is limited to the proximal epithelium of anagen hair follicles. During anagen, melanogenesis is activated in the hair bulb and suggests that hair follicle melanocyte autoantigens play a key role as potential immune targets [28, 31].

The hair follicle IP is maintained by several factors [32]:

- Downregulation of MHC class I expression in the proximal ORS and matrix cells.
- Local production of potent immunosuppressants like TGF-β1, IL-10 and α-MSH.
- Functional deterioration of antigen presenting cells.
- Absence of lymphatics.
- Establishment of extracellular matrix barriers to hinder immune cell trafficking.
- Expression of non-classical MHC class 1.
- Expression of fas ligand.

3.6. Pigmentation of hair follicle

Hair shaft pigmentation ensures multiple benefits including UV protection, thermoregulation and sexual perceptions. Furthermore, the hair pigment, melanin, is a potent free-radical scavenger. Melanin production inside the active anagen hair bulb may, therefore, help to buffer cell stress induced by reactive oxygen species.

In contrast to the continuous melanogenesis observed in epidermal melanocytes, follicular melanogenesis is a cyclic phenomenon. It is ceased in early the anagen-catagen transition, restarted with the down-regulation of key enzymes of melanogenesis, followed by hair follicle melanocyte apoptosis.

Hair follicle melanocytes and their precursors reside in the hair matrix and along the outer root sheath of anagen hair follicles. However, production of hair pigment (black eumelanin and/or the reddish pheomelanin) only occurs in the specialized hair follicle pigmentary unit, located above and around the dermal papilla during anagen III–VI. Melanin synthesis is established in lysosome-related organelles named melanosomes. In the precortical matrix, these melanosomes are transferred to the hair shaft keratinocytes and formed a pigmented hair shaft. The hair follicle also contains melanocyte stem cells, which are located in the bulge and in the secondary hair [33–35].

4. Physiology of the hair

4.1. Hair growth cycle

Hair development is a continuous cyclic process and all mature follicles go through a growth cycle consisting of growth (anagen), regression (catagen), rest (telogen) and shedding (exogen) phases (**Figure 3**). The duration of the phases changes based on the location of the hair and also personal nutritional and hormonal status and age [15, 33].

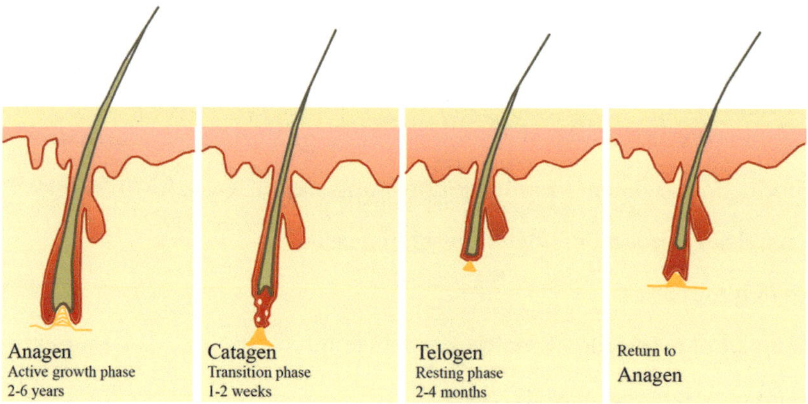

Figure 3. The hair cycle.

4.1.1. Anagen

The inception of anagen phase is presented by the onset of the mitotic activity in the secondary epithelial germ located between the club hair and dermal papilla in telogen hair follicle [5, 16]. The anagen is the active growth phase in which the follicle enlarges and takes the original shape and the hair fiber is produced. Almost 85–90% of all scalp hairs are in anagen.

Six portion of the anagen stage is demonstrated. Through the anagen I–V, hair stem cells proliferate, encloses the dermal papilla, grow downwards to the skin and begin to proliferate hair shaft and IRS, respectively. Subsequently, hair matrix melanocytes begin to develop pigment and the form of the hair shaft begins to arise; in anagen VI, hair bulb and adjacent the dermal papilla formation is realized and the new hair shaft appears from the skin. This phase can last up to 6–8 years in hair follicles [1, 11, 18].

Hair shaft synthesis and pigmentation only take place in anagen [11]. The degree of axial symmetry within the hair bulb determines the curvature of the final hair structure [35]. Fiber length is often dependent on the duration of the anagen or actively growing phase of the follicle [17]. The featured regulatory proteins in anagen phase are BMPs, sonic hedgehog, several WNT proteins and receptors. Insulin like growth factor-1 (IGF-1), fibroblast growth factor-7 hepatic growth factor (HGF), and vascular endothelial growth factor (VEGF) are thought to be important for anagen maintenance [36].

4.1.2. Catagen

At the end of anagen, mitotic activity of the matrix cells is diminished and the follicle enters a highly controlled involutionary phase known as catagen. Catagen lasts approximately 2 weeks in humans, regardless of the site and follicle type [37]. During catagen the proximal of the hair shaft is keratinized and forms the club hair, whereas the distal part of the follicle is involuted by apoptosis [16, 38].

Catagen phase is consisted of eight different stages. The first sign of catagen is the termination of melanogenesis in the hair bulb. Follicular epithelium, mesenchyme, neuroectodermal cell populations and also perifollicular vascular and neural systems demonstrates cyclic changes in differentiation and apoptosis. However, any apoptosis is occurred in dermal papilla due to the expression of suppressor bcl-2 [11].

Catagen is a process of bulbar involution. The perifollicular sheath collapses and vitreous membrane thickens. Eventually, the lower hair follicle becomes reduced to an epithelial strand, bringing the dermal papilla into close proximity of the bulge [36]. The epithelial strand begins to elongate and finally reaches to just below the insertion of pilar muscle. After the keratinization of the presumptive club hair, the epithelial strands begin to involute and shorten progressively followed by the papilla which condenses, moves upward and locates to rest below the bulge. The column eventually reduces to a nipple and forms secondary hair germ below the club. The club hair itself is formed from cortical and cuticle cells only, and it is characterized by a lack of pigmentation [2, 37]. The presence of hairless gene mutation contributes to the failure of dermal papilla migration toward the bulge area in catagen phase [3]. FGF5 is a key inducer of catagen and FGF5-deficient mice have a prolonged anagen phase. In addition to FGF5, TGF-β1, IL-1b, the neurotrophins NT-3, NT-4 and BMP2/4 and TNF-α have been described to induce catagen [36].

4.1.3. Telogen

The telogen stage is defined as the duration between the completion of follicular regression and the onset of the next anagen phase. Telogen stage lasts for 2–3 months. Approximately 10–15% of all hair is in telogen stage. During the telogen stage, the hair shaft is transformed to club hair and finally shed. The follicle remains in this stage until the hair germ which is responsive to anagen initiating signals from the dermal papilla, starts to show enhanced proliferative and transcriptional activity in late telogen, leading to the initiation of anagen [2, 39].

Telogen is one of the main targets of hair cycle which is influenced by several modulatory agents like androgens, prolactin, ACTH, retinoids and thyroid hormones [40]. No unique molecular markers associated with the telogen follicle are determined yet; however, estrogen receptor expression is reported to be limited to the telogen papilla fibroblasts. Germ cells of telogen follicles also express basonuclin and FGF-5 [33]. The bone morphogenic protein-4 (BMP-4) as a growth factor plays an essential role in suppressing follicular growth and differentiation at telogen stage [16].

The macro-environment surrounding the hair follicle also takes part in regulating cycle transitions. BMPs in the subcutaneous fat are capable of maintaining follicles in a "refractory" telogen, and cessation of this inhibitory activity by BMPs enables the follicle to progress to a "competent" telogen with a hair germ that is responsive to anagen-initiation signals and capable of entering a new anagen phase [2, 41].

4.1.4. Exogen

There is less interest for the mechanism of the hair shedding but from the patient's perspective it is probably the most important part of the hair growth. It is not unusual for human telogen hairs to be retained from more than one follicular cycle and this suggests that anagen and exogen phases are independent. The shedding period is believed to be an active process and independent of telogen and anagen thus this distinct shedding phase is named exogen [16, 33].

4.2. Hair cycle clock

Based on the observations: the hair follicle has no need for intact innervation, vascularization or other extrafollicular components to maintain cycling, and the basic oscillator system which controls hair cycling is located presumably in the follicle [42]. The principal challenge is to define the underlying "oscillator" system. Probably, the hair cycle clock is controlled by regulating the balance of the interactions between the follicle epithelium and the surrounding mesenchyme. This might be provided by the rhythmic secretions of growth/modulatory signals from follicle epithelium or mesenchyme as well as the rhythmic alterations in the expressions of corresponding receptors [40].

5. Conclusion

In this chapter, the basic anatomy and the amazing and complicated biology of the hair follicle is reviewed. Enhanced knowledge on the normal dynamics of the hair provides understanding the basis of how the follicle behaves during a disease. However recent progress in our understanding of the biology and pathology of hair follicles should lead more effective therapies for hair disorders.

Acknowledgements

I very much thank Seda Bilir Aksu for the excellent work of the figures in this chapter.

Author details

Bilgen Erdoğan

Address all correspondence to: bcakil@hotmail.com

Bakırköy Dr. Sadi Konuk Research and Training Hospital, İstanbul, Turkey

References

[1] Buffoli B, Rinaldi F, Labanca M et al. The human hair: from anatomy to physiology. Int J Dermatol 2014;53: 331–341.

[2] De Berker D, Higgins CA, Jahoda C et al. Biology of hair and nails. In: Bolognia JL, Jorrizzo JL, Schaffer JV, editors. Dermatology. 3 ed. Elsevier Saunders Ltd. 2012. pp. 1075–1092.

[3] Cotseralis G, Botchkarev V. Biology of hair follicle. In: Wollf K, Goldsmith LA, Katz SI, editors. Fitzpatrik's Dermatology in General Medicine. 7th ed. New York: Mc Graw Hill. 2008. pp. 739–749.

[4] Hardy MH. The secret life of the hair follicle. Trends Genet 1992;8:55–61.

[5] Paus R, Cotsarelis G. The biology of hair follicle. N Engl J Med 1999;341:491–497.

[6] Miller SE. Molecular mechanisms regulating hair follicle development. J Invest Dermatol 2002;118:216–225.

[7] Andl T, Reddy ST, Gaddapara T et al. WNT signals are required for the initiation of hair follicle development. Dev Cell 2002;2:643–653.

[8] Headon DJ, Overbeek PA. Involvement of a novel Tnf receptor homologue in hair follicle induction. Nat Genet 1999; 22:370–374.

[9] Laurikkala J, Pispa J, Jung HS et al. Regulation of hair follicle development by the TNF signal ectodysplasin and its receptor Edar. Development. 2002;129:2541–2553.

[10] Botchkarev VA, Botchkareva NV, Sharov AA et al. Modulation of BMP signaling by noggin is required for induction of the secondary (nontylotrich) hair follicles. J Invest Dermatol 2002;118:3–10.

[11] Krause K, Foitzik K. Biology of hair follicle: the basics. Semin Cutan Med Surg 2006;25:2–10.

[12] De La Mettrie R, Saint-Leger D, Loussouarn G et al. Shape variability and classification of human hair: a worldwide approach. Hum Biol 2007;79:265–281.

[13] Otberg N, Richter H, Schaefer H et al. Variation of hair follicle size and distribution in different body sites. J Invest Dermatol 2004;122:14–19.

[14] Sperling LC: Hair anatomy for the clinician. J Am Acad Dermatol 1991;25:1–17.

[15] Wolfram LJ. Human hair: a unique physicochemical composite. J Am Acad Dermatol 2003;48:S106–S114.

[16] Messenger AG, De Berker DAR, Sinclair RD. Disorders of hair. In: Burns T, Breathnach S, Cox N, editors. Rook's Textbook of Dermatology. 8 ed. Oxford: Wiley-Blackwell. 2010. pp. 66.1–66.16.

[17] Jones LN. Hair structure anatomy and comparative anatomy. Dermatol Clin 2001;19:95–103.

[18] Randal VA, Botchkareva NV. The biology of hair growth. In: Ahluwalia GS, editor. Cosmetic Application of Laser and Light based system. Norwich, NY: William Andrew Inc. 2009. pp. 3–35.

[19] Blume-Peytavi U, Vogt A. Human hair follicle: reservoir function and selective targeting. Br J Dermatol 2011;165:13–17.

[20] Oshima H, Rochat A, Kedzia C et al. Morphogenesis and renewal of hair follicles from adult multipotent stem cells. Cell 2001;104:233–245.

[21] Ito M, Kizawa K, Hamada K et al. Hair follicle stem cells in the lower bulge form the secondary germ, a biochemically distinct but functionally equivalent progenitor cell population, at the termination of catagen. Differentiation 2004;72:548–557.

[22] Cotseralis G, Sun TT, Lavker RM. Label-retaining cells reside in the bulge area of pilosebaceous unit: implications for follicular stem cells, hair cycle, and skin carcinogenesis. Cell 1990;61:1329–1337.

[23] Rothnagel JA, Roop DR. Hair follicle companion layer: reacquainting an old friend. J Invest Dermatol 1995; 104: 42S–43S.

[24] Rogers MA, Langbein L, Praetzer-Wundel S et al. Human hair keratin associated proteins (KAPs). Int Rev Cytol 2006;251:209–263.

[25] Jankovic SM, Jankovic SV. The control of hair growth. Dermatol Online J 1998;4:2.

[26] Jahoda CA, Reynolds AJ. Dermal-epidermal interactions. Adult follicle derived cell populations and hair growth. Dermatol Clin 1996;14:573–583.

[27] Paus R, Müller-Röver S, Botchkarev VA. Chronobiology of the hair follicle: hunting the "hair cycle clock". J Invest Dermatol Symp Proc 1999;4:338–345.

[28] Peus D, Pittelkow MR. Growth factors in hair organ development and the hair growth cycle. Dermatol Clin 1996;14:559–572.

[29] Roger GE. Hair follicle differantiation and regulation. Int J Dev Biol 2004;48:163–170.

[30] Christoph T, Müller-Röver S, Audring H et al. The human hair follicle immun system: cellular compositon and immun privilage. Br J Dermatol 2000;142:862–873.

[31] Ito T. Hair follicle is a target of stress hormone and autoimmune reactions. J Dermatol Sci 2010;60:67–73.

[32] Paus R, Ito N, Takigawa M et al. The hair follicle and immune privilege. J Investig Dermatol Symp Proc 2003;8:188–194.

[33] Stenn KS, Paus R. Controls of hair follicle cycling. Physiol Rev 2001;81:449–494.

[34] Slominski A, Wortsman J, Plonka PM et al. Hair follicle pigmentation. J Invest Dermatol 2005; 124: 13–21.

[35] Thibaut S, Gaillard O, Bouhanna P et al. Human hair shape is programmed from the bulb. Br J Dermatol 2005;152:632–638.

[36] Schneider MR, Schmidt-Ulrich R, Paus R. The hair follicle as a dynamic miniorgan. Curr Biol 2009;19:R132–R142.

[37] Kligman AM. The human hair cycle. J Invest Dermatol 1959;33:307–316.

[38] Paus R, Foitzik K. In search of the "hair cycle clock": a guided tour. Differentiation 2004;72:489–511.

[39] Greco V, Chen T, Rendl M et al. A two-step mechanism for stem cell activation during hair regeneration. Cell Stem Cell 2009;4:155–169.

[40] Paus R. Principles of hair cycle control. J Dermatol 1998;25:793–802.

[41] Plikus MV, Mayer JA, de la Cruz D et al. Cyclic dermal BMP signalling regulates stem cell activation during hair regeneration. Nature 2008;451:340–344.

[42] Sten KS, Nixon J, Jahoda CAB et al. What controls hair follicle cycling? Exp Dermatol 1999; 8:229–233.

Chapter 3

Mechanism of Hair Loss from the Point of View of Epidermal Cell Polarity

Shin-Ichi Osada

Additional information is available at the end of the chapter

http://dx.doi.org/10.5772/66735

Abstract

The epidermis and hair follicle epithelium have a polarized stratified architecture, and epidermal homeostasis is maintained by stem cell and progenitor populations present in the basal layer of the interfollicular epidermis and in different compartments of the hair follicle. Atypical protein kinase Cs (aPKCs—a subgroup of the PKC family) are localized to tight junctions and regulate the apico-basal epithelial polarity in simple epithelia. In the stratified epidermis, aPKCs are expressed in the basal layer and are implicated in the regulation of oriented cell division by localizing to the apical pole of basal cells during mitosis. Mutant mice harboring epidermis-specific deletion of aPKCλ showed progressive hair loss, abnormal hair cycling, an increase of asymmetric cell division in the epidermis and hair follicles, and a gradual decrease in the hair follicle stem cell (HFSC) population. Lineage tracing analysis has demonstrated that mutant HFSCs lose their stemness and become more committed proliferating progenitors. Moreover, the expressions of quiescence-inducing factors (Bmp6 and Fgf18) were suppressed in the mutant hair follicles. These results clarify a novel function of aPKCλ in maintaining the quiescence of HFSCs and suggest that epidermal cell polarity is a new clue to understanding the pathogenesis of hair loss.

Keywords: cell polarity, atypical protein kinase C, hair follicle stem cell, quiescence, alopecia, hair cycle, conditional knockout mouse

1. Introduction

The stimulus-induced turnover of membrane lipids is an important event during cell signaling. The protein kinase C (PKC) family is a group of serine/threonine kinases that mediate intracellular signaling activated by growth factor receptors, G-protein-coupled receptors, and tyrosine kinase receptors through lipid-derived secondary messengers [1]. The PKC family members share a highly conserved carboxy-terminal kinase domain, and differences in their requirements for lipids and calcium for activation are attributed to structural differences in the amino-terminal regulatory domain [2]. In mammals, the PKC family is composed of the following three structurally and functionally distinct subgroups: conventional PKCs (cPKC; α, βI/II, and γ), novel PKCs (nPKC; δ, ε, η, and θ), and atypical PKCs (aPKC; ζ and ι/λ: λ in mice) (**Figure 1**) [2, 3]. The cPKCs have a prototypic regulatory domain consisting of the following two conserved regions: C1 and C2. The C1 region serves as a binding site for diacylglycerol (DAG) and phospholipids, whereas the C2 region serves as a binding site for calcium. The C1 domain also acts as a target for tumor-promoting phorbol esters [4]. The nPKCs are similarly activated by DAG, phospholipids, and phorbol esters, but are not activated by calcium because of the lack of calcium-binding loops in the C2-like region [2]. The aPKCs have an atypical C1 domain and do not depend on DAG or calcium for activation [5, 6]. The activity of aPKCs is primarily regulated by protein-protein interactions through a Phox/Bem1 (PB1) domain located at the amino-terminus, which interacts with other PB1 domain-containing proteins, such as PAR 6 (see below) [7, 8].

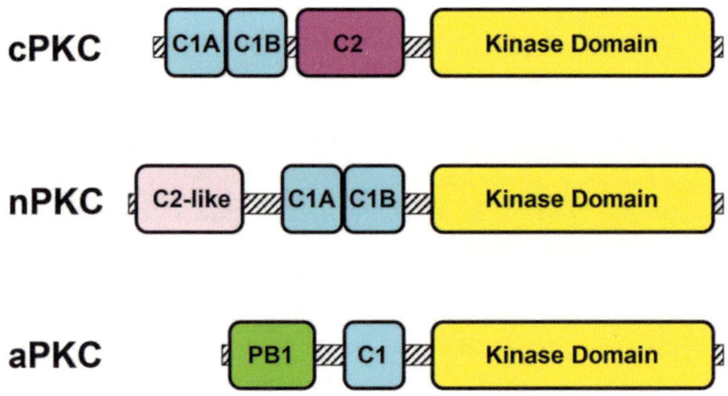

Figure 1. Schematic presentation of the PKC family. In mammals, the PKC family is composed of the following three structurally and functionally distinct subgroups: conventional PKCs (cPKCs; α, βI/II, and γ), novel PKCs (nPKCs; δ, ε, η, and θ), and atypical PKCs (aPKCs; ζ and ι/λ: λ in mice). aPKC (a regulator of epithelial cell polarity) lacks the prototypic regulatory domain composed of C1 and C2 regions.

Among the PKC family members, aPKCs play essential roles in establishing epithelial cell polarity by interacting with partition-defective (Par) proteins [9, 10]. The par genes were first identified in genetic screening for regulators of asymmetric division in the early embryo of *Caenorhabditis elegans* (*C. elegans*) [11, 12]. Par3 (a mammalian ortholog of *C. elegans* par-3) has been rediscovered as an aPKC-interacting protein [13]. Depletion of PKC-3 (an aPKC ortholog in *C. elegans*) using RNA interference results in a phenotype similar to that of par-3 and par-6 mutants [14, 15], leading to the discovery of physical and functional interactions among PKC-3, par-3, and par-6. Both Par3 and Par6 are PDZ domain-containing proteins and act as scaffold proteins. Indeed, Par6 and aPKCs form a stable heterodimer through their respective PB1 domains [7, 8]. Subsequently, Par6 serves as an adaptor protein for Rho family GTPases, Rac1, and Cdc42, in the activation of the Par6-aPKC heterodimer [16, 17]. The active form of Par6-aPKC, in turn, binds to Par3, which is mediated by the kinase domain of aPKCs and the

PDZ domain of Par6. This aPKC-Par3-Par6 ternary complex is evolutionarily conserved and is implicated in a variety of cell polarity events [9, 10, 18].

Although in mammalian simple epithelia, the aPKC-Par complex is located at tight junctions and regulates apicobasal epithelial polarity, in the stratified epidermis, tight junctions are present only in the stratum granulosum [19, 20]. The aPKCs are expressed in the multilayered epidermis; aPKCλ, a predominant aPKC isoform in the epidermis, is distributed throughout the epidermis, whereas aPKCζ is present in basal cells [21]. These distributions suggest that the aPKCs have unidentified functions in the stratified epidermis, where epithelial polarity is established across different cell layers, and proliferation and differentiation are strictly regulated.

To clarify the functions of aPKCs in the stratified epidermis, two groups, including my group, have generated mutant mice harboring epidermis-specific deletion of aPKC [22, 23], using the transgenic mouse line expressing Cre recombinase under the control of the keratin 5 (K5) or keratin 14 (K14) promoter [24, 25]. These mice show essentially the same phenotypes: progressive hair loss, abnormal hair cycling, hyperplasia of the epidermis and sebaceous gland, loss of the hair follicle stem cell (HFSC) quiescence, and a gradual decrease in HFSC in population. In this article, I discuss how these various phenotypes are related with one another and present the mechanism of hair loss from the point of view of epidermal cell polarity.

2. Progressive hair loss

Whole-body inactivation of aPKCλ results in embryonic lethality, which hampers further examination of the role of the aPKCλ-Par complex in epidermal homeostasis. To overcome this problem, two groups, including my group, generated mutant mice with epidermis-specific loss of aPKCλ using K5-Cre or K14-Cre mice [22, 23]. Although, in a strict sense, the distribution of K14-Cre transgene activity differs from that of K5-Cre transgene activity in the epidermis and hair follicle [25, 26], both mutant mice showed similar skin phenotypes. Thus, hereafter, when referring to findings common to both conditional knockout (cKO) mice, the term mutant mice or aPKCλ cKO mice is used, and when referring to findings obtained in the mutant mice associated with K5-Cre or K14-Cre individually, the term K5-cKO or K14-cKO mice is used, respectively.

Although aPKCλ cKO mice showed no gross anomalies at birth, they were easily distinguished from their control counterparts by the thinning of pledge hair from around postnatal day (P) 14 onward. The hair loss was progressive, and one-year-old mutant mice exhibited total alopecia (**Figure 2**) [22, 23]. The vibrissae were also shortened or were lost in the mutant mice [23].

K14-cKO mice showed impaired hair morphology. Scanning electron microscopy demonstrated that the regular cuticle pattern was lost in the mutant hair shafts. Consistent with this finding, the expressions of hair keratins in the inner root sheath (K28), cuticle (K35, K82, K85), cortex (K35, K81, K85), medulla (K28, K6, K75), and companion layer (K75, K6) were severely reduced [22].

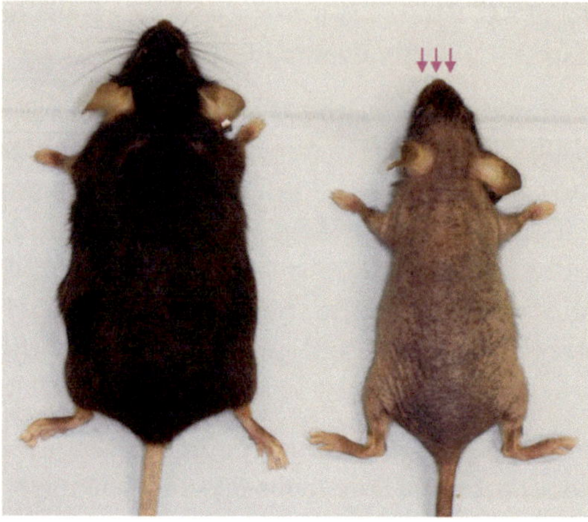

Figure 2. Hair loss phenotype of mutant mice. Macroscopic presentation of a one-year-old control (left) and a K5-cKO mouse (right). Note that the vibrissae were lost in the mutant mouse (arrows).

3. Abnormal hair cycling

During postnatal morphogenesis stages (P0–P16), the hair cycling of mutant hair follicles appeared to proceed normally, although the mutant integument became histologically noticeable with a thickened interfollicular epidermis (IFE) and enlarged sebaceous glands [22, 23]. However, entry into the first postnatal telogen (resting phase, normally starts around P18) was delayed in the mutant hair follicles. At P28, when control hair follicles entered into the first anagen (growth phase), they still had a long epithelial strand, a characteristic structure of catagen (regression phase) [27], and were positive for placental cadherin (P-cadherin), a marker for the epithelial strand. As a result, the start of the first anagen was delayed until P37 in the K5-cKO mice. In the K14-KO mice, the percentages of hair follicles that properly entered into catagen, telogen, and anagen were significantly reduced.

Moreover, mutant hair follicles were morphologically abnormal. They exhibited hyperkeratotic plugs and cyst-like structures with an expanded infundibulum and isthmus. Strikingly, these severely deformed mutant hair follicles regrew and entered into the second anagen much later than the control hair follicles. However, the mutant hair follicles in anagen did not proceed further into the second catagen or telogen. Instead, they started to degenerate, as revealed by the shrinking hair bulbs and reduced expressions of Ki67 and Lef1 [23]. In one-year-old mutant mice, the number of hair follicles was severely diminished.

Fibroblast growth factor 18 (Fgf18) is expressed in hair follicles and colocalized with keratin 15 (K15) and CD34 [28, 29], both of which are expressed in the bulge region at telogen. Fgf18 shows a cyclic expression pattern in hair follicles; its levels are low in anagen and high throughout telogen [29]. In mutant mice with epidermis-specific loss of Fgf18, the length of telogen was short, resulting in rapid succession of hair cycling [29]. Interestingly, the expression of Fgf18 was severely suppressed in the K5-cKO mice during hair morphogenesis and hair development [23]. Although precise molecular mechanisms associated with abnormal hair cycling in cKO mice remain to be elucidated, these results suggest that aPKCλ controls hair follicle cycling through Fgf18 signaling.

4. Hyperplasia of the epidermis and sebaceous gland

In aPKCλ cKO mice, the IFE and sebaceous glands were affected [22, 23]. The thickness of the IFE of the dorsal skin increased in the mutant mice, as revealed by significant expansion of the expression domain for loricrin (a marker for terminal differentiation) and keratin 10 (K10, a marker for spinous cells). Moreover, the sebaceous glands were enlarged in the cKO mice. Accordingly, immunostaining for adipose differentiation-related protein (ADFP, a marker for the surface of lipid droplets) and stearoyl-CoA desaturase 1 (SCD1, a marker for mature sebocytes), and Nile red staining showed remarkable increases in the sebaceous glands of the mutant mice.

Importantly, the expression domain of Lrig1 was expanded in the mutant mice [22, 23]. Lrig1 marks the junctional zone between the infundibulum and the sebaceous gland, and Lrig1-expressing cells contribute to the IFE and sebaceous glands [30]. Thus, this bipotent activity of Lrig1 is thought to be implicated in hyperplasia of these tissues.

5. Dysregulation of HFSC marker expression

The hair follicle at telogen is composed of several compartments, including the interfollicular epidermis, infundibulum, isthmus, bulge, and hair germ. Recent studies have identified multiple new stem cell and progenitor populations in each compartment, which exhibits unique marker expression profiles (**Figure 3**) [31, 32].

5.1. Bulge

In the skin, label-retaining cells (LRCs) having a highly proliferative activity reside in the bulge region of the hair follicle [33], and LRCs in the bulge are multipotent [34, 35]. Since the first identification of K15 as a bulge marker [36], several factors have been demonstrated to be expressed in the bulge region at telogen, such as CD34 [37], leucine-rich repeat-containing G protein-coupled receptor 5 (Lgr5) [38], and transcriptional factors Sox9 [39, 40], Tcf3 [41], Lhx2 [42, 43], and nuclear factor of activated T cells c1 (Nfatc1) [44]. CD34, a hematopoietic stem and progenitor cell marker, colocalizes with LRCs and K15 expression in the bulge region [37]. Lgr5 marks the lower bulge and secondary hair germ during telogen, and contributes to all hair lineages, but not to the epidermis and sebaceous glands [38]. Sox9-expressing cells also contribute to all skin epithelial lineages [39, 40]. Tcf3 and Tcf4 are downstream targets of Wnt signaling, and in Tcf3/Tcf4-null mice, hair follicle formation was initiated, but further development was severely impaired [45]. Lhx2 maintains the HFSC character downstream of Wnt and Shh signaling [43]. Nfatc1 colocalizes with other bulge stem cell markers, including CD34, Sox9, Tcf3, and Lhx2 [44]. Nfatc1 mediates HFSC quiescence by transcriptionally suppressing cyclin-dependent kinase 4 (CDK4) expression upstream of BMP4 signaling [44].

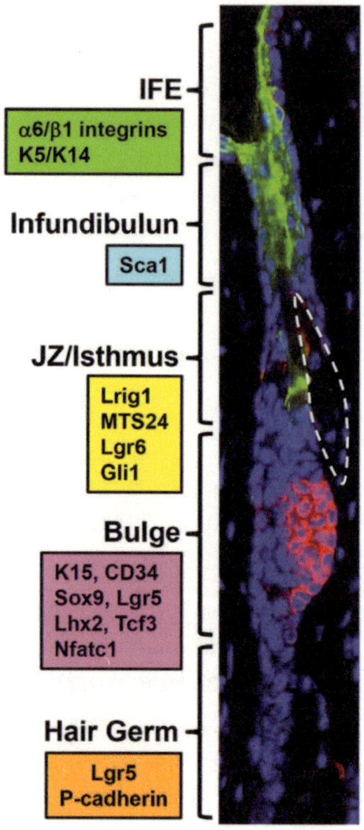

Figure 3. Distinct stem cell populations in the hair follicle. The hair follicle is divided into the interfollicular epidermis (IFE), infundibulum, junctional zone (JZ)/isthmus, sebaceous gland, bulge, and hair germ. The expressions of proposed stem cell markers at telogen are indicated. Note that the expression domains of these markers dynamically change during hair cycling. A murine hair follicle in telogen is immunostained for keratin 10 (a marker for suprabasal cells, green) and keratin 15 (a marker for bulge stem cells, red). Nuclei are counterstained with 4′, 6-diamidino-2-phenylindole. The dotted area indicates the sebaceous gland.

Comparison of the expression profiles of these bulge stem cell markers between the early and late stages in mutant mice demonstrated that the expressions of these markers diminished at later stages or were mislocalized to areas outside the bulge [22, 23]. These results indicate that aPKCλ regulates the expression and localization of HFSCs.

5.2. Junctional zone/isthmus

Markers that recognize distinct cell populations of the upper (junctional zone) and lower bulge regions have been identified. As mentioned above, Lrig1 is a marker for the junctional zone/isthmus, which is located between the sebaceous gland and the bulge [30]. Lrig1-expressing cells have a bipotent activity in the steady state, and give rise to the IFE and sebaceous glands [30]. The cell-surface glycoprotein MTS24 is another marker for the isthmus/junctional zone [46]. MTS24-expressing cells do not express CD34 or keratin 15, and LRCs are infrequently observed among them. Lgr6 is expressed in a distinct population between the upper K5- and CD34-expressing cells and lower MTS24- and Lrig1-expressing cells in the bulge region [47]. Although prenatal Lgr6-positive cells contribute to the IFE, sebaceous glands, and hair follicles, the contribution to the hair follicles diminishes with age. In mutant hair follicles, the expression domains for Lrig1 and MTS24 were considerably expanded.

6. Depletion of HFSCs

HFSCs can be identified as α6-integrin and CD34 double-positive cells with fluorescence-activated cell sorting (FACS) analysis [48]. Consistent with the decrease in the expression of the bulge stem cell markers at later stages, quantitative FACS analysis demonstrated that the number of α6-integrin/CD34 double-positive cells gradually decreased in aPKCλ cKO mice as the mice aged [22, 23]. Moreover, LRCs in BrdU pulse-chase labeling experiments were severely reduced in the bulge region of the mutant hair follicles [22, 23]. Conversely, the number of Lrig1- or MTS24-expressiong cells was gradually increased [22]. These results indicate that in aPKCλ cKO mice a decrease in quiescent HFSCs is accompanied by an increase of progenitor cells committed to the junctional zone/isthmus and infundibulum.

7. Loss of HFSC quiescence

Mutant mice analyses have identified intrinsic and paracrine mechanisms to clarify the loss of HFSC quiescence caused by epidermis-specific inactivation of aPKCλ.

7.1. Intrinsic mechanism: oriented cell division

Oriented cell division is crucial for tissue morphogenesis and homeostasis [49, 50]. Basal cells in the epidermis show the following two types of cell division: symmetric cell division (SCD) and asymmetric cell division (ACD). SCD, in which alignment of the mitotic spindle is parallel to the basement membrane, results in two equivalent daughter cells, whereas ACD, in which alignment of the mitotic spindle is perpendicular to the basement membrane, results in two daughter cells with different fates (one basal cell and one more differentiation-committed suprabasal cell) (**Figure 4**).

In the epidermis, a balance between SCD and ACD is important for coordinated proliferation and differentiation. A shift from SCD to ACD in basal cells of the developing epidermis coincides with the onset of stratification [51]. At embryonic day 12.5 (E12.5), most of the murine epidermis is single-layered, and the majority of cell divisions (>90%) are symmetric, whereas at E14.5–18.5, more than 70% of cell divisions are perpendicular to the basement membrane [51]. ACD promotes Notch signaling, leading to epidermal differentiation [52]. During SCD and ACD, the aPKC-Par complex localizes at the apical surface in a β1-integrin- and α-catenin-dependent manner [51]. Thus, in the β1-integrin KO and α-catenin KO epidermis, apical localization of the aPKC and Par3-LGN-inscuteable complex is abolished. Niessen et al. demonstrate that epidermal loss of aPKCλ induced a shift toward ACD not only in the IFE but also in the bulge stem cells and the junctional zone/isthmus region, leading to an expansion of progenitor cell populations committed to epidermal cell fate [22].

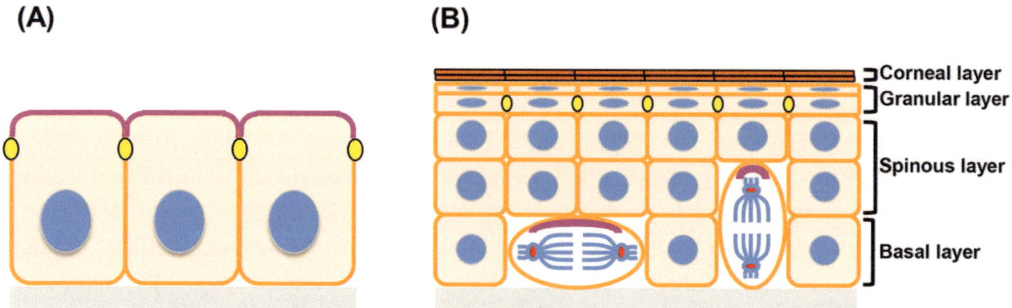

Figure 4. Localization of aPKC in the simple epithelium and multilayered epidermis. (A) In the simple epithelium, aPKC forms a ternary complex with Par3 and Par6 and is localized to the apical surface of the cell and tight junctions (yellow circles). (B) In the stratified epidermis, tight junctions are only present in the granular layer. During symmetric cell division, in which alignment of the mitotic spindle is parallel to the basement membrane (gray), and during asymmetric cell division, in which alignment of the mitotic spindle is perpendicular to the basement membrane, aPKC (pink) is localized to the apical surface of the cell.

Lineage tracing analysis using Lgr5-Cre mice confirmed that epidermal loss of aPKCλ changes the fate of a bulge stem cell to an epidermal lineage [22]. In telogen, Lgr5-positive cells resided in the lower bulge and hair germ, as described above. During anagen, Lgr5 progeny exclusively contributed to down-growing hair follicles, whereas upon loss of aPKCλ, Lgr5-positive cells contributed to the upper junctional zone/isthmus and the IFE, as well as the lower-growing hair follicles. Consistent with this the expression domains for Lig1 and MTS24 increased. These findings indicate that aPKCλ regulates oriented cell division and thereby controls epidermal stem cell behavior and cell fate decisions.

7.2. Paracrine mechanism

HFSCs remain quiescent during telogen. Near the end of telogen, the HFSCs become activated to elicit the growth phase of the hair cycle. Basically, Bmp signaling induces quiescence and Wnt signaling activates HFSCs. However, the molecular mechanism underlying the cyclic inhibition and activation of HFSCs has recently started to be elucidated. Three types of Bmps from different sources induce quiescence in HFSCs: Bmp2 from subcutaneous adipocytes, Bmp4 from dermal fibroblasts [53], and Bmp6 from the inner layer of the bulge (**Figure 5**) [54]. Bmp antagonism is one of the key concepts to understand morphogenesis. In the telogen to anagen transition, the dermal papilla secretes HFSC-activating factors, Fgf7, Fgf10, Wnts, and

http://dx.doi.org/10.5772/66735

Tgfβ2 [55], and Bmp inhibitors, such as noggin [53, 56], overcome the inhibitory effects of Bmps to activate HFSCs (**Figure 5**) [57].

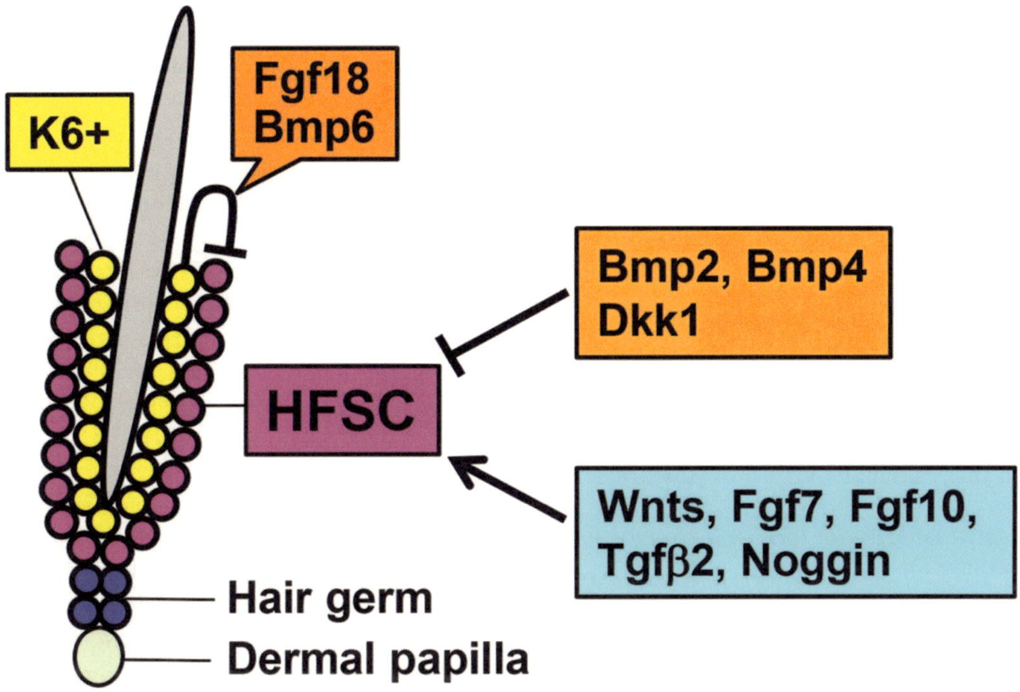

Figure 5. Current model for the maintenance of HFSC quiescence. A hair follicle at telogen is presented. K6-positive cells mark the inner layer of the bulge, from which quiescence-inducing Bmp6 and Fgf18 are produced. The HFSCs are kept quiescent by Bmp2 from subcutaneous adipocytes and Bmp4 from dermal fibroblasts. At the telogen to anagen transition, HFSC-activating factors, such as Fgf7, Fgf10, Wnts, Noggin (Bmp antagonist), and Tgfβ2, antagonize the inhibitory effects of quiescence-inducing factors.

The inner layer of the bulge has attracted attention as a source of the quiescence-inducing factors Bmp6 and Fgf18 [54]. Although induction of K6 expression is closely associated with hyperproliferative conditions [58, 59], such as psoriasis and squamous cell carcinoma, a recent study has clarified that during telogen, K6 is strongly expressed in the inner layer of the bulge and K6-positive bulge cells secrete Bmp4 and Fgf18 to inhibit proliferation of the CD34-positive outer bulge stem cells [54]. Thus, upon the ablation of K6-positive bulge cells, HFSCs become prematurely activated and enter a new cycle of hair growth [54]. In the K5-cKO mice, K6 expression in the inner bulge cells was abolished, and the expressions of Bmp6 and Fgf18 were suppressed at the mRNA and protein levels [23], suggesting that aPKCλ regulates HFSC quiescence upstream of Bmp6 and Fgf18. Moreover, because K6-positive bulge cells are also involved in intercellular junctions that anchor the old hair shaft [54], a decrease in the expression of K6 in the inner layer of the mutant bulge may be involved in the falling-off of hair shafts in mutant hair follicles.

8. The roles of other components of the aPKC-Par complex in hair loss

8.1. aPKC

In the epidermis, aPKCζ, another isoform of aPKC, localizes in the cytoplasm and nucleus of basal cells, although its expression level is much lower than that of aPKCλ in the skin of newborns and adults (40-fold and 10-fold, respectively) [21]. Although the activity of aPKCζ in epithelial polarity in vitro is distinguishable from that of aPKCλ, mice lacking aPKCζ at the whole-body level were viable and showed no obvious skin phenotypes [60]. This may be attributed to the low expression of aPKCζ in the epidermis, and aPKCλ may compensate for the loss of aPKCζ. However, these results do not exclude the possibility that aPKCλ and aPKCζ synergistically regulate epithelial cell polarity, oriented cell division, epidermal differentiation, and HFSC maintenance. Indeed, the combined deletion of the aPKCλ/ι and aPKCζ isoforms in podocytes leads to defective glomerular maturation with incomplete capillary formation and mesangiolysis, and causes severe proteinuria and perinatal death [61]. Thus, studies on mutant mice with simultaneous epidermal inactivation of aPKCλ and aPKCζ would help provide further information on the synergism between the two.

8.2. Junctional aPKC vs non-junctional aPKC

Because aPKCs are localized to tight junctions, in aPKCλ cKO mice, the aPKCλ-Par6-Par3 complex at tight junctions was supposed to be absent or impaired in the granular layer. However, in the mutant mice, the overall multilayered architecture of the epidermis appeared to be normal, or rather hyperplasic [22, 23], suggesting that in contrast to simple epithelia, junctional aPKCλ is dispensable for establishing the polarity of the stratified epidermis, and that aPKCλ localized to the apical surface of basal cells during mitosis is more critical for maintaining epidermal homeostasis. Par6 and aPKCs form a stable heterodimer through their respective Phox/Bem1 (PB1) domains [7, 8], and aPKC-mediated phosphorylation is required for the dissociation of Par3 from the ternary complex. Thus, analysis of the dynamics of Par6 and Par3 or the Par6-Par3 complex in the absence of aPKCλ is helpful to understand the role of junctional aPKCλ.

The difference between junctional and non-junctional aPKC has been demonstrated by two-step chemical skin carcinogenesis experiments using epidermis-specific Par3 knockouts [62]. The epidermal loss of Par3 reduced papilloma formation and promoted keratoacanthoma formation, indicating that Par3 acts as a tumor promoter for papilloma and as a tumor suppressor for keratoacanthoma. In the absence of Par3, the aPKC-Par6 complex localized to the cytoplasm [62]. These results imply that the junctional aPKC-Par6 complex with Par3 is involved in papilloma formation, whereas the non-junctional, cytoplasmic aPKC-Par6 complex without Par3 is involved in keratoacanthoma formation.

8.3. Par proteins

The role of other components of the aPKC-Par complex (Par3 and Par6) in HFSC maintenance is unknown. Par3 is expressed throughout the interfollicular epidermis and the hair follicles, and it interacts with aPKCλ to colocalize at keratinocyte tight junctions [62]. However, no hair abnormalities were described in epidermis-specific Par3-deleted mice [62]. During SCD and ACD in the basal layer, Par3 was localized to the apical surface of the cell as a component of the Par3-LGN-inscuteable complex [51]. It would be useful to examine whether a shift from SCD to ACD in the hair follicle and subsequent HFSC depletion occurs in Par3-deficient mice as seen in aPKCλ cKO mice. Additionally, it would be interesting to investigate whether Par6 knockouts show similar phenotypes to those of aPKCλ knockouts. To the best of my knowledge, Par6 knockouts have not yet been reported. The presence of three isoforms of Par6 in mammals might make it difficult to reveal the phenotypes of Par6 inactivation.

9. aPKC and aging

Is alopecia observed in aPKCλ cKO mice relevant to human diseases? As few inflammatory cells were present around the hair follicles of mutant mice, the mutant mice model is unlikely to be a disease model for alopecia areata, which involves perifollicular T cell infiltration and autoimmune responses to hair antigens. Progressive hair loss in aPKCλ cKO mice was similar to alopecia observed in collagen XVII (COL17A1/BP180/BPAG2, a structural component of the hemidesmosome) knockout mice and aged mice. In humans, COL17A1 deficiency causes a subtype of congenital junctional epidermolysis bullosa [63]. The patients also show premature hair loss (alopecia) with hair follicle atrophy [64, 65], suggesting that COL17A1 plays a role in hair follicle homeostasis. Consistent with this finding, *Col17a1*-deficient mice also show premature hair loss [66]. Mouse Col17a1 is preferentially localized along the dermal-epidermal junction of bulge keratinocytes, and loss of Col17a1 prevents the expression of HFSC markers, such as K15, CD34, and α6-integrin [67]. Similar to aPKCλ cKO mice, *Col17a1*-deficient mice showed progressive hair loss, hair follicles in sustained anagen, HFSC depletion, and deficient stemness of the HFSC population [67], indicating that Col17a1 is essential for HFSC maintenance. In addition, *Col17a1*-deficient HFSCs coexpress K15 and K1 in the bulge, and show increased K1 expression in the upper junctional zone and IFE, implying that the fate of HFSCs changes to epidermal differentiation.

A recent study clarified that accumulation of DNA damage in HFSCs leads to proteolysis of COL17A1 that triggers HFSC aging [68]. Importantly, aged HFSCs lose their stem cell signature and commit to epidermal differentiation, and they are finally eliminated from the epidermis [68]. The progressive depletion of HFSCs and the cell fate change observed in aPKC cKO mice are similar to aged mice. Thus, it would be interesting to examine whether the expression of Col17a1 is decreased in mutant mice and whether aPKCλ is involved in the induction and maintenance of Col17a1.

10. Concluding remarks

Analyses of mutant mice with epidermal loss of aPKCλ have clarified a novel function of aPKCλ in HFSC maintenance. aPKCλ influences HFSC maintenance through the regulation of oriented cell division among HFSCs in the bulge (intrinsic mechanism) and the regulation of the expression of quiescence-inducing Fgf18 and Bmp6 (paracrine mechanism). Identification and evaluation of the downstream effectors of aPKCλ in HFSC maintenance will provide further insight into the mechanism of hair loss.

Author details

Shin-Ichi Osada

Address all correspondence to: osada0130@gipc.akita-u.ac.jp

Department of Dermatology & Plastic Surgery, Akita University Graduate School of Medicine, Akita, Japan

References

[1] Nishizuka Y. Protein kinase C and lipid signaling for sustained cellular responses. FASEB J. 1995;9(7):484–496.

[2] Steinberg SF. Structural basis of protein kinase C isoform function. Physiol Rev. 2008;88(4):1341–1378. DOI: 10.1152/physrev.00034.2007

[3] Ohno S, Nishizuka Y. Protein kinase C isotypes and their specific functions: prologue. J Biochem. 2002;132(4):509–511.

[4] Castagna M, Takai Y, Kaibuchi K, Sano K, Kikkawa U, Nishizuka Y. Direct activation of calcium-activated, phospholipid-dependent protein kinase by tumor-promoting phorbol esters. J Biol Chem. 1982;257(13):7847–7851.

[5] Ono Y, Fujii T, Ogitat K, Kikkawat U, Igarashi K, Nishizukat Y. Protein kinase C ζ subspecies from rat brain: its structure, expression, and properties. Biochemistry. 1989;86:3099–3103.

[6] Akimoto K, Mizuno K, Osada SI, Hirai SI, Tanuma SI, Suzuki K, et al. A new member of the third class in the protein kinase C family, PKCλ, expressed dominantly in an undifferentiated mouse embryonal carcinoma cell line and also in many tissues and cells. J Biol Chem. 1994;269(17):12677–12683.

[7] Suzuki A, Yamanaka T, Hirose T, Manabe N, Mizuno K, Shimizu M, et al. Atypical protein kinase C is involved in the evolutionarily conserved par protein complex and plays a critical role in establishing epithelia-specific junctional structures. J Cell Biol. 2001;152(6):1183–1196.

[8] Moscat J, Diaz-Meco MT, Albert A, Campuzano S. Cell signaling and function organized by PB1 domain interactions. Mol Cell. 2006;23(5):631–640. DOI: 10.1016/j.molcel.2006.08.002

[9] Suzuki A, Ohno S. The PAR-aPKC system: lessons in polarity. J Cell Sci. 2006;119(Pt 6): 979–987. DOI: 10.1242/jcs.02898

[10] Goldstein B, Macara IG. The PAR proteins: fundamental players in animal cell polarization. Dev Cell. 2007;13(5):609–622. DOI: 10.1016/j.devcel.2007.10.007

[11] Kemphues KJ, Priess JR, Morton DG, Cheng NS. Identification of genes required for cytoplasmic localization in early *C. elegans* embryos. Cell. 1988;52(3):311–320.

[12] Kemphues K. PARsing embryonic polarity. Cell. 2000;101(4):345–348. DOI: 10.1016/S0092-8674(00)80844-2

[13] Izumi Y, Hirose T, Tamai Y, Hirai S, Nagashima Y, Fujimoto T, et al. An atypical PKC directly associates and colocalizes at the epithelial tight junction with ASIP, a mammalian homologue of *Caenorhabditis elegans* polarity protein PAR-3. J Cell Biol. 1998;143(1): 95–106.

[14] Watts JL, Etemad-Moghadam B, Guo S, Boyd L, Draper BW, Mello CC, et al. par-6, a gene involved in the establishment of asymmetry in early *C. elegans* embryos, mediates the asymmetric localization of PAR-3. Development. 1996;122(10):3133–3140.

[15] Tabuse Y, Izumi Y, Piano F, Kemphues KJ, Miwa J, Ohno S. Atypical protein kinase C cooperates with PAR-3 to establish embryonic polarity in *Caenorhabditis elegans*. Development. 1998;125(18):3607–3614.

[16] Lin D, Edwards AS, Fawcett JP, Mbamalu G, Scott JD, Pawson T. A mammalian PAR-3-PAR-6 complex implicated in Cdc42/Rac1 and aPKC signalling and cell polarity. Nat Cell Biol. 2000;2(8):540–547. DOI: 10.1038/35019582

[17] Yamanaka T, Horikoshi Y, Suzuki A, Sugiyama Y, Kitamura K, Maniwa R, et al. PAR-6 regulates aPKC activity in a novel way and mediates cell-cell contact-induced formation of the epithelial junctional complex. Genes Cells. 2001;6(8):721–731.

[18] Rosse C, Linch M, Kermorgant S, Cameron AJM, Boeckeler K, Parker PJ. PKC and the control of localized signal dynamics. Nat Rev Mol Cell Biol. 2010;11(2):103–112. DOI: 10.1038/nrm2847

[19] Furuse M, Hata M, Furuse K, Yoshida Y, Haratake A, Sugitani Y, et al. Claudin-based tight junctions are crucial for the mammalian epidermal barrier: a lesson from claudin-1-deficient mice. J Cell Biol. 2002;156(6):1099–1111. DOI: 10.1083/jcb.200110122

[20] Yoshida K, Yokouchi M, Nagao K, Ishii K, Amagai M, Kubo A. Functional tight junction barrier localizes in the second layer of the stratum granulosum of human epidermis. J Dermatol Sci. 2013;71(2):89–99. DOI: 10.1016/j.jdermsci.2013.04.021

[21] Helfrich I, Schmitz A, Zigrino P, Michels C, Haase I, le Bivic A, et al. Role of aPKC isoforms and their binding partners Par3 and Par6 in epidermal barrier formation. J Invest Dermatol. 2007;127(4):782–791. DOI: 10.1038/sj.jid.5700621

[22] Niessen MT, Scott J, Zielinski JG, Vorhagen S, Sotiropoulou PA, Blanpain C, et al. aPKCλ controls epidermal homeostasis and stem cell fate through regulation of division orientation. J Cell Biol. 2013;202(6):887–900. DOI: 10.1083/jcb.201307001

[23] Osada S-I, Minematsu N, Oda F, Akimoto K, Kawana S, Ohno S. Atypical protein kinase C isoform, aPKCλ, is essential for maintaining hair follicle stem cell quiescence. J Invest Dermatol. 2015;135(11):2584–2592. DOI: 10.1038/jid.2015.222

[24] Tarutani M, Itami S, Okabe M, Ikawa M, Tezuka T, Yoshikawa K, et al. Tissue-specific knockout of the mouse Pig-a gene reveals important roles for GPI-anchored proteins in skin development. Proc Natl Acad Sci U S A. 1997;94(14):7400–7405. DOI: 10.1073/pnas.94.14.7400

[25] Hafner M, Wenk J, Nenci A, Pasparakis M, Scharffetter-Kochanek K, Smyth N, et al. Keratin 14 Cre transgenic mice authenticate keratin 14 as an oocyte-expressed protein. Genesis. 2004;38(4):176–181. DOI: 10.1002/gene.20016

[26] Adolphe C, Nieuwenhuis E, Villani R, Li ZJ, Kaur P, Hui CC, et al. Patched 1 and patched 2 redundancy has a key role in regulating epidermal differentiation. J Invest Dermatol. 2014;134(7):1981–1990. DOI: 10.1038/jid.2014.63

[27] Müller-Röver S, Handjiski B, van der Veen C, Eichmüller S, Foitzik K, McKay IA, et al. A comprehensive guide for the accurate classification of murine hair follicles in distinct hair cycle stages. J Invest Dermatol. 2001;117(1):3–15. DOI: 10.1046/j.0022-202x.2001.01377.x

[28] Kawano M, Komi-Kuramochi A, Asada M, Suzuki M, Oki J, Jiang J, et al. Comprehensive analysis of FGF and FGFR expression in skin: FGF18 is highly expressed in hair follicles and capable of inducing anagen from telogen stage hair follicles. J Invest Dermatol. 2005;124(5):877–885. DOI: 10.1111/j.0022-202X.2005.23693.x

[29] Kimura-Ueki M, Oda Y, Oki J, Komi-Kuramochi A, Honda E, Asada M, et al. Hair cycle resting phase is regulated by cyclic epithelial FGF18 signaling. J Invest Dermatol. 2012;132(5):1338–1345. DOI: 10.1038/jid.2011.490

[30] Jensen KB, Collins CA, Nascimento E, Tan DW, Frye M, Itami S, et al. Lrig1 expression defines a distinct multipotent stem cell population in mammalian epidermis. Cell Stem Cell. 2009;4(5):427–439. DOI: 10.1016/j.stem.2009.04.014

[31] Plikus MV, Gay DL, Treffeisen E, Wang A, June R, Cotsarelis G. Epithelial stem cells and implications for wound repair. Semin Cell Dev Biol. 2012;23(9):946–953. DOI: 10.1016/j.semcdb.2012.10.001.Epithelial

[32] Rompolas P, Greco V. Stem cell dynamics in the hair follicle niche. Semin Cell Dev Biol. 2014;25–26:34–42. DOI: 10.1016/j.semcdb.2013.12.005

[33] Cotsarelis G, Sun TT, Lavker RM. Label-retaining cells reside in the bulge area of pilosebaceous unit: implications for follicular stem cells, hair cycle, and skin carcinogenesis. Cell. 1990;61(7):1329–1337.

[34] Taylor G, Lehrer MS, Jensen PJ, Sun TT, Lavker RM. Involvement of follicular stem cells in forming not only the follicle but also the epidermis. Cell. 2000;102(4):451–461. DOI: 10.1016/S0092-8674(00)00050-7

[35] Oshima H, Rochat A. Morphogenesis and renewal of hair follicles from adult multipotent stem cells. Cell 2001;104:233–245.

[36] Lyle S, Christofidou-Solomidou M, Liu Y, Elder DE, Albelda S, Cotsarelis G. The C8/144B monoclonal antibody recognizes cytokeratin 15 and defines the location of human hair follicle stem cells. J Cell Sci. 1998;111:3179–3188.

[37] Trempus CS, Morris RJ, Ehinger M, Elmore A, Bortner CD, Ito M, et al. CD34 expression by hair follicle stem cells is required for skin tumor development in mice. Cancer Res. 2007;67(9):4173–4181. DOI: 10.1158/0008-5472.CAN-06-3128

[38] Jaks V, Barker N, Kasper M, van Es JH, Snippert HJ, Clevers H, et al. Lgr5 marks cycling, yet long-lived, hair follicle stem cells. Nat Genet. 2008;40(11):1291–1299. DOI: 10.1038/ng.239

[39] Nowak JA, Polak L, Pasolli HA, Fuchs E. Hair follicle stem cells are specified and function in early skin morphogenesis. Cell Stem Cell. 2008;3(1):33–43. DOI: 10.1016/j.stem.2008.05.009

[40] Vidal VPI, Chaboissier MC, Lützkendorf S, Cotsarelis G, Mill P, Hui CC, et al. Sox9 is essential for outer root sheath differentiation and the formation of the hair stem cell compartment. Curr Biol. 2005;15(15):1340–1351. DOI: 10.1016/j.cub.2005.06.064

[41] Merrill BJ, Gat U, DasGupta R, Fuchs E. Tcf3 and Lef1 regulate lineage differentiation of multipotent stem cells in skin. Genes Dev. 2001;15(13):1688–1705. DOI: 10.1101/gad.891401

[42] Mardaryev AN, Meier N, Poterlowicz K, Sharov AA, Sharova TY, Ahmed MI, et al. Lhx2 differentially regulates Sox9, Tcf4 and Lgr5 in hair follicle stem cells to promote epidermal regeneration after injury. Development. 2011;138(22):4843–4852. DOI: 10.1242/dev.070284

[43] Rhee H, Polak L, Fuchs E. Lhx2 maintains stem cell character in hair follicles. Science. 2006;312(5782):1946–1949. DOI: 10.1126/science.1128004

[44] Horsley V, Aliprantis AO, Polak L, Glimcher LH, Fuchs E. NFATc1 balances quiescence and proliferation of skin stem cells. Cell. 2008;132(2):299–310. DOI: 10.1016/j.cell.2007.11.047

[45] Nguyen H, Merrill BJ, Polak L, Nikolova M, Rendl M, Shaver TM, et al. Tcf3 and Tcf4 are essential for long-term homeostasis of skin epithelia. Nat Genet. 2009;41(10):1068–1075. DOI: 10.1038/ng.431

[46] Nijhof JGW, Braun KM, Giangreco A, van Pelt C, Kawamoto H, Boyd RL, et al. The cell-surface marker MTS24 identifies a novel population of follicular keratinocytes with characteristics of progenitor cells. Development. 2006;133(15):3027–3037. DOI: 10.1242/dev.02443

[47] Snippert HJ, Haegebarth A, Kasper M, Jaks V, van Es JH, Barker N, et al. Lgr6 marks stem cells in the hair follicle that generate all cell lineages of the skin. Science. 2010;327(5971):1385–1389. DOI: 10.1126/science.1184733

[48] Trempus CS, Morris RJ, Bortner CD, Cotsarelis G, Faircloth RS, Reece JM, et al. Enrichment for living murine keratinocytes from the hair follicle bulge with the cell surface marker CD34. J Invest Dermatol. 2003;120(4):501–511. DOI: 10.1046/j.1523-1747.2003.12088.x

[49] Williams SE, Fuchs E. Oriented divisions, fate decisions. Curr Opin Cell Biol. 2013;25(6):749–758. DOI: 10.1016/j.ceb.2013.08.003

[50] Tellkamp F, Vorhagen S, Niessen CM. Epidermal polarity genes in health and disease. Cold Spring Harb Perspect Med. 2014;4(12):a015255. DOI: 10.1101/cshperspect.a015255

[51] Lechler T, Fuchs E. Asymmetric cell divisions promote stratification and differentiation of mammalian skin. Nature. 2005;437(7056):275–280. DOI: 10.1038/nature03922

[52] Williams SE, Beronja S, Pasolli HA, Fuchs E. Asymmetric cell divisions promote Notch-dependent epidermal differentiation. Nature. 2011;470(7334):353–358. DOI: 10.1038/nature09793

[53] Plikus MV, Mayer JA, de la Cruz D, Baker RE, Maini PK, Maxson R, et al. Cyclic dermal BMP signalling regulates stem cell activation during hair regeneration. Nature. 2008;451(7176):340–344. DOI: 10.1038/nature06457

[54] Hsu YC, Pasolli HA, Fuchs E. Dynamics between stem cells, niche, and progeny in the hair follicle. Cell. 2011;144(1):92–105. DOI: 10.1016/j.cell.2010.11.049

[55] Oshimori N, Fuchs E. Paracrine TGF-β signaling counterbalances BMP-mediated repression in hair follicle stem cell activation. Cell Stem Cell. 2012;10(1):63–75. DOI: 10.1016/j.stem.2011.11.005

[56] Botchkarev VA, Botchkareva NV, Roth W, Nakamura M, Chen LH, Herzog W, et al. Noggin is a mesenchymally derived stimulator of hair-follicle induction. Nat Cell Biol. 1999;1(3):158–164. DOI: 10.1038/11078

[57] Hsu YC, Fuchs E. A family business: stem cell progeny join the niche to regulate homeostasis. Nat Rev Mol Cell Biol. 2012;13(2):103–114. DOI: 10.1038/nrm3272

[58] Weiss RA, Eichner R, Sun TT. Monoclonal antibody analysis of keratin expression in epidermal diseases: a 48- and 56-kdalton keratin as molecular markers for hyperproliferative keratinocytes. J Cell Biol. 1984;98(4):1397–1406.

[59] Stoler A, Kopan R, Duvic M, Fuchs E. Use of monospecific antisera and cRNA probes to localize the major changes in keratin expression during normal and abnormal epidermal differentiation. J Cell Biol. 1988;107(2):427–446.

[60] Leitges M, Sanz L, Martin P, Duran A, Braun U, García JF, et al. Targeted disruption of the zetaPKC gene results in the impairment of the NF-kappaB pathway. Mol Cell. 2001;8(4):771–780.

[61] Hartleben B, Widmeier E, Suhm M, Worthmann K, Schell C, Helmstädter M, et al. aPKCλ/ι and aPKCζ contribute to podocyte differentiation and glomerular maturation. J Am Soc Nephrol. 2013;24(2):253–267. DOI: 10.1681/ASN.2012060582

[62] Iden S, van Riel WE, Schäfer R, Song JY, Hirose T, Ohno S, et al. Tumor type-dependent function of the Par3 polarity protein in skin tumorigenesis. Cancer Cell. 2012;22(3):389–403. DOI: 10.1016/j.ccr.2012.08.004

[63] McGrath JA, Gatalica B, Christiano AM, Li K, Owaribe K, McMillan JR, et al. Mutations in the 180-kD bullous pemphigoid antigen (BPAG2), a hemidesmosomal transmembrane collagen (COL17A1), in generalized atrophic benign epidermolysis bullosa. Nat Genet. 1995;11(1):83–86. DOI: 10.1038/ng0995-83

[64] Darling TN, Bauer JW, Hintner H, Yancey KB. Generalized atrophic benign epidermolysis bullosa. Adv Dermatol. 1997;13:87–119.

[65] Hintner H, Wolff K. Generalized atrophic benign epidermolysis bullosa. Arch Dermatol. 1982;118(6):375–384.

[66] Nishie W, Sawamura D, Goto M, Ito K, Shibaki A, McMillan JR, et al. Humanization of autoantigen. Nat Med. 2007;13(3):378–383. DOI: 10.1038/nm1496

[67] Tanimura S, Tadokoro Y, Inomata K, Binh NT, Nishie W, Yamazaki S, et al. Hair follicle stem cells provide a functional niche for melanocyte stem cells. Cell Stem Cell. 2011;8(2): 177–187. DOI: 10.1016/j.stem.2010.11.029

[68] Matsumura H, Mohri Y, Binh NT, Morinaga H, Fukuda M, Ito M, et al. Hair follicle aging is driven by transepidermal elimination of stem cells via COL17A1 proteolysis. Science. 2016;351(6273):1–14. DOI: 10.1126/science.aad4395

Chapter 4

Hair Follicle Reconstruction and Stem Cells

Ekaterina P. Kalabusheva, Elina S. Chermnykh,
Vasily V. Terskikh and Ekaterina A. Vorotelyak

Additional information is available at the end of the chapter

http://dx.doi.org/10.5772/66707

Abstract

De novo hair follicle (HF) formation in embryonic skin and hair growth in postnatal skin are the result of epithelial-mesenchymal interactions between specialized mesenchymal dermal papilla (DP) and epithelial stem cells that give rise to hairs. Adult HF is a valuable source of different lineages of stem cells (SCs) with morphogenetic potential. Epithelial stem cells are residing in the special compartment of HF (the bulge) and can be mobilized to regenerate the new follicle with each hair cycle and to reepithelialize epidermis during wound repair. This review summarizes the current knowledge on key characteristics of HF SC populations in terms of regenerative potential. General biological principles that govern the mesenchymal-epithelial interactions within the HF and the signaling pathways that control HF development are discussed. The main focus is on recent approaches to reconstruct folliculogenesis *in vitro* and perspectives of the tissue engineering in alopecia therapy.

Keywords: epidermis, hair follicle, morphogenesis, stem cells, hair follicle reconstruction, dermal papilla

1. Introduction

Alopecia is a growing health problem in the world, and the age of patients tends to decrease [1]. Dermatologists and trichologists have an increasing list of young patients including women, at the age of 25–30 years or even teenagers. At the same time, there are only few really effective remedies in the field. Achievements in cell biology and biotechnology propose novel products to solve these problems. One of the promising and reasonable ways to develop cell products for hair loss treatment is to obtain trichogenic cells and then to grow small follicle-like structures. To develop effective strategies of hair follicle (HF) reconstruction we need to have a deep insight into cellular and molecular mechanisms of HF development and regeneration. The research on HF is a rapidly developing area of skin biology. This mini-organ can be successfully used for a wide range of studies into the mechanisms of morphogenesis, stem cell behavior, cell differentiation, and apoptosis [2–4]. Moreover, as mentioned above, HF investigations can provide invaluable insights into the possible causes of human hair disorders and provide conditions for development of HF restoration technologies.

2. Hair follicle: structure, cycling and stem cells

HF is a skin appendage with very complex structure undergoing lifelong periods of morphogenesis. The major part of HF is produced by the epithelium. Highly proliferative matrix cells in HF bulb gradually move upwards in the course of differentiation. They are progenitors for the inner and outer root sheaths and hair shaft later on. Mesenchymal portion of HF includes dermal papilla (DP) and HF connective tissue sheath. DP is located inside the bulb and is separated from the matrix cells by a basement membrane. In a lower part of the bulb, DP contacts with the dermal sheath that surrounds the entire follicle. This structure is maintained throughout the hair-growth phase – anagen. With time, when HF transits into the destructive phase–catagen–the lower two-thirds of the HF epithelial strand degenerate and the hair shaft production stops. DP also becomes smaller but its losses are much less significant and are mainly caused by reduced content of an extracellular matrix [5] and migration of cells between the DP and the adjacent dermal sheath [6]. During catagen, HF is reduced to a tiny epidermal strand surrounded by a basement membrane. As it retracts, the DP is pulled upward to the upper permanent portion of the HF containing bulge stem cells [7].

Then HF enters the resting phase – telogen. The transition from telogen to anagen is the beginning of a new HF cycle, a process that continues throughout life. In mice, the lengths of anagen and catagen phases are similar from one cycle to the next, while each telogen becomes longer than the previous one. This results in progressive asynchrony in HF cycling with age [8].

Now it is quite clear that the regeneration cycle is maintained by activity of HF stem cells. HF is considered to be a valuable source of adult stem cells (SCs) with morphogenetic potential. SCs may be isolated from epidermal and mesenchymal compartments of HF. Additionally neural crest-derived cells are found in HF, at least in the facial skin [9, 10]. Matrix cells had been thought to be stem cells for a long time as they proliferate very intensively at the beginning of the growth phase. However in experiments with murine HFs, Cotsarelis and co-authors discovered special population of cells at the bottom of a permanent portion of the HF known as the bulge [11]. These cells retained thymidine DNA label after 4 weeks of chase period unlike matrix cells which lost the label as early as 1 week after cessation of labeling. From these pioneering experiments, the bulge has been proved in many studies to be the main reservoir of SCs in HF. It contains morphologically undifferentiated and slow-cycling under the normal conditions of cells. The bulge is a swelling and contiguous part of outer root sheath. As many HFs lack anatomically well-defined bulge region, the term 'bulge' is often referred loosely to the permanent region of the follicle below the sebaceous gland [12, 13]. The bulge region is also the point of attachment of the arrector pilorum muscles [11]. SCs of melanocyte lineage are located in close proximity of the bulge epithelial SCs. Melanocyte proliferation and differentiation is strongly coordinated with the HF cycle. In fact, both types of SCs occupy the same niche or two partially overlapping niches [14, 15]. The arrector pilorum muscle is tightly connected with the bulge region. Epithelial SCs of the outer root sheath deposit nefronectin onto underlying basement membrane and regulate adhesion of mesenchymal cells expressing the receptor to nefronectin. Thus, bulge SC create the niche for smooth muscle cells and participate in regulation of the arrector pilorum muscle [16].

Epithelial and mesenchymal SCs of HF are not only a source of cell mass during HF regrowth phase, but they are also key regulators of hair cycle. Both pools of SCs produced multiple growth factors and cytokines regulating cellular proliferation, differentiation, and HF morphogenesis. Key regulators of hair cycle belong to Wnt, TGFbeta, FGF, and some other signaling pathway families [17, 18].

Bulge cells remain dormant during telogen. The DP plays a pivotal role in initiation of the next cycle of HF formation and hair growth [19–21]. This is associated with bulge cell migration and proliferation in the hair germ to generate the highly proliferative cells at the base of the follicle [7, 22]. Hair germ likely represents a special subpopulation of bulge descendants capable of quick recruitment into intensively proliferating state [7]. The authors suggest that the crosstalk between hair germ and DP via FGF7 signaling contributes significantly to the early steps of hair cycle activation.

3. Dermal papilla cells and their inductive properties

Dermal papilla cells represent mesenchymal cell subpopulation with stem properties. According to their specific features, they may be attributed to classical fibroblast-like cells with special functions. At the same time, DP cells meet stem cell criteria. In a number of works, including those coming from our lab, it was demonstrated that DP cells, according to their characteristics, may be attributed to mesenchymal stem cells along with those derived from bone marrow and adipose tissue [23–26]. These characteristics are widely accepted criteria for mesenchymal stem cells including fibroblastic morphology, ability to adhere and to differentiate into osteogenic, chondrogenic, and adipogenic lineages [24, 27, 28]. It should be mentioned that DP differentiation abilities are often pronounced not to the same extent as those of classical mesenchymal stem cells [23]. As other lineages of differentiation were demonstrated some authors believe DP cells to be multipotent [28]. In laboratory animals, it was demonstrated that this type of cells is able to incorporate into skin structures by grafting [29] and stimulate hair growth and angiogenesis. As it was found in detail during the last 20 years, the ability to induce and regulate HF morphogenesis has been considered to be the main characteristic and core biological function of DP cells. They are indispensable component for embryonic development of HF and postnatal cycling [30]. They serve as the niche for providing signals to matrix progenitors in specifying the size, shape, and pigmentation of hair fiber [5, 31]. Multiple pathways and molecules regulating epithelio-mesenchymal interactions were discovered [32]. Using double reporter Lef1-RFP/K14-H2BGFP mice, Rendl with co-authors discovered detailed genetic signature of isolated mouse DP cells [33].

In ontogenesis, DP first appears as cell condensates on the dermis. As HF develops, epidermal cells proliferate actively and envelope the dermal condensates [34]. Exposed to these new niche conditions, DP cells acquire the expression of BMP-4, its inhibitor noggin, and the surface markers N-CAM and p-75. Additionally, they secret specific extracellular matrix protein versican and show a high level of alkaline phosphatase activity.

Inducing capacity of DP cells, i.e., their ability to induce HF development in embryogenesis and regulate postnatal HF cycling, is the most interesting and intriguing trait of these cells. It is noteworthy that not only DP but also skin dermis on the whole has an ability to regulate differentiation of integumental epithelia. As an example, keratinocytes of the palmoplantar thick skin exclusively express keratin 9 [35]. Recombination of the epidermis from different body sites with palmoplantar dermis caused onset of keratin 9 expression and differentiation of keratinocytes into thick skin [36]. Later it was shown that paleness and thickness of the palmoplantar skin is determined by Wnt signaling. Fibroblasts present in thick skin secrete Wnt inhibitor Dikkopf1, which causes thickening of the epidermis and decreases pigmentation both *in vivo* and *in vitro* [37]. HFs and, thus, DPs are distributed over the entire surface of the mammal body. In spite of different embryological origin of DPs from different sites of the body, their functional properties are quite similar. Analysis of global gene expression using microarrays demonstrated a very high degree of similarity between facial and trunk dermal hair-associated cells indicating phenotypic convergence within HF niche [38].

DP cells have been quite profoundly investigated but their isolation and long-term cultivation is not a trivial task yet. They quickly lose intrinsic biological characteristics, especially hair inductive capacity, with passaging [39–41]. This process correlates with decrease in expression of DP markers including alkaline phosphatase, versican, Wnt5a, and some others [42–45].

A number of studies reported various approaches to maintain innate properties in cultured DP cells. Earlier approach implied cocultivation with keratinocytes or addition of keratinocyte-derived factors [46, 47] based on close interaction of DP cells with keratinocytes in their natural niche. Another group of studies considers specific signaling pathways participating in hair growth activation and epithelial-mesenchymal interactions. Wnt and BMP signaling were shown to play a key role in HF morphogenesis [18, 44, 48, 49]. Wnt proteins demonstrated high effectiveness in respect of DP maintenance [50, 51]. Shimizu and Morgan found that Wnt 3a can maintain the hair-inductive properties of DP cells when they are cultured *in vitro* [49]. The medium containing recombinant Wnt-10b protein promoted the proliferation of DP cells, which successfully maintained their ability to induce HFs up to at least 10 serial passages [52]. Noteworthy, Wnt10b has been shown to be expressed in developing HFs, with the earliest and most marked localization in placodes [53] while Wnt10b-producing cells promoted hair folliculogenesis [54]. Canonical Wnt pathway in cultured DP cells was shown to be modulated by several compounds: ciprofloxacin [55], valproic acid [56, 57], and glycogen synthase kinase (GSK)-3 –inhibitors [43, 58]. Addition of vitamin D3 to culture medium upregulated expression of Wnt10b and TGF-β2 in murine DP cell providing significantly enhanced hair growth in hemivascularized sandwich assay [59].

Members of TGFbeta signaling pathway, Bmp 4 and Bmp 6 were used successfully to maintain specific characteristics of DP cells in culture [44, 48]. EGF and VEGF demonstrated stimulation of DP proliferation [60, 61]. However, these factors failed to maintain specific DP markers (unpublished data). It is not surprising as cell proliferation may necessarily correlate with hair inductive activity. On the other hand, combination of FGF and PDGF-AA promoted DP growth in culture and increased *de novo* HF induction in chamber assay using treated DP cells [62].

Ohyama and co-authors studied molecular signature of freshly dissected human DP cells and found gene expression profiles that distinguish intact human DP from conventionally cultured human DP cells and fibroblasts. Because the bioinformatics analysis performed by the authors implied the involvement of Wnt, BMP, and FGF signaling pathways in the maintenance of specific DP properties they used the mixture of recombinant proteins and small molecules for stimulation of BMP, FGF, and Wnt pathways, respectively. This approach allowed them to maintain or even restore innate DP gene expression profile and trichogenic properties demonstrated in an *in vivo* hair induction assay [43].

Recently it was shown that systemically administered pharmacological inhibitors of Janus kinase (JAK) family of protein tyrosine kinases, as downstream effectors of the IFN-γ and γc cytokine receptors, prevented the development of alopecia areata in a mouse model reducing the accumulation of effector T cells in the skin [63]. During the course of the study, the authors noticed unexpected regrowth of HFs after topical treatment with JAK-STAT inhibitors. They checked it in a separate study and were able to demonstrate direct stimulation of HFs growth both in mice, and the human xenografts and HF organ culture model [64]. Moreover, treatment of human DP spheres with the inhibitor of JAK1/3 signaling tofacitinib enhanced inductivity of human DP cells grown in spheres significantly which resulted in larger and significantly greater numbers of HFs obtained in the patch assay.

Another way to get closer to native DPs is to cultivate DP cells in spheres. It has been noticed long ago that DP cells demonstrate aggregative behavior in culture [65]. This may be readily used for creation of three-dimensional (3D) environment by hanging drop or non-adherent biomaterial culture systems. This approach can partially recover expression of core markers in human DP cultures [66]. Cells in spheres stop to proliferate and establish multiple cell-cell contacts that may enhance Wnt signaling. They returned to a more native state judged by alpha-smooth muscle actin expression. It is noteworthy that not all strains demonstrated this behavior indicating large differences between cultures derived from different donors. Nevertheless, many studies with DP cells have been conducted recently using 3D cultivation [31, 64, 67, 68]. They showed prolongation of specific markers expression and enhancement of hair inductive capacity after preliminary DP cell aggregation [42, 43, 66].

Taking into account complex natural HF niche it seems quite reasonable to introduce elements of this niche into DP culture systems. Huang with co-authors [68] combined DP with SCs derived from the adipose tissue (ASC) which normally surrounds HF and is shown to influence HF cycling presumably via PDGF signaling [69]. It was found that core-shell patterning of combined spheres with DP cells inside and ASC outside had a beneficial effect on DP markers expression (Hey 1 and Versican) and the rate of hair formation in *in vivo* patch assay. Mature adipocytes incorporated into the same type of spheres had no impact on these processes. A simple mixture of cells within spheres without the formation of core-shell structures yielded much worse results [68]. The authors assume that the mixture of ASCs and DPs in simple mixed spheres interrupted the direct cell-cell interactions and association in DP cells or diluted the signals from ASCs to the DP sphere. It was reported that extracts and conditioned medium from neural stem cells were able to stimulate keratinocyte growth and enhanced hair growth compared to minoxidil [70].

Further search for suitable factors and conditions for effective cultivation and propagation of DP cells will allow one to elucidate mechanism of their self-maintenance and develop large-scale culture technologies.

4. Hair follicle reconstruction

Regeneration ability of organs and even tissues is significantly limited in humans. At the same time, loss of teeth, hair, and even mammary glands due to different reasons is quite abundant. These organs are comparable by their ontogenetic epithelial-mesenchymal origin i.e., like almost all organs in the body, they arise from organ germs which undergo subsequent stages of reciprocal epithelial-mesenchymal crosstalk and close interactions. In adult human body, reproduction of these interactions in the right order and availability of germ-initiating cells to regenerate the entire architecture of multicomponent tissues and organs seems to be impossible or at least dramatically impeded. Development of novel technologies proposes a new hope for people. Tissue engineering is a promising approach to replace the lost tissues and organs. However, the problem how to obtain complex structures which can imitate an organ or develop the organ after grafting is far from solution. In many cases, practical technologies imply transplantation of specialized cells in suspension or sheets. More complicated structures are much more difficult to grow.

Reconstruction of folliculogenesis *in vitro* has been in the minds of scientists for a long period of time taking into account vast knowledge and impressive progress in skin biology beginning from the pioneering works on cultivation of epidermal cells [71] and the epidermis being one of the first tissues that has been reconstructed using tissue engineering [72]. Skin comprises epithelial and mesenchymal components which form body coverage and multiple skin appendages like HF and different types of glands. Since it became possible to reconstruct and reconstitute damaged skin, the problem of HF and gland reconstruction emerged for proper functioning of skin grafts as well as for fundamental studies. It has become especially attractive because a new direction of tissue engineering and regenerative medicine has been developed which utilized the ability of pluripotent cells to self-organize in culture into organ-like structures reproducing functional activity of the corresponding organ [73]. However postnatal cells represent quite a different story.

During recent decades, HF biology was profoundly studied. As mentioned above, HF in mammals is the only organ which in normal physiological condition undergoes degeneration (catagen) to small aggregates of resting cells (telogen) with subsequent full regeneration leading to complete restoration of multicellular organ generating corneal shaft (anagen). Multiple mechanisms regulating organogenesis and physiological regeneration of HFs are found, the

http://dx.doi.org/10.5772/66707

cellular structure of HF is studied in detail, properties and functions of cell subpopulations are elucidated [74–78].

Numerous studies utilized the ability of epithelial and mesenchymal cells of different organs to produce mutual influence even in culture conditions in attempts to reproduce morphogenetic processes. After both compartments were determined in HF, this approach was applied to reconstruct folliculogenesis *in vitro*. It was proved that DP cells affect interfollicular keratinocytes in many aspects. Coculturing of keratinocytes and DP cells in Transwell system stimulated expression of follicular markers in keratinocytes [79]. Direct contact between cells of different types enhances this interaction [80].

Due to specific inducing properties of DP cells morphogenesis of HF may be reproduced in culture. While keratinocytes possess intrinsic ability to form structures resembling different stages of HF morphogenesis, HF mesenchyme regulates and intensifies this process. DP-conditioned medium stimulates morphogenesis in keratinocyte culture demonstrating high rate of tube formation in the collagen gel [81]. However, production of fully functional HFs from postnatal cells is still challenging.

Scientists tried to improve effectiveness of HF morphogenesis using more potent cells including keratinocytes from HFs or embryonic cells. As it can be predicted, embryonic tissues demonstrate higher potential to develop organs after inoculation into culture. Significant portion of studies were performed using embryonic tissues in order to avoid roadblocks of postnatal conditions. Mouse embryonic skin explants may successfully develop HFs in culture [82]. Dissociated cells from embryonic tissues aggregate and form the organ germs which can develop into mature primordium and then into a functioning organ. Such results were demonstrated for tooth and hair germs. Buds from dissociated skin of murine embryos developed into mature HFs in culture or after transplantation to immunocompromised animals [83–85]. However, it is quite difficult to reproduce this type of experiments using postnatal HF cells. Long-term cultivation of HFs from postnatal skin is usually completed with gradual degradation of the structure and degeneration of HF. Even in optimized conditions, HFs begin to degenerate after 20 days in culture, on average, while apoptotic cells appear approximately on day 5 [86]. HFs maintained *in vitro* are unable to keep cycling [87, 88]. In the study on rat HFs cultured on gelfoam supports, Philpott and Kealey were able to demonstrate signs of cycling but all follicles appeared to remain blocked in pro-anagen [89]. Non-follicular keratinocytes failed to reconstruct HFs in combination with DP cells but the latter improved significantly the quality of engineered skin grafts applied onto acute skin defects in nude mice [90]. Human DP cells used in skin equivalent together with epidermal cells enriched with HF keratinocytes could generate HF bud 14 days after transplantation into nude mice but further development was impeded [91]. Interestingly, the authors also noticed a quality improvement in composite skin substitutes containing DP cells as compared to dermal fibroblasts, these substitutes more accurately mimicked a well-ordered epithelium. More impressive results in terms of folliculogenesis were reported in xenogenic equivalents combining human foreskin keratinocytes and murine dermal cells [92, 93]. Six weeks after grafting, the authors recorded bulbous pegs and HFs, which however lacked sebaceous glands and were not able to erupt through the epidermal surface. These experiments declare the development of skin substitutes with a high degree of homology to native skin as a long-term objective. At the same time, such an approach may be a useful tool to elaborate an effective technique for HF production. To overcome problems with HF eruption through the epithelial sheet and prevent epithelial cyst formation, a nylon thread was used as a guide for the infundibulum direction via insertion into the bioengineered germ [94]. This method showed perfect results in terms of the shaft formation after transplantation onto nude mice. Both mouse and human HF germs were reconstructed in the study. Human bioengineered HF germ was composed of the bulge region-derived epithelial cells and scalp HF-derived intact DPs of an androgenetic alopecia patient. These germs developed pigmented hair shafts within 21 days after intracutaneous transplantation into the back skin of nude mice [94].

Inamatsu with colleagues compared the process of neofolliculogenesis after intracutaneous transplantation of postnatal DP cells and embryonic dermal condensate in mice [95]. They showed that the dermal condensate-triggered development of HFs is similar to that in embryogenesis. Postnatal DP induced formation of new follicles by a different way, it induces the onset of the anagen-like stage without embryonic-like development.

Nevertheless, a number of studies have demonstrated successful reconstruction of follicle-like structures from cells cultivated *in vitro*. They are focused on development of these structures into HF after transplantation as it was discussed above. This is achieved by two ways: skin equivalents with cells capable of hair follicle induction or aggregates made of keratinocytes and trichogenic mesenchyme with subsequent transplantation. Zheng and co-authors [96, 97] used DP and keratinocyte suspension to inject into mice. It was shown that keratinocytes aggregated first, DP cells stimulated their proliferation enlarging hair follicle primordium and then the shaft began to grow into the cavity which had been formed in the aggregate. It was found that the way of cell combination affects epithelio-mesenchymal interactions. In mixed culture, aggregates were smaller; keratinocytes proliferated better and escaped apoptosis [98]. In the study by Havlickova with co-authors, human keratinocytes of the outer root sheath and DP were placed into specially constructed pseudodermis comprising collagen matrix and dermal fibroblasts. The authors found that cells preserved viability, expressed specific markers, and supported proliferation. They were also able to produce specific reaction on substances stimulating or inhibiting hair growth [99]. However, the appropriate architecture of hair follicle bud was lost. Thus, authors supposed to use the model for drug testing. They think such model should (1) imitate at least one typical feature of the human HF; (2) manifest the predicted reaction to the known modulators of HF cycle and development; and (3) exhibit the reactions which are reproducible *in vivo* [99]. Scientists from Technical University in Berlin reported the production of microfollicles *in vitro* by mixing DP aggregates with the basement membrane components and the outer root sheath keratinocytes [100]. They found expression of HF markers such as vimentin, cytokeratins, trichohyalin, and chondroitin sulfate. Remarkably, they observed hair-like fibers sprouting from the nascent microfollicles. Different types of free aggregates present another modification of culture conditions. Cells may be placed on partially-adhesive substrates [101]. Being seeded on poly(ethylene-co-vinyl alcohol), DP cells first aggregate in this model and then are

http://dx.doi.org/10.5772/66707

covered with keratinocytes. The authors found keratinocytes expressed keratin 6 and, thus, underwent differentiation.

Another way to closely reproduce HF morphogenesis *in vitro* may involve specialized HF cells derived from the pluripotent cells. For example, the derivation of functional DP-like cells from human embryonic stem cells was recently reported [102]. Derivation of multipotent progenitors of the epithelial lineage [103, 104] gives an opportunity to combine trichogenic cells at their early stages of commitment with hopefully better results.

Using the advantage of induced pluripotency Yang with colleagues [105] obtained folliculogenic CD200+/ITGA6+ epidermal stem cells from human fibroblast-derived induced pluripotent cells. Patch *in vivo* assay demonstrated the ability of these cells to generate all HF lineages including the hair shaft, and the inner and outer root sheaths. The regenerated HFs possessed a stem cell population and produced hair shafts expressing hair specific keratins. The ability of pluripotent cells to self-organize and spontaneously differentiate into all cell lineages was used by Takagi and colleagues [106] who carefully selected conditions that enabled direct derivation of HFs from induced pluripotent cells through embryoid bodies using the clustering-dependent embryoid body transplantation method.

Currently, there are a number of ongoing clinical trials using cultured cells to treat alopecia [107]. It is noteworthy that interfollicular unspecialized cells are used in many cases, put it simply, dermal fibroblasts and epidermal keratinocytes. Therapeutic mechanisms of such preparations are unclear and positive effect depends on patient's remaining HFs. However, the latter are absent in many cases. Therefore, modern approaches to HF restoration are badly needed for severe cases of hair loss or alopecia. Taking into account great progress in skin and HF biology, biotechnology, and tissue engineering we hope to meet highly effective methods of HF production in the nearest future.

Acknowledgements

The work was funded by the Russian Science Foundation (Project No. 16-14-00204).

Author details

Ekaterina P. Kalabusheva[1,2,*], Elina S. Chermnykh[1,2], Vasily V. Terskikh[1] and Ekaterina A. Vorotelyak[1,2]

*Address all correspondence to: vorotelyak@yandex.ru

1 N.K. Koltzov Institute of Developmental Biology, Russian Academy of Sciences, Moscow, Russia

2 Pirogov Russian National Research Medical University, Moscow, Russia

References

[1] Miteva M, Tosti A. Treatment options for alopecia: an update, looking to the future. Expert Opin Pharmacother. 2012;13(9):1271–1281. DOI: 10.1517/14656566.2012.685160

[2] Shimomura Y. Journey toward unraveling the molecular basis of hereditary hair disorders. J Dermatol Sci. 2016. DOI: 10.1016/j.jdermsci.2016.08.006

[3] Zheng Y, Hsieh J-C, Escandon J, Cotsarelis G. Isolation of mouse hair follicle bulge stem cells and their functional analysis in a reconstitution assay. Methods Mol Biol. 2016;1453:57–69. DOI: 10.1007/978-1-4939-3786-8_8

[4] Rippa A, Terskikh V, Nesterova A, Vasiliev A, Vorotelyak E. Hair follicle morphogenesis and epidermal homeostasis in we/we wal/wal mice with postnatal alopecia. Histochem Cell Biol. 2015;143(5):481–496. DOI: 10.1007/s00418-014-1291-1

[5] Elliott K, Messenger AG, Stephenson TJ. Differences in hair follicle dermal papilla volume are due to extracellular matrix volume and cell number: implications for the control of hair follicle size and androgen responses. J Invest Dermatol. 1999;113(6):873–877. DOI: 10.1046/j.1523-1747.1999.00797.x

[6] Tobin DJ, Magerl M, Gunin A, Paus R. Plasticity and cytokinetic dynamics of the hair follicle mesenchyme during the hair growth cycle: implications for growth control and hair follicle transformations. J Investig Dermatology Symp Proc. 2003;8(1):80–86. DOI: 10.1046/j.1523-1747.2003.12177.x

[7] Greco V, Chen T, Rendl M, Schober M, Pasolli HA, Stokes N, et al. A two-step mechanism for stem cell activation during hair regeneration. Cell Stem Cell. 2009;4(2):155–169. DOI: 10.1016/j.stem.2008.12.009

[8] Müller–Röver S, Foitzik K, Paus R, Handjiski B, van der Veen C, Eichmüller S, et al. A comprehensive guide for the accurate classification of murine hair follicles in distinct hair cycle stages. J Invest Dermatol. 2001;117(1):3–15. DOI: 10.1046/j.0022-202x.2001.01377.x

[9] Sieber-Blum M, Grim M, Hu YF, Szeder V. Pluripotent neural crest stem cells in the adult hair follicle. Dev Dyn. 2004;231(2):258–269. DOI: 10.1002/dvdy.20129

[10] Amoh Y, Li L, Katsuoka K, Penman S, Hoffman RM. Multipotent nestin-positive, keratin-negative hair-follicle bulge stem cells can form neurons. Proc Natl Acad Sci U S A. 2005;102(15):5530–5534. DOI: 10.1073/pnas.0501263102

[11] Cotsarelis G, Sun T-T, Lavker RM. Label-retaining cells reside in the bulge area of pilosebaceous unit: implications for follicular stem cells, hair cycle, and skin carcinogenesis. Cell. 1990;61(7):1329–1337. DOI: 10.1016/0092-8674(90)90696-C

[12] Morris RJ, Potten CS. Slowly cycling (label-retaining) epidermal cells behave like clonogenic stem cells in vitro. Cell Prolif. 1994;27(5):279–289.DOI: 10.1111/j.1365-2184.1994.tb01425.x

[13] Stenn KS, Paus R. Controls of hair follicle cycling. Physiol Rev. 2001;81(1):449–494.

[14] Chang C-Y, Pasolli HA, Giannopoulou EG, Guasch G, Gronostajski RM, Elemento O, et al. NFIB is a governor of epithelial-melanocyte stem cell behaviour in a shared niche. Nature. 2013;495(7439):98–102. DOI: 10.1038/nature11847

[15] Nishimura EK, Jordan SA, Oshima H, Yoshida H, Osawa M, Moriyama M, et al. Dominant role of the niche in melanocyte stem-cell fate determination. Nature. 2002;416(6883):854–860. DOI: 10.1038/416854a

[16] Fujiwara H, Ferreira M, Donati G, Marciano DK, Linton JM, Sato Y, et al. The basement membrane of hair follicle stem cells is a muscle cell niche. Cell. 2011;144(4):577–589. DOI: 10.1016/j.cell.2011.01.014

[17] Schneider MR, Schmidt-Ullrich R, Paus R. The hair follicle as a dynamic miniorgan. Curr Biol. 2009;19(3):R132–142. DOI: 10.1016/j.cub.2008.12.005

[18] Botchkarev VA, Paus R. Molecular biology of hair morphogenesis: development and cycling. J Exp Zool. 2003;298(1):164–180. DOI: 10.1002/jez.b.33

[19] Blanpain C, Lowry WE, Geoghegan A, Polak L, Fuchs E. Self-renewal, multipotency, and the existence of two cell populations within an epithelial stem cell niche. Cell. 2004;118(5):635–648. DOI: 10.1016/j.cell.2004.08.012

[20] Morris RJ, Liu Y, Marles L, Yang Z, Trempus C, Li S et al. Capturing and profiling adult hair follicle stem cells. Nat Biotechnol. 2004; 22:411–417. DOI: 10.1038/nbt950

[21] Tumbar T, Guasch G, Greco V, Blanpain C, Lowry WE, Rendl M, et al. Defining the epithelial stem cell niche in skin. Science. 2004;303(5656):359–363. DOI: 10.1126/science.1092436

[22] Zhang Y V, Cheong J, Ciapurin N, McDermitt DJ, Tumbar T. Distinct self-renewal and differentiation phases in the niche of infrequently dividing hair follicle stem cells. Cell Stem Cell. 2009;5(3):267–278. DOI: 10.1016/j.stem.2009.06.004

[23] Kiseleva EV, Chermnykh ES, Vorotelyak EA, Volozhin AI, Vasiliev AV, Terskikh VV. Differentiation capacity of stromal fibroblast-like cells from human bone marrow, adipose tissue, hair follicle dermal papilla and derma. Cell Tissue Biol. 2009;3(1):42–49.

[24] Bobis S, Jarocha D, Majka M. Mesenchymal stem cells: characteristics and clinical applications. Folia Histochem Cytobiol. 2006;44(4):215–230.

[25] Ross FP, Christiano AM. Nothing but skin and bone. J Clin Invest. 2006;116(5):1140–1149. DOI: 10.1172/JCI28605

[26] Lorenz K, Sicker M, Schmelzer E, Rupf T, Salvetter J, Schulz-Siegmund M, et al. Multilineage differentiation potential of human dermal skin-derived fibroblasts. Exp Dermatol. 2008;17(11):925–932. DOI: 10.1111/j.1600-0625.2008.00724.x

[27] Zuk PA, Zhu M, Ashjian P, De Ugarte DA, Huang JI, Mizuno H, et al. Human adipose tissue is a source of multipotent stem cells. Mol Biol Cell. 2002;13:4279–4295. DOI: 10.1091/mbc.E02-02-0105

[28] Driskell RR, Clavel C, Rendl M, Watt FM. Hair follicle dermal papilla cells at a glance. J Cell Sci. 2011;124(Pt 8):1179–1182. DOI: 10.1242/jcs.082446

[29] Chermnykh ES, Vorotelyak EA, Vasilev AV, Terskikh VV, Radyukhina NV, Rutkevich PN, et al. Capability of cultivated human hair-follicle cells to integrate with skin structure in vivo. Cell Tissue Biol. 2010;4(3):245–250

[30] Morgan BA. The dermal papilla: an instructive niche for epithelial stem and progenitor cells in development and regeneration of the hair follicle. Cold Spring Harb Perspect Med. 2014;4(7):a015180. DOI: 10.1101/cshperspect.a015180

[31] Huang Y-C, Chan C-C, Lin W-T, Chiu H-Y, Tsai R-Y, Tsai T-H, et al. Scalable production of controllable dermal papilla spheroids on PVA surfaces and the effects of spheroid size on hair follicle regeneration. Biomaterials. 2013;34(2):442–451. DOI: 10.1016/j.biomaterials.2012.09.083

[32] Balañá ME, Charreau HE, Leirós GJ. Epidermal stem cells and skin tissue engineering in hair follicle regeneration. World J Stem Cells. 2015;7(4):711–727. DOI: 10.4252/wjsc.v7.i4.711.

[33] Rendl M, Lewis L, Fuchs E. Molecular dissection of mesenchymal-epithelial interactions in the hair follicle. PLoS Biol. 2005;3(11):e331. DOI: 10.1371/journal.pbio.0030331

[34] Schmidt-Ullrich R, Paus R. Molecular principles of hair follicle induction and morphogenesis. Bioessays. 2005;27(3):247–261. DOI: 10.1002/bies.20184

[35] Knapp AC, Franke WW, Heid H, Hatzfeld M, Jorcano JL, Moll R. Cytokeratin No. 9, an epidermal type I keratin characteristic of a special program of keratinocyte differentiation displaying body site specificity. J Cell Biol. 1986;103(2):657–667.

[36] Yamaguchi Y, Itami S, Tarutani M, Hosokawa K, Miura H, Yoshikawa K. Regulation of keratin 9 in nonpalmoplantar keratinocytes by palmoplantar fibroblasts through epithelial–mesenchymal interactions. J Invest Dermatol. 1999;112(4):483–488. DOI: 10.1046/j.1523-1747.1999.00544.x

[37] Yamaguchi Y, Passeron T, Hoashi T, Watabe H, Rouzaud F, Yasumoto K, et al. Dickkopf 1 (DKK1) regulates skin pigmentation and thickness by affecting Wnt/beta-catenin signaling inkeratinocytes. FASEB J. 2008;22(4):1009–1020. DOI: 10.1096/fj.07-9475com

[38] Jinno H, Morozova O, Jones KL, Biernaskie JA, Paris M, Hosokawa R, et al. Convergent genesis of an adult neural crest-like dermal stem cell from distinct developmental origins. Stem Cells. 2010;28(11):2027–2040. DOI: 10.1002/stem.525

[39] Horne KA, Jahoda CAB, Oliver RF. Whisker growth induced by implantation of cultured vibrissa dermal papilla cells in the adult rat. J Embryol Exp Morphol. 1986;97(1):111–124.

[40] Lichti U, Weinberg WC, Goodman L, Ledbetter S, Dooley T, Morgan D, et al. In vivo regulation of murine hair growth: insights from grafting defined cell populations onto nude mice. J Invest Dermatol. 1993;101(1 Suppl):124S–129S.

[41] Weinberg WC, Goodman L V., George C, Morgan DL, Ledbetter S, Yuspa SH, et al. Reconstitution of hair follicle development in vivo: determination of follicle formation, hair growth, and hair quality by dermal cells. J Invest Dermatol. 1993;100(3):229–236. DOI: 10.1111/1523-1747.ep12468971

[42] Higgins CA, Chen JC, Cerise JE, Jahoda CA, Christiano AM. Microenvironmental reprogramming by three-dimensional culture enables dermal papilla cells to induce de novo human hair-follicle growth. Proc Natl Acad Sci U S A. 2013;110:19679–19688. DOI: 10.1073/pnas.1309970110

[43] Ohyama M, Kobayashi T, Sasaki T, Shimizu A, Amagai M. Restoration of the intrinsic properties of human dermal papilla in vitro. J Cell Sci. 2012;125(Pt 17):4114–4125. DOI: 10.1242/jcs.105700

[44] Rendl M, Polak L, Fuchs E. BMP signaling in dermal papilla cells is required for their hair follicle-inductive properties. Genes Dev. 2008;22(4):543–557. DOI: 10.1101/gad.1614408

[45] Inoue K, Kato H, Sato T, Osada A, Aoi N, Suga H, et al. Evaluation of animal models for the hair-inducing capacity of cultured human dermal papilla cells. Cells Tissues Organs. 2009;190(2):102–110. DOI: 10.1159/000178021

[46] Reynolds A, Jahoda C. Hair matrix germinative epidermal cells confer follicle-inducing capabilities on dermal sheath and high passage papilla cells. Development. 1996;122(10):3085–3094.

[47] Kobayashi T, Fujisawa A, Amagai M, Iwasaki T, Ohyama M. Molecular biological and immunohistological characterization of canine dermal papilla cells and the evaluation of culture conditions. Vet Dermatol. 2011;22(5):414–422. DOI: 10.1111/j.1365-3164.2011.00964.x

[48] Kishimoto J, Burgeson RE, Morgan BA. Wnt signaling maintains the hair-inducing activity of the dermal papilla service Wnt signaling maintains the hair-inducing activity of the dermal papilla. Genes Dev. 2000;14(10):1181–1185. DOI: 10.1101/gad.14.10.1181

[49] Shimizu H, Morgan BA. Wnt signaling through the beta-catenin pathway is sufficient to maintain, but not restore, anagen-phase characteristics of dermal papilla cells. J Invest Dermatol. 2004;122(2):239–245. DOI: 10.1046/j.0022-202X.2004.22224.x

[50] Ouji Y, Nakamura-Uchiyama F, Yoshikawa M. Canonical Wnts, specifically Wnt-10b, show ability to maintain dermal papilla cells. Biochem Biophys Res Commun. 2013;438(3):493–499. DOI: 10.1016/j.bbrc.2013.07.108

[51] Ouji Y, Yoshikawa M. Maintenance of dermal papilla cells by Wnt-10b in vitro. Methods Mol Biol. 2016;1516:269–277. DOI: 10.1007/7651_2016_319

[52] Ouji Y, Ishizaka S, Yoshikawa M. Dermal papilla cells serially cultured with wnt-10b sustain their hair follicle induction activity after transplantation into nude mice. Cell Transplant. 2012;21(10):2313–2324. DOI: 10.3727/096368912X636867

[53] Reddy S, Andl T, Bagasra A, Lu MM, Epstein DJ, Morrisey EE, et al. Characterization of Wnt gene expression in developing and postnatal hair follicles and identification of Wnt5a as a target of sonic hedgehog in hair follicle morphogenesis. Mech Dev. 2001;107(1):69–82. DOI: 10.1016/S0925-4773(01)00452-X

[54] Ouji Y, Yoshikawa M, Shiroi A, Ishizaka S. Promotion of hair follicle development and trichogenesis by Wnt-10b in cultured embryonic skin and in reconstituted skin. Biochem Biophys Res Commun. 2006;345(2):581–587. DOI: 10.1016/j.bbrc.2006.04.142

[55] Kiratipaiboon C, Tengamnuay P, Chanvorachote P. Ciprofloxacin Improves the Stemness of Human Dermal Papilla Cells. Stem Cells Int. 2016. DOI: 10.1155/2016/5831276

[56] Lee S-H, Yoon J, Shin SH, Zahoor M, Kim HJ, Park PJ, et al. Valproic acid induces hair regeneration in murine model and activates alkaline phosphatase activity in human dermal papilla cells. PLoS One. 2012;7(4):e34152. DOI: 10.1371/journal.pone.0034152

[57] Jo SJ, Choi S-J, Yoon S-Y, Lee JY, Park W-S, Park P-J, et al. Valproic acid promotes human hair growth in in vitro culture model. J Dermatol Sci. 2013;72(1):16–24. DOI: 10.1016/j.jdermsci.2013.05.007

[58] Yamauchi K, Kurosaka A. Inhibition of glycogen synthase kinase-3 enhances the expression of alkaline phosphatase and insulin-like growth factor-1 in human primary dermal papilla cell culture and maintains mouse hair bulbs in organ culture. Arch Dermatol Res. 2009;301(5):357–365. DOI: 10.1007/s00403-009-0929-7

[59] Aoi N, Inoue K, Chikanishi T, Fujiki R, Yamamoto H, Kato H, et al. 1α,25-dihydroxyvitamin D3 modulates the hair-inductive capacity of dermal papilla cells: therapeutic potential for hair regeneration. Stem Cells Transl Med. 2012;1:615–626. DOI: 10.5966/sctm.2012-0032

[60] Zhang H, Nan W, Wang S, Zhang T, Si H, Wang D, et al. Epidermal growth factor promotes proliferation of dermal papilla cells via Notch signaling pathway. Biochimie. 2016;127:10–18. DOI: 10.1016/j.biochi.2016.04.015

[61] Li W, Man X-Y, Li C-M, Chen J-Q, Zhou J, Cai S-Q, et al. VEGF induces proliferation of human hair follicle dermal papilla cells through VEGFR-2-mediated activation of ERK. Exp Cell Res. 2012;318(14):1633–1640. DOI: 10.1016/j.yexcr.2012.05.003

[62] Kiso M, Hamazaki TS, Itoh M, Kikuchi S, Nakagawa H, Okochi H. Synergistic effect of PDGF and FGF2 for cell proliferation and hair inductive activity in murine vibrissal dermal papilla in vitro. J Dermatol Sci. 2015;79(2):110–118. DOI: 10.1016/j.jdermsci.2015.04.007

[63] Xing L, Dai Z, Jabbari A, Cerise JE, Higgins CA, Gong W, et al. Alopecia areata is driven by cytotoxic T lymphocytes and is reversed by JAK inhibition. Nat Med. 2014;20(9):1043–1049. DOI: 10.1038/nm.3645

[64] Harel S, Higgins CA, Cerise JE, Dai Z, Chen JC, Clynes R, et al. Pharmacologic inhibition of JAK-STAT signaling promotes hair growth. Sci Adv. 2015;1(9):e1500973. DOI: 10.1126/sciadv.1500973

[65] Jahoda CA, Reynolds AJ, Chaponnier C, Forester JC, Gabbiani G. Smooth muscle alpha-actin is a marker for hair follicle dermis in vivo and in vitro. J Cell Sci. 1991;99(3):627–636.

[66] Higgins CA, Richardson GD, Ferdinando D, Westgate GE, Jahoda CAB. Modelling the hair follicle dermal papilla using spheroid cell cultures. Exp Dermatol. 2010;19(6):546–548. DOI: 10.1111/j.1600-0625.2009.01007.x

[67] Lin B, Miao Y, Wang J, Fan Z, Du L, Su Y, et al. Surface tension guided hanging-drop: producing controllable 3D spheroid of high-passaged human dermal papilla cells and forming inductive microtissues for hair-follicle regeneration. ACS Appl Mater Interfaces. 2016;8(9):5906–5916. DOI: 10.1021/acsami.6b00202

[68] Huang C-F, Chang Y-J, Hsueh Y-Y, Huang C-W, Wang D-H, Huang T-C, et al. Assembling composite dermal papilla spheres with adipose-derived stem cells to enhance hair follicle induction. Sci Rep. 2016;6:26436. DOI: 10.1038/srep26436

[69] Festa E, Fretz J, Berry R, Schmidt B, Rodeheffer M, Horowitz M, et al. Adipocyte lineage cells contribute to the skin stem cell niche to drive hair cycling. Cell. 2011;146(5):761–771. DOI: 10.1016/j.cell.2011.07.019

[70] Hwang I, Choi K, Park H, Jeong H, Kim J. Neural stem cells restore hair growth through activation of the hair follicle niche. Cell Transplant. 2016;25(8):1439–1451. DOI: 10.3727/096368916X691466

[71] Rheinwatd JG, Green H. Seria cultivation of strains of human epidemal keratinocytes: the formation keratinizin colonies from single cell is. Cell. 1975;6(3):331–343.

[72] De Luca M, Albanese E, Bondanza S, Megna M, Ugozzoli L, Molina F, et al. Multicentre experience in the treatment of burns with autologous and allogenic cultured epithelium, fresh or preserved in a frozen state. Burns. 1989;15(5):303–309.

[73] Sasai Y. Next-generation regenerative medicine: organogenesis from stem cells in 3D culture. Cell Stem Cell. 2013;12(5):520–530. DOI: 10.1016/j.stem.2013.04.009

[74] Botchkarev VA, Botchkareva NV, Roth W, Nakamura M, Chen L-H, Herzog W, et al. Noggin is a mesenchymally derived stimulator of hair-follicle induction. Nat Cell Biol. 1999;1(3):158–164. DOI: 10.1038/11078

[75] Blanpain C, Fuchs E. Epidermal stem cells of the skin. Annu Rev Cell Dev Biol. 2006;22:339–373. DOI: 10.1146/annurev.cellbio.22.010305.104357

[76] Sharov AA, Sharova TY, Mardaryev AN, Tommasi di Vignano A, Atoyan R, Weiner L, et al. Bone morphogenetic protein signaling regulates the size of hair follicles and modulates the expression of cell cycle-associated genes. Proc Natl Acad Sci U S A. 2006;103(48):18166–18171. DOI: 10.1073/pnas.0608899103

[77] Fuchs E. Scratching the surface of skin development. Nature. 2007;445(7130):834–842. DOI: 10.1038/nature05659

[78] Samuelov L, Sprecher E, Tsuruta D, Bíró T, Kloepper JE, Paus R. P-Cadherin regulates human hair growth and cycling via canonical Wnt signaling and transforming growth factor-β2. J Invest Dermatol. 2012;132(10):2332–2341. DOI: 10.1038/jid.2012.171

[79] Roh C, Tao Q, Lyle S. Dermal papilla-induced hair differentiation of adult epithelial stem cells from human skin. Physiol Genomics. 2004;19(2):207–217. DOI: 10.1152/physiolgenomics.00134.2004

[80] Chan CC, Fan SM, Wang WH, Mu YF, Lin SJ. A Two-stepped culture method for efficient production of trichogenic keratinocytes. Tissue Eng Part C Methods. 2015;21(10):1070–1079. DOI: 10.1089/ten.TEC.2015.0033

[81] Chermnykh ES, Vorotelyak EA, Gnedeva KY, Moldaver MV, Yegorov YE, Vasiliev AV, et al. Dermal papilla cells induce keratinocyte tubulogenesis in culture. Histochem Cell Biol. 2010;133(5):567–576. DOI: 10.1007/s00418-010-0691-0

[82] Hardy MH. The development of mouse hair in vitro with some observations on pigmentation. J Anat. 1949;83(4):364–384, 3 pl.

[83] Qiao J, Turetsky A, Kemp P, Teumer J. Hair morphogenesis in vitro: formation of hair structures suitable for implantation. Regen Med. 2008;3(5):683–692. DOI: 10.2217/17460751.3.5.683

[84] Nakao K, Morita R, Saji Y, Ishida K, Tomita Y, Ogawa M, et al. The development of a bioengineered organ germ method. Nat Meth. 2007;4(3):227–230. DOI: 10.1038/nmeth1012

[85] Ihara S, Watanabe M, Nagao E, Shioya N. Formation of hair follicles from a single-cell suspension of embryonic rat skin by a two-step procedure in vitro. Cell Tissue Res. 1991;266(1):65–73. DOI: 10.1007/BF00678712

[86] Lu Z, Hasse S, Bodo E, Rose C, Funk W, Paus R. Towards the development of a simplified long-term organ culture method for human scalp skin and its appendages under serum-free conditions. Exp Dermato. 2007;16(1):37–44. DOI: 10.1111/j.1600-0625.2006.00510.x

[87] Li L, Margolis LB, Paus R, Hoffman RM. Hair shaft elongation, follicle growth, and spontaneous regression in long-term, gelatin sponge-supported histoculture of human scalp skin. Proc Natl Acad Sci U S A. 1992;89(18):8764–8768.

[88] Magerl M, Paus R, Farjo N, Müller-Röver S, Peters EMJ, Foitzik K, et al. Limitations of human occipital scalp hair follicle organ culture for studying the effects of minoxidil as a hair growth enhancer. Exp Dermatol. 2004;13(10):635–642. DOI: 10.1111/j.0906-6705.2004.00207.x

[89] Philpott MP, Kealey T. Cyclical changes in rat vibrissa follicles maintained in vitro. J Invest Dermatol. 2000;115(6):1152–1155. DOI: 10.1046/j.1523-1747.2000.00183.x

[90] Qi S-H, Liu P, Xie J-L, Shu B, Xu Y-B, Ke C-N, et al. Experimental study on repairing of nude mice skin defects with composite skin consisting of xenogeneic dermis and epidermal stem cells and hair follicle dermal papilla cells. Burns. 2008;34(3):385–392. DOI: 10.1016/j.burns.2007.04.003

[91] Leirós GJ, Kusinsky AG, Drago H, Bossi S, Sturla F, Castellanos ML, et al. Dermal papilla cells improve the wound healing process and generate hair bud-like structures in grafted skin substitutes using hair follicle stem cells. Stem Cells Transl Med. 2014;1:1209–1219. DOI: 10.5966/sctm.2013-0217

[92] Sriwiriyanont P, Lynch KA, Maier EA, Hahn JM, Supp DM, Boyce ST. Morphogenesis of chimeric hair follicles in engineered skin substitutes with human keratinocytes and murine dermal papilla cells. Exp Dermatol. 2012;21(10):783–785. DOI: 10.1111/exd.12003

[93] Sriwiriyanont P, Lynch KA, McFarland KL, Supp DM, Boyce ST. Characterization of hair follicle development in engineered skin substitutes. PLoS One. 2013;8(6):e65664. DOI: 10.1371/journal.pone.0065664

[94] Toyoshima K, Asakawa K, Ishibashi N, Toki H, Ogawa M, Hasegawa T, et al. Fully functional hair follicle regeneration through the rearrangement of stem cells and their niches. Nat Commun. 2012;3:784. DOI: 10.1038/ncomms1784

[95] Inamatsu M, Tochio T, Makabe A, Endo T, Oomizu S, Kobayashi E, et al. Embryonic dermal condensation and adult dermal papilla induce hair follicles in adult glabrous epidermis through different mechanisms. Dev Growth Differ. 2006;48(2):73–86. DOI: 10.1111/j.1440-169X.2006.00848.x

[96] Zheng Y, Du X, Wang W, Boucher M, Parimoo S, Stenn KS. Organogenesis from dissociated cells: generation of mature cycling hair follicles from skin-derived cells. J Invest Dermatol. 2005;124(5):867–876. DOI: 10.1111/j.0022-202X.2005.23716.x

[97] Zheng Y, Nace A, Chen W, Watkins K, Sergott L, Homan Y, et al. Mature hair follicles generated from dissociated cells: a universal mechanism of folliculoneogenesis. Dev Dyn. 2010;239(10):2619–2626. DOI: 10.1002/dvdy.22398

[98] Havlickova B, Bíró T, Mescalchin A, Arenberger P, Paus R. Towards optimization of an organotypic assay system that imitates human hair follicle-like epithelial-mesenchymal interactions. Br J Dermatol. 2004;151(4):753–765. DOI: 10.1111/j.1365-2133.2004.06184.x

[99] Havlickova B, Bíró T, Mescalchin A, Tschirschmann M, Mollenkopf H, Bettermann A, et al. A human folliculoid microsphere assay for exploring epithelial–mesenchymal interactions in the human hair follicle. J Invest Dermatol. 2009;129(4):972–983. DOI: 10.1038/jid.2008.315

[100] Lindner G, Horland R, Wagner I, Ataç B, Lauster R. De novo formation and ultrastructural characterization of a fiber-producing human hair follicle equivalent in vitro. J Biotechnol. 2011;152(3):108–112. DOI: 10.1016/j.jbiotec.2011.01.019

[101] Yen C-M, Chan C-C, Lin S-J. High-throughput reconstitution of epithelial–mesenchymal interaction in folliculoid microtissues by biomaterial-facilitated self-assembly of dissociated heterotypic adult cells. Biomaterials. 2010;31(15):4341–4352. DOI: 10.1016/j.biomaterials.2010.02.014

[102] Gnedeva K, Vorotelyak E, Cimadamore F, Cattarossi G, Giusto E, Terskikh VV, et al. Derivation of hair-inducing cell from human pluripotent stem cells. PLoS One. 2015;10(1):e0116892. DOI: 10.1371/journal.pone.0116892

[103] Selekman JA, Lian X, Palecek SP. Generation of epithelial cell populations from human pluripotent stem cells using a small-molecule inhibitor of Src family kinases. Methods Mol Biol. 2016;1307:319–327. DOI: 10.1007/7651_2014_70

[104] Lian X, Selekman J, Bao X, Hsiao C, Zhu K, Palecek SP. A small molecule inhibitor of SRC family kinases promotes simple epithelial differentiation of human pluripotent stem cells. PLoS One. 2013;8(3):e60016. DOI: 10.1371/journal.pone.0060016

[105] Yang R, Zheng Y, Burrows M, Liu S, Wei Z, Nace A, et al. Generation of folliculogenic human epithelial stem cells from induced pluripotent stem cells. Nat Commun. 2014;5:3071. DOI: 10.1038/ncomms4071

[106] Takagi R, Ishimaru J, Sugawara A, Toyoshima K -e., Ishida K, Ogawa M, et al. Bioengineering a 3D integumentary organ system from iPS cells using an in vivo transplantation model. Sci Adv. 2016;2(4):e1500887–e1500887. DOI: 10.1126/sciadv.1500887

[107] Clinical trials of alopecia. Available from: https://clinicaltrials.gov/ct2/results?term=alopecia+AND+cells&Search=Search [Accessed: 2016-08-10]

Section 3

Hair Examination Techniques

Chapter 5

The Histological Mechanisms of Hair Loss

Vsevolodov Eduard Borisovich

Additional information is available at the end of the chapter

http://dx.doi.org/10.5772/67275

Abstract

The growing hair resists pulling out of the skin in particular site, where the keratinization of hair cortex and hair cuticle cells as well as the cells of the hair inner root sheath (IS) (being in tight contact) are advanced enough to make them rather strong but lower the level where the hair separates from the hair inner root sheath. The hair which does not grow is kept for some time within the skin by the direct contact of the keratinized hair cortex cells with the cells of the hair outer root sheath. Such contact is absent at the phase of growing hair and even in the case of proliferation inhibition in the follicle bulb causing the lack of hair resistance to pulling it out of the skin several days after inhibition induction.

Keywords: hair matrix dysplasia, hair break, hair upward promotion, cell proliferation/evacuation balance

1. Introduction

First of all let us remember most briefly the histological structure of the hair follicle (F) (**Figure 1**) in the phase of stable hair growth [1–3]. The lowest (innermost) part of the hair F is presented by hair bulb including its cambium zone ("matrix"), which consists of cells dividing all the time while the hair grows. These cells do not seem to differ from each other. Their division does not cause the increase of the matrix volume while hair growth is stable because the number of newly produced cells equals the number of the cells leaving matrix and starting to differentiate into the layers of the hair (medulla, cortex, and hair cuticle) and hair root inner sheath (inner sheath cuticle, Huxley layer, and Henle layer). All six layers move upward (toward the skin surface). In the course of differentiation, the cells of all these layers stop dividing and start to synthesize several types of keratins (K) or "keratin-like" (Kl) proteins [2]. The sets of these proteins are different in the medulla, cortex, and cuticle of the

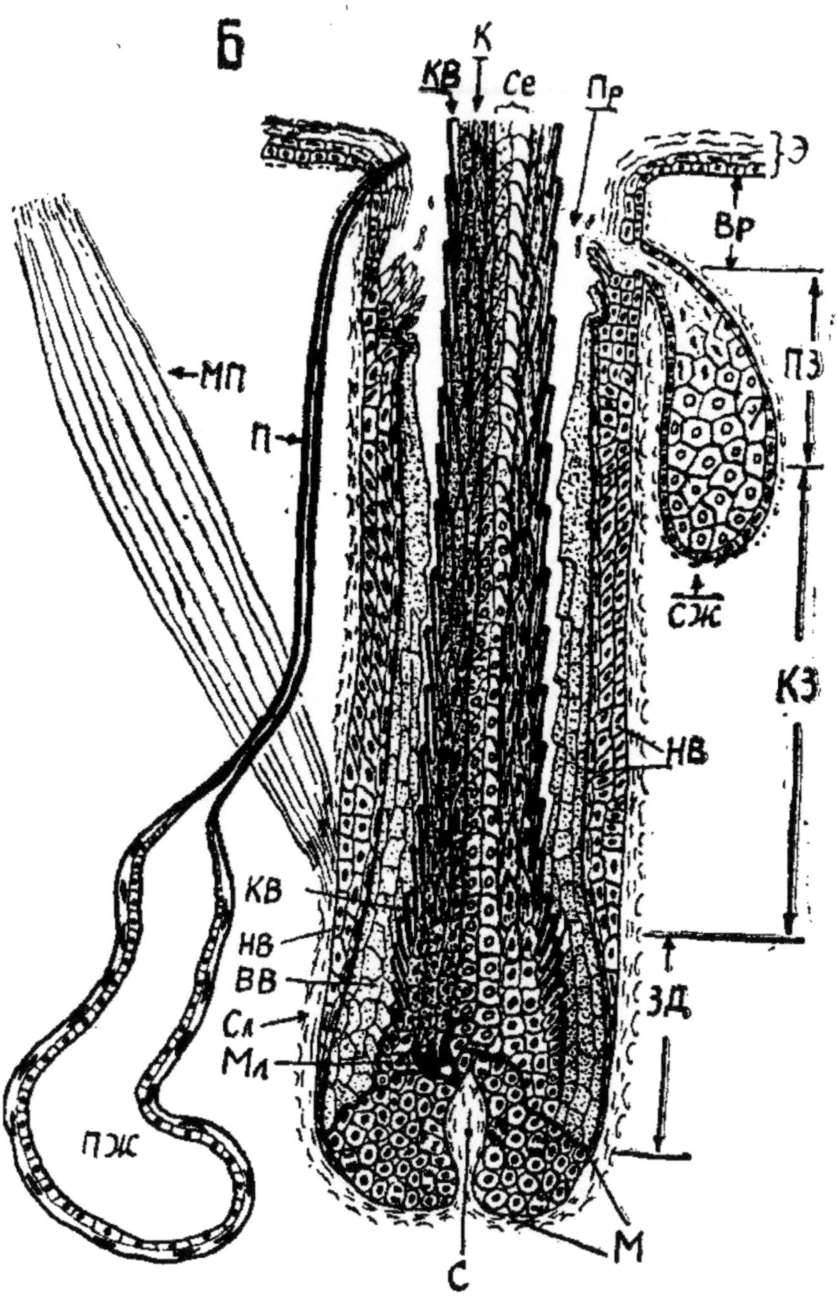

Figure 1. General scheme of the hair follicle in the phase of stable hair growth. М, matrix (cambium zone); С, connective tissue papilla; ЗД, zone of differentiation; КЗ, zone of keratinization; ПЗ, postkeratogenic zone; Вр, hair follicle infundibulum; Э, interfollicular epidermis; СЖ, sebaceous gland; ПЖ, sweat gland; Се, hair medulla; К, hair cortex; Кв, hair cuticle; ВВ, hair inner root sheath; НВ, hair outer root sheath; Сл, connective tissue sheath around the hair follicle ("vitreous membrane"); and Мл, melanocyte (melanin-producing cell). МП, musculus arrector pili; П, sweat gland duct; and Пр, the pilary lumen (the fissure separating hair from inner root sheath by the end of differentiation).

http://dx.doi.org/10.5772/67275

hair. The morphological features of these layers are also very different. The main hair layer is the cortex. Its cells have spindle-like form with their long axes parallel to hair length. Almost all cell volume is filled with K fibers when the K synthesis is over. The neighboring cortex cells are agglutinated by the strong intercellular glue capable to resist the water.

The outermost hair layer—the cuticle—has no fiber structures. The cell has the somewhat curved plate-like form as the cell "tries" to surround the hair (**Figure 2**). The upper ends of the hair cuticle cells lie over the lower parts of the preceding (more distal) cuticle cells of the hair so that the general pattern resembles the piling (**Figure 3**). So the upper ends of cuticle cells stick out of the hair surface like the dents of gear wheel. This pattern is imprinted on the inner root sheath (IS) cuticle surface, and the dents of the hair cuticle are inserted between the corresponding dents of IS cuticle like the dents of a joint gear wheel pair (**Figures 4** and **5**).

Hair cortex and cuticle K contain some sulfur-rich proteins preventing K destruction by proteases because the sulfur-containing amino acids bind molecules of K with each other or the

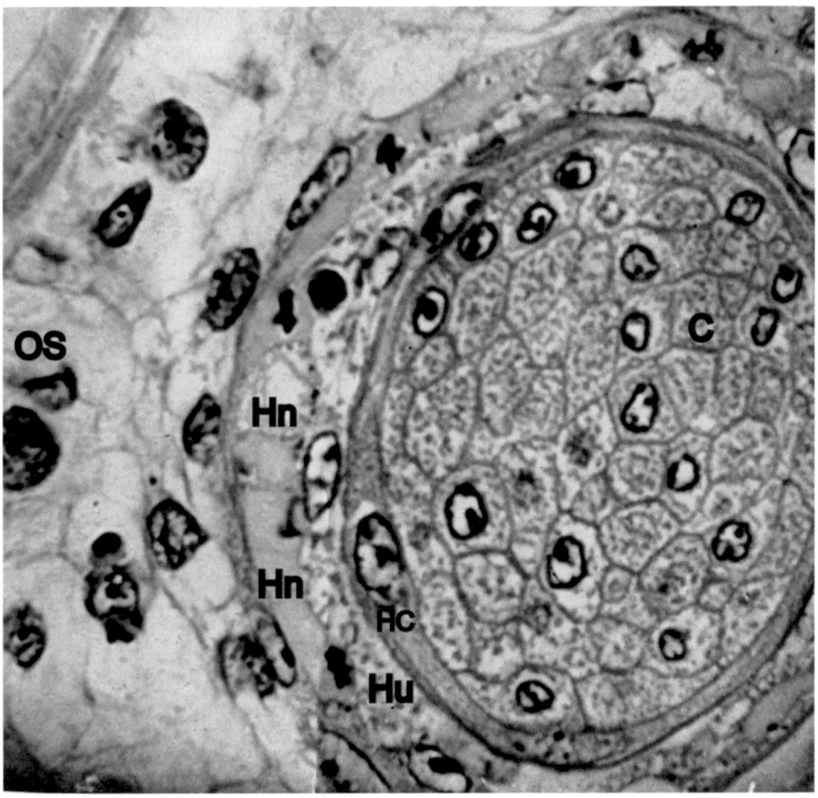

Figure 2. A transversal section of fine-wool sheep hair follicle (no medullar layer is present). C, the cell of cortex layer. The visible cell borders are "underlined" by keratin layer on the inner side of cytomembranes as well as in central parts of the cytoplasm. The nuclei are present only in the cells which were cut across in the middle part of spindle-like cell where the nucleus is located. HC, hair cuticle. This plate-like cell "tries" to surround the hair root. Hn and Hu, Henle and Huxley layers of inner hair root sheath. OS, hair outer root sheath. Hematoxylin + eosin.

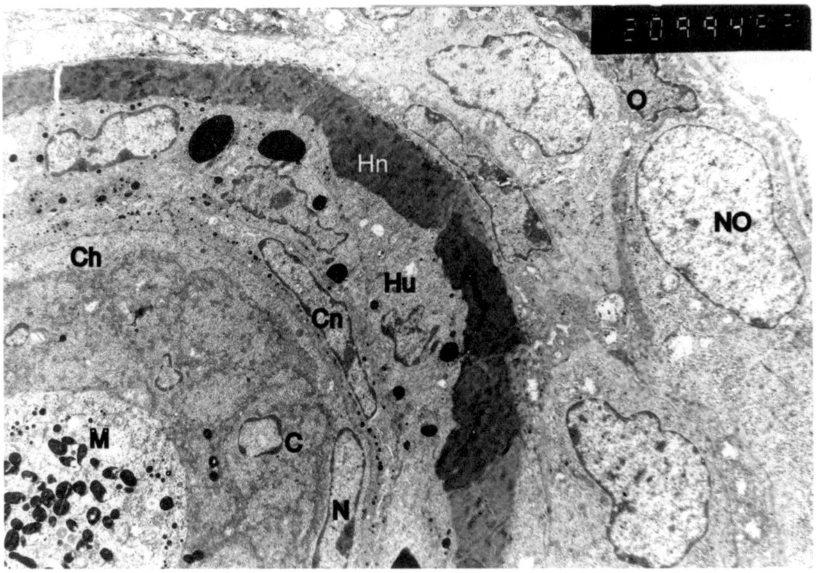

Figure 3. The electron microscopic photo of the transversal section of mouse hair follicle on the level of keratogenic zone. M, hair medulla containing larger black particles corresponding to melanosomes (diameters about 0.5 mcm) and with much less diameters (trichohyalin-like material). C, hair cortex. N, nucleus of the hair cuticle—very flat cells of the hair outer layer lacking trichohyalin. Cn, the nucleus of the inner hair root sheath cuticle including little black particles of the trichohyalin. Both cuticles are lying close to each other fixing the hair within the hair follicle. Hu, middle layer of the inner sheath, including some very large black trichohyalin granules. He, outer layer of the inner sheath which unlike Huxley layer is already keratinized. NO, the nucleus of nonmigrating cell of the outer layer of outer hair root sheath. O, the cell of the same layer but starting migration toward Henle layer, forming long pseudopodium for this purpose.

parts within the same molecules by many disulfide "bridges" (–S–S–) which do not allow large protease molecules to reach the proper sites of K molecules to hydrolyze them.

The most obvious feature of the hair medulla cells is rather poor keratinization (**Figures 3** and **4**). When this process is over, very high proportion of the cell volume is filled by the air. So the cells seem to be "half empty." Some Kl material usually is present under the cell membrane, and some other Kl materials cross the cell as rather rare fibers (in sheep hair), but we must take into account that medulla cells' morphology is extremely polymorphic when we compare different taxons.

The Kl material of the inner root sheath (IS) does not contain much sulfur and is partly hydrolyzed by proteases in the upper segment of the F. The chemical nature of the Kl material in all three layers of the IS does not seem to differ much. But morphologically they can be easily distinguished in the lower part of the follicle thanks to heterochrony of their keratinization process. In the outer layer (Henle) of the IS, the synthesis of Kl material begins earlier (lower) than in other F layers, progresses faster, and becomes the first solid structure on the way from the F bottom to the skin surface (**Figures 3** and **4**). The same phases of Kl material synthesis take place later (on the higher level of the F) in IS cuticle and especially in the middle (Huxley) layer.

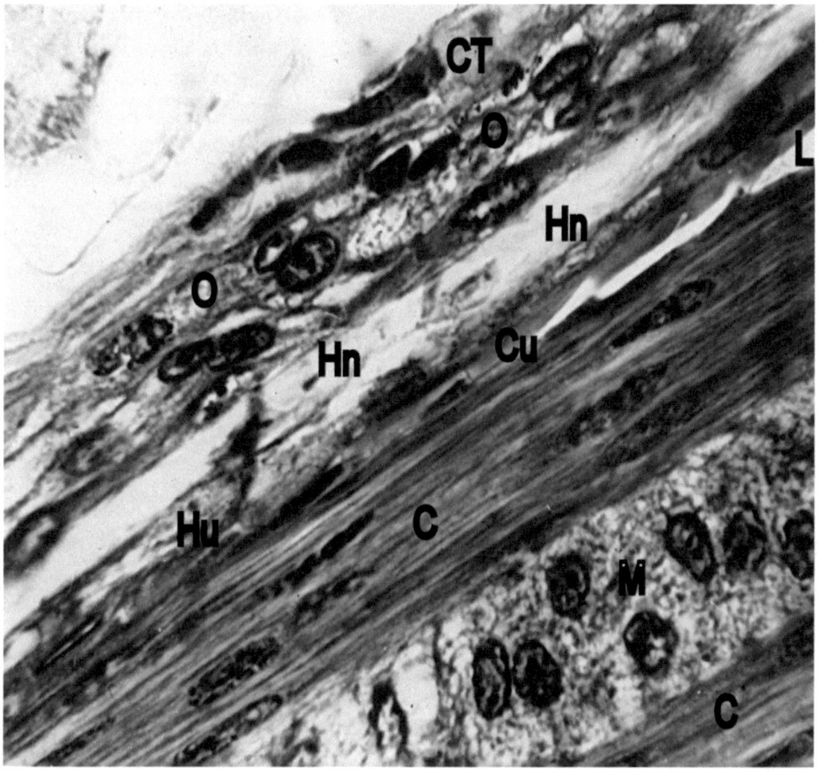

Figure 4. Longitudinal section of a sheep hair follicle on the level close to the end of keratogenesis. C, hair cortex; M, medulla; Hn, Henle and Huxley layers; O, outer root sheath; and CT, connecting tissue surrounding the hair follicle. Cu, two cuticles (hair cuticle and inner root sheath cuticle) starting to separate by pilary lumen —L—(right half of the photo) and tightly bind lower (left half of the photo where no lumen is present). Slightly projecting out of hair surface "dents" of upper hair cuticle edges that are imprinted in inner root sheath cuticle cells. So these dents of the hair cuticle are inserted into indentations of inner root sheath cuticle like the dents of a gear wheel into indentations of another gear wheel.

The hair outer root sheath (OS) surrounds the IS and even matrix. Its cells do not originate from the matrix, and at least outer layer cells of the OS do not move upward like the cells of the hair and IS [4]. Outer layer cells of the OS can move downward toward the bottom of the matrix, penetrate into it, and renew its proliferation potential after its decrease after some damages or as Hayflick limit [5] being exhausted. OS outer layer contains stem cells of the hair F, and its cambium cells are located in the OS outer layer over the hair F bulb. The cells produced by this cambium zone migrate from the outer layer of OS into the inner ("companion") layer which, unlike cells of the OS outer layer cells, move permanently upward together with IS and hair cells [6].

The structure of the OS is very different depending upon the F level (from matrix bottom to the skin surface). On the deepest level around the matrix, the outer and inner cell layers are presented each by the single row of very flattened cells having the thickness less than 1 mcm except the sites close to the nuclei of the cells. Over the bulb the OS becomes much thicker than around the matrix and consists of three and more rows of cells which are not flat but cubic or cylindrical (except the inner OS layer cells which are rather flat). Some of the outer layer cells proliferate and display the inward amoeboid movement toward IS wedging between the already present companion cells arrived from below. Then these cells become new elements of companion layer and take part in its upward movement together with the IS and hair [4, 7].

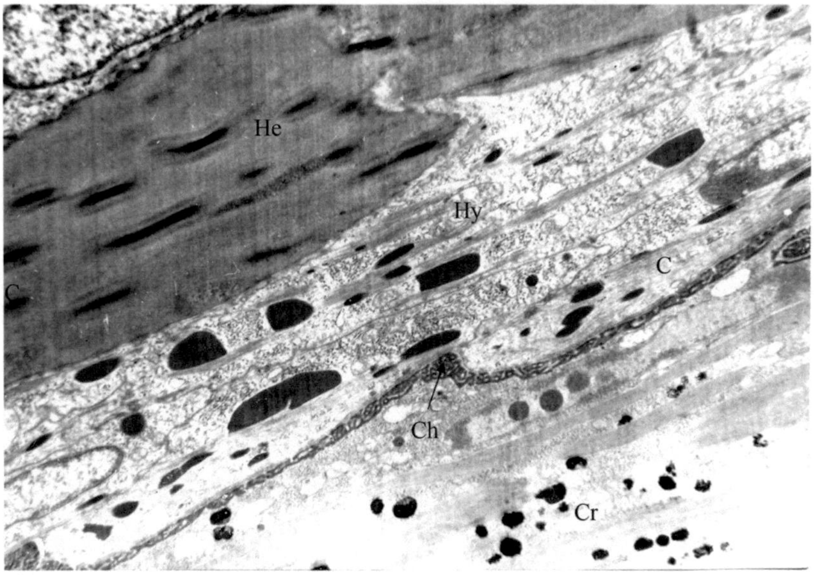

Figure 5. Electron microscopic photo of the part of longitudinal section of the keratinization zone sheep hair follicle on the border of the hair and hair inner root sheath. The hair growth direction is from low left to upper right. Cr, cortex of the hair with melanosomes. Ch, cuticle of the hair. The long apoptotic nucleus of the hair cuticle cell is just to the right from Ch letters. Arrow, "labyrinth-like" epicuticular layer of the immature hair cuticle. C, hair root inner sheath cuticle cell with trichohyalin black granules. Its lower end protrudes into the hair, and the hair cuticle protrudes bellow it to the inner sheath arranging gear wheel-like indentations. Hy, Huxley layer with large black trichohyalin granules. He, keratinized Henle layer folded in the course of cutting.

The uppermost portion of the OS—the hair F infundibulum—has the same structure as the interfollicular epidermis of the skin surface. It produces the keratinized squamous cells and lays them around the fully differentiated hair. Neither IS nor companion layer are present in the infundibulum as no ascending cell flow exists there. So rather quick upward movement of partly hydrolyzed IS and companion layer is stopped running against this obstacle. New and new portions of the IS and companion layer arrive and form folds projecting into the pilary lumen (**Figure 6**). By this moment partly hydrolyzed IS starts to destroy and the companion layer cells finish their keratinization [8]. These keratinized cells do not seem to hydrolyze like the IS. Their K must be of the different nature and can resist enzyme hydrolysis. Keratinized cell processes of the companion layer cells penetrate into nonkeratinized cells of OS middle layer cells (**Figure 6**) which may stabilize the folds for some time, and destruction and exit of arriving from below companion layer cells into the pilary lumen are postponed for some time.

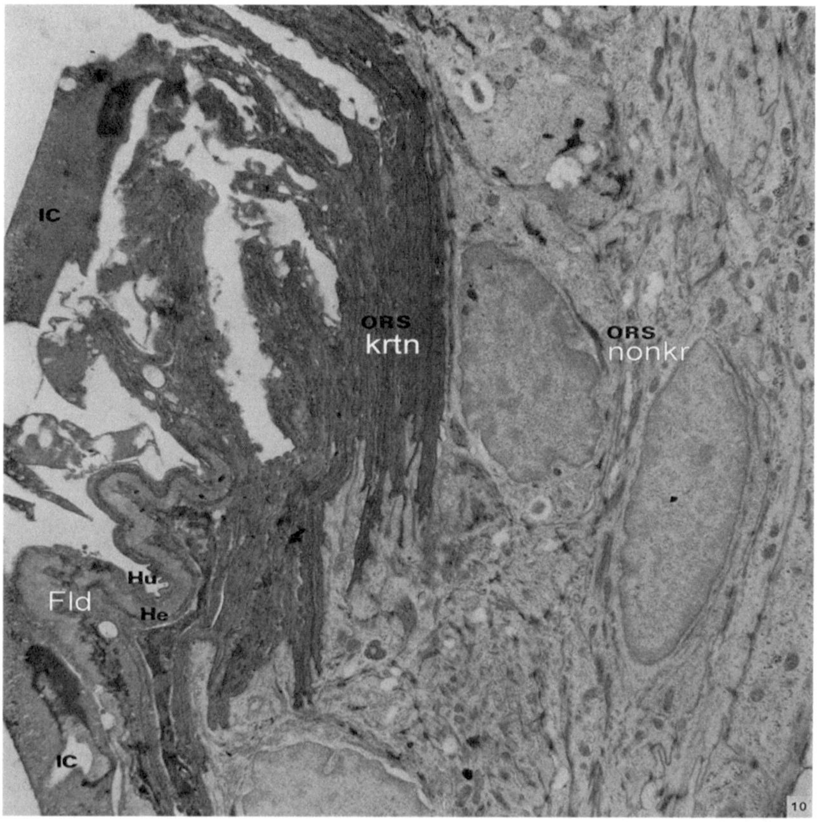

Figure 6. Most informative electron microscopic photo of the pattern of the sheep hair follicle wall at the level just under the sebaceous gland orifice made by Gemmel and Chapman [8]. Anagen VI phase of hair growth cycle. Fld, folds are formed by three layers of the hair follicle inner hair root sheath (IC, cuticle; Hu, Huxley; Hn, Henle) and keratinized companion layer of the outer sheath (ORS krtn). The long keratinized processes of the companion layer are inserted into the nonkeratinized outer sheath cells (ORS nonkr) which seem to retard the desquamation of keratinized companion cells.

The hair F is surrounded by the condensed connective tissue (vitreous membrane) which like peninsula intrudes into the matrix (papilla). The vitreous membrane includes the layers of collagen fibers oriented longitudinally and circularly (around the F). The basal membrane is present on the border of the F epithelium and surrounding connective tissue including the papilla.

We must realize how the hair is normally fixed in the skin while it grows. Once I could see how my assistant caught rather large crossbred ram grasping from behind two portions of wool on both sides of its body holding them in his clenched fists. The ram pulled my assistant forward and the heels of his boots made a deep long furrow in the soil before my assistant could stop the ram.

So hairs are fixed in the skin strongly enough. It does not seem to be easily expected after the preliminary analysis of hair follicle histologic structure. Indeed the keratinized hair upper part consists of rather strong composite material including protein filaments agglutinated by nonfibrous proteins. In the upper part of the F, the hair is separated by the fissure from the surrounding tissue layers which makes it impossible for upper part of the hair to resist pulling out of the skin (**Figure 4**). Following deeper along the less and less "mature" hair, we reach after all the cambium zone ("matrix") of the F where cells divide providing new and new cell material for hair growth. Permanently dividing cells cannot include hard materials which would make impossible to produce two equal daughter cells. So the lack of hard materials in the matrix means it is practically liquid substance and cannot resist pulling the hair out of the skin. It would be as expecting the water in the vase to resist pulling out a bouquet from a vase. Even immediately over matrix where the cell division stops and hair cortex and hair cuticle keratinization is in the very beginning, hair root does not differ much from the matrix in its capacity to resist pulling out of the skin.

Where the hair is really fixed strongly in the F? This position is over the level of start of keratinization but below the level of hair separation from the surrounding F layers (more exactly from the inner layer of the IS—the cuticle of the IS). As we mention above, the dents of the hair cuticle are inserted between the corresponding dents of IS cuticle like the dents of a joint gear wheel pair. When we try to pull the hair out of the skin, our exertion is transmitted from the mature (fully keratinized) hair to the portion of the hair essentially keratinized, then through the hair cuticle dents to the dents of the IS cuticle, and further to almost fully keratinized IS then to the OS and to some extent to connective tissue vitreous membrane. The exertion of pulling out the hair is supposed to be transferred along the following trajectory: mature (fully keratinized) hair → essentially but not fully keratinized hair → its cuticle dents → the dents of IS dents—almost fully keratinized IS → OS → to some extent to connective tissue vitreous membrane. The pulling exertion will cause upward moving of the hair and outward folding of the IS and OS which will be limited by almost unstretchable vitreous membrane. So the folding will squeeze the hair and will not allow the hair to leave the F easily. So the hair is pulled out only with some portions of IS and OS. The regrowth of the hair in the follicle from which the growing hair was pulled out starts almost immediately. If we change rather careful pulling the hair out of the skin for very abrupt jerking out, then even the bulb with the matrix can be extracted from the skin and no hair regeneration will follow.

So rather strong fixation of the growing hair within the skin seems to be based on the impossibility of hair slipping against the IS caused by interdigitating gear wheel-like dents on the hair and IS surfaces. This obstacle for free sliding exists only on the definite level of the F. As the hair and IS cells move up from this level, the hair separates from the IS, but by this moment, new portions of maturing to proper state hair and IS cells take their place and support growing hair "anchoring" function.

The phase of stable hair growth (anagen VI) is interrupted after some time of hair growth by the phase of no growth (telogen). Depending upon the position on the site of the body surface, specious peculiarity, and some other factors, the transition of an F to telogen phase happens after a few weeks of hair growth and up to several years of growth. The daily increase of the hair length in the phase of anagen VI varies usually within the range of 0.3–1.0 mm/day. So the hair length about 1 m (scalp region) of the human can be obtained by the hair growth for approximately 5–6 years, and the hair length about 5 mm (brows) can be obtained by the hair

http://dx.doi.org/10.5772/67275

growth for approximately 2 weeks. The transition from anagen VI to telogen occurs through the phase named the catagen. In the course of it, cell division decreases and stops. The IS is not produced. There appears the hair proximal end looking like the brush with the keratinized cortex most proximal cells sticking out apart and contacting directly with OS companion layer cells as the IS is absent and does not isolate hair cortex from the OS (**Figure 7**). The upward movement of the hair and companion layer goes on even when no proliferation in the disappearing matrix takes place. Its mechanism is based on the active OS cell migration. The upward movement stops below the sebaceous gland orifice. The hair keratinized brush-like end cells keep for some time (several days or months) their tight binding to also keratinized

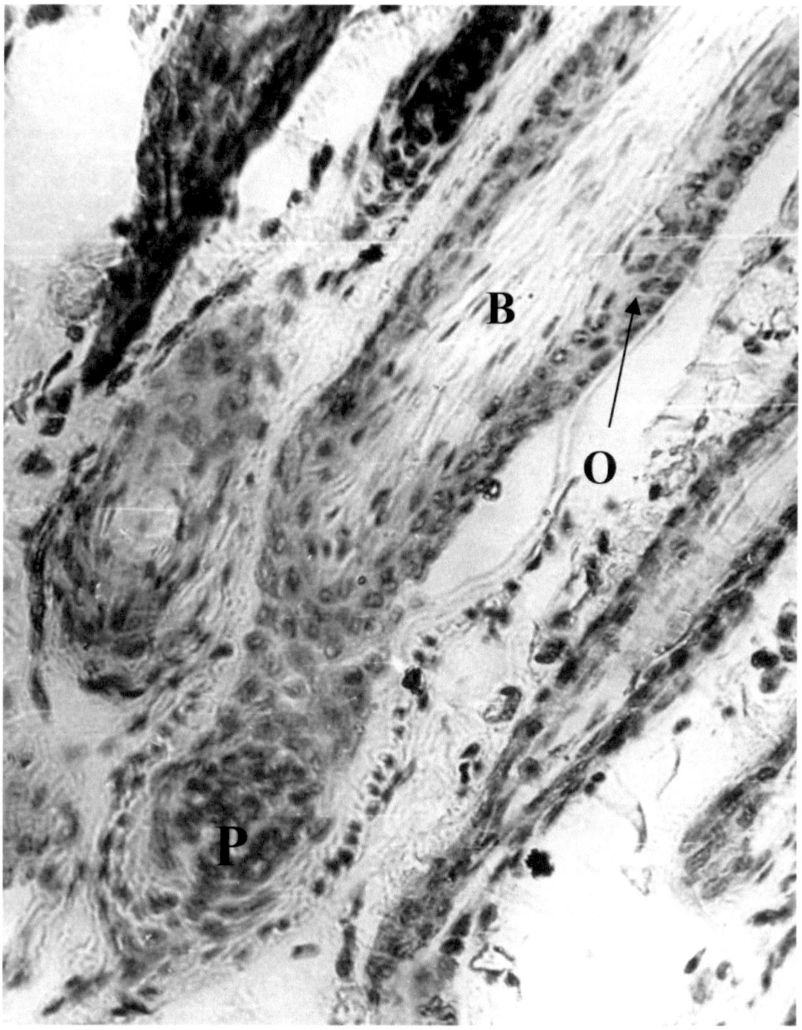

Figure 7. A telogen phase hair follicle of sheep. P, hair follicle papilla ascended upward after the brash-like (B) lower hair end ("club") which is directly connected with outer hair root sheath (O) unlike anagen phase (growing hair) follicle where the hair is separated from the outer sheath by the inner sheath. Hematoxylin + eosin.

by this moment OS inner layer cells surrounded by the cells of nonkeratinized outer layers of the OS. In such a way, the nongrowing hair is anchored in the skin. Its loss from the skin is postponed after stopping the growth up to the moment when the keratinized companion layer cells will be peeled into the pilary lumen, and the hair will be shed out of the skin perhaps because the intercellular "glue" is destroyed between keratinized cells like between peeling cells of the interfollicular epidermis.

After some period of anchoring, the new matrix and bulb regenerate and the new hair starts to grow in this follicle. In such species as mice, one follicle in the early postnatal period can produce four generations of hairs all being kept anchored and allowing new hair to grow past them.

2. The hair follicle sites of resistance to hair pulling out of the skin

So let us list the histological conditions necessary to keep the clearly visible hair shaft within the skin:

(1) The hair shaft must not be too thin and short and rare (like on the cheek of a girl), or such underdeveloped hair most probably would be interpreted as hair loss (**Figure 8**).

(2) There must not be extreme local thinnings of hair shafts caused by the short temporary action of mitostatic agents (stress—hydrocortisone, short time ionizing irradiation). Hairs can be easily broken in these thin sites and hair loss will take place (**Figure 9**).

(3) The keratinization of the hair cortex cells must be perfect enough not to allow the hair to break easily especially after these cells leave the skin in the course of hair growth. The defects of the keratin can be caused by the parasitic organisms or genetic mutations or the lack of some nutrients.

(4) When the hair grows, its fixation in the F is possible when the correct proportion of IS and hair cuticle layers are produced and their interaction takes place.

(5) When the hair stops growing, its fixation in the skin for some time is possible only when the IS is not produced and cannot isolate the modified hair cortex cells of the brush-like proximal club-hair end from companion layer cells. Direct contact between the hair brush-like end and keratinized companion cells seems to be the main mechanism of telogen hair temporary fixation in the skin and postponing of the hair shedding.

(6) Unlike the events in the "planned" catagen phase where the IS production is stopped and brush-like proximal hair shaft end is produced, the mitostatic agents do not stop IS formation, and nothing like brush-like proximal hair end is formed (merely thinning pointed end) (**Figure 10**). So the hair shedding is not postponed and is not fixed in the skin 8 days after any type of mitostatic action in the proper dose.

(7) Relatively high proportion of hair F entered into telogen phase at any moment means that the hair will be neither long nor dense. Even postponed shedding will still in-

volve rather many hairs in shedding process at any moment and all these features will be interpreted as hair loss. So the hair loss can be partly decreased by the regulatory mechanisms prolonging anagen VI phase and lowering the proportion of F in the telogen phase.

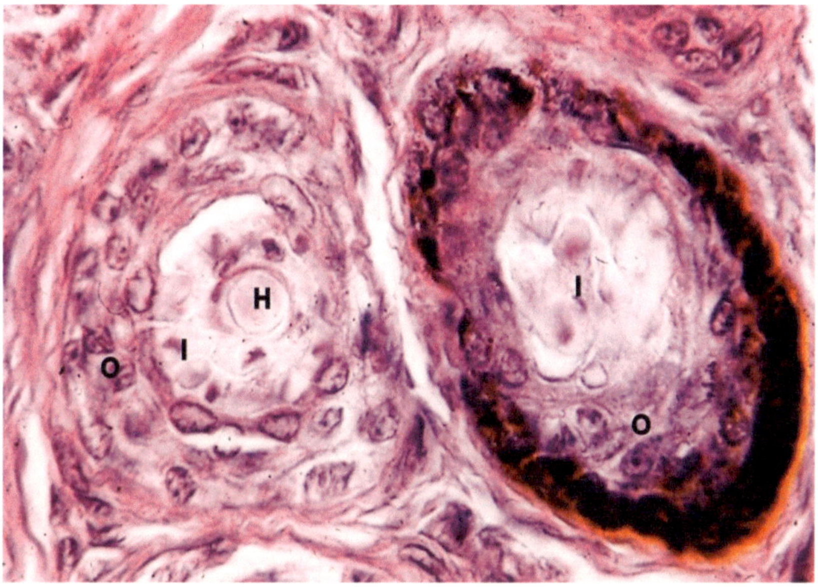

Figure 8. Transverse histological sections of neighbor hair follicles of nude goat supposedly with nude mutation causing underdevelopment of hairs. The left follicle produced very thin hair (H) as well as rather developed hair root inner sheath (I). The right follicle produced only inner sheath (I) and no hair at all. O, well developed outer hair root sheaths. The right one includes some melanocytes producing melanin. Hematoxylin + eosin.

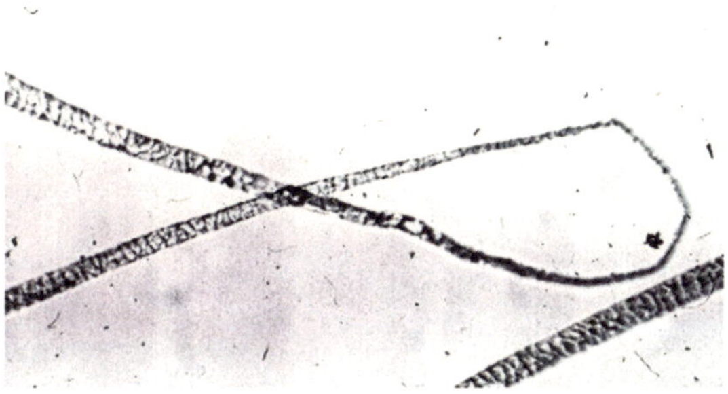

Figure 9. Hair dysplasia caused by the local fine-wool sheep skin X-irradiation by subepilation doze (300 sZv). The left and higher hair segment was formed before the irradiation. This segment is followed by one with some disturbance of normal structure (3 days after irradiation) and progressive thinning of the wool fiber. In the course of further growth, the restoration of original hair diameter took place (lower left hair segment).

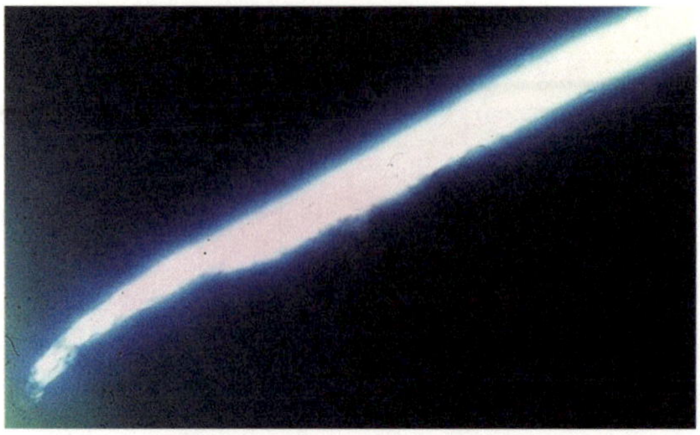

Figure 10. Polarization microscopy picture of the lower end of the sheep hair which appeared as the result of local X-irradiation of the skin by epilation doze (500 sZv). No "club" or brush-like structures could be seen. White "shining" is caused by the capacity of the very dense keratin regular structure to turn the plane of light polarization between two crossed polaroids (dark background) of "NU" Carl Zeiss microscope.

Abbreviations

F	Hair follicle
K	Keratins
Kl	"Keratin-like" proteins
IS	Hair inner root sheath
OS	Hair outer root sheath

Author details

Vsevolodov Eduard Borisovich

Address all correspondence to: eduardvsevolodov@mail.ru

Faculty of Biology and Biotechnology, Al-Farabi Kazakh National University, Almaty, Kazakhstan

References

[1] Vsevolodov, E.B., Volosyanye follikuly (Hair Follicles), Alma-Ata: Nauka, 1979, pp. 1-190.

[2] Rogers, G.E., Hair follicle differentiation and regulation, Int. J. Dev. Biol., 2004, vol. 48, pp. 163-170.

[3] Oh, J.W., et al., A guide to studying human hair follicle cycling in vivo, J. Invest. Dermatol., 2015, pp. 1-124.

http://dx.doi.org/10.5772/67275

[4] Vsevolodov, E.B., Golichenkov, V.A., and Latypov, I.F., Cellular dynamics of the outer layers of the hair follicle of fine-wool sheep during the phase of stable hair growth, Russ. J. Dev Biol., 2014, vol. 45, no. 6, pp. 342-350, ISSN 1062-3604.

[5] Hayflick, L., Aging under glass, Exp. Gerontol., 1970, vol. 5, pp. 291-303.

[6] Orwin, D.F.G., Cell differentiation in the lower outer sheath of the Romney wool follicle; a companion cell layer, Aust. J. Biol. Sci., 1971, vol. 24, pp. 989-999.

[7] Chapman, R.E., Cell migration in wool follicles of sheep, J. Cell Sci., 1971, vol. 9, pp. 791-803.

[8] Gemmel, R.T., and Chapman, R.E., Formation and breakdown of the inner root sheath and features of the pilary canal epithelium in the wool follicle, J. Ultrastruct. Res., 1971, vol. 36, pp. 355-366.

Chapter 6

Trichoscopy and Trichogram

Melike Kibar

Additional information is available at the end of the chapter

http://dx.doi.org/10.5772/66836

Abstract

Hair and scalp examination techniques can be classified into three categories: noninvasive methods (clinical history, general examination, photography, hair count, weighing shed hair, pull test, global hair counts, dermoscopy, electron microscopy, laser scanning microscopy, etc.); semi-invasive methods (the trichogram, unit areatrichogram); and invasive methods (biopsies in cicatritial alopecia). Scalp dermoscopy or trichoscopy is one of thenoninvasive techniques for the evaluation of patients with hair loss that allows for magnified visualization of the hair and scalp skin. It may be performed with a manual dermoscope (10× magnification) or a videodermoscope (up to 1000× magnification). This method is simple, quick, and easy to perform, is well-accepted by patients, and is useful for monitoring treatment, determining severity of the disease and follow-up. It is a simple, minimally invasive and rapid technique for measuring hair follicle activity. Trichogram represents a semi-invasive technique for the evaluation of patients with hair loss that allows the microscopic examination of hairs plucked from the scalp and provides information about the state of the proximal end of the hair shaft and the distal end. The trichogram is a useful complementary tool for clinical evaluation, diagnosis, and the monitoring of treatment response.

Keywords: trichoscopy, trichogram, scalp dermoscopy, dermoscopy, dermatoscopy, hair loss, cicatritial alopecia, noncicatritial alopecia, alopecia, alopecia areata, androgenetic alopecia, discoid lupus erythematosus, frontal fibrosing alopecia, lichen planopilaris, telogen effluvium

1. Introduction

Hair loss is the most common hair disease and diagnosis of the type of alopecia may sometimes be challenging. Methods commonly used to investigate can be classified as either invasive (e.g., biopsies in scarring alopecia), semi-invasive (trichogram, unit areatrichogram), or noninvasive (e.g., hair count, weighing shed hair, pull test, global hair counts, dermoscopy, phototrichogram, electron microscopy, laser scanning microscopy) methods. In this chapter, I will try to explain the basics of trichoscopy and trichogram.

2. Trichoscopy

Scalp dermoscopy is a simple and noninvasive instrument for appraising a number of hair and scalp disorders. Scalp dermoscopy, which may be defined as "trichoscopy" [1–3] is widely used in dermatology for the evaluation of pigmented skin lesions, represents a valuable, noninvasive, and rapid technique for the assessment of patients with hair loss that allows for a magnified visualization of the hair and scalp skin [4–7]. Trichoscopy allows for magnified observation of the following: hair shafts, hair follicle openings, the perifollicular epidermis, and blood vessels. In particular, trichoscopy may be useful for the diagnosis, prognosis and follow-up of androgenetic alopecia (AGA), alopecia areata (AA), telogen effluvium (TE), trichotillomania, congenital triangular alopecia, tinea capitis, cicatritial alopecias, and hair shaft disorders [8, 9]. Dermoscopy may be performed with a manual dermoscope (10× magnification) or videodermoscope (up to 1000× magnification) [10]. Both polarized and nonpolarized light may be used, with or without the use of immersion oil (dry dermoscopy).

2.1. Trichoscopy equipment

Both handheld dermatoscope and videodermatoscope is suitable to perform trichoscopy. Handheld dermatoscopes allow for tenfold magnification, while the magnification of digital dermatoscopes is ranging from tenfold to 50-fold and higher. Handheld dermatoscopes have the advantage of being both time and cost-effective. On the other hand, digital dermatoscopes have the superiority of taking easier photography and having higher magnifications [5]. I prefer using videodermatoscope that allows vascular structures more obvious [8, 9]. Water, ultrasound gels, aqueous gels, liquid paraffin, alcohol, and oil can be used to enhance clarity and visualization [11]. The choice of a particular device and fluid immersion is a matter of individual preference.

Trichoscopy images can be used to assess hair shaft thickness by folliscope [12] or analyzing hair growth by trichoscan [13] while trichoscan has been criticized by some dermatologists for the need of shaving and dying hair in the analyzed area [14, 15]. These images may be used to obtain optimal areas for scalp biopsy in cicatricial alopecia [16].

2.2. Trichoscopy structures and patterns

2.2.1. Scalp without any complaint

Normal scalp is characterized by the presence of follicular units containing about 2–4 terminal hairs and 1 or 2 vellus hairsof uniform thickness and color [17–20]. The mean thickness of normal hair was about 0.06 mm [19]; however, up to 10% of hairs are represented by vellus hairs which lack the medulla [6, 21, 22]. A normal terminal hair is uniform in thickness and color throughout its length, however, vellus hairsare lightly pigmented [21, 22]. Simple, fine red loops, which represent capillaries within the dermal papillae, are generally visible among hairs, and the subpapillary plexus is visible as linear arborizing vessels. In dark-skinned individuals, a perifollicular pigmented network (honeycomb pattern) is usually appreciated over the scalp which is accentuated over sun-exposed areas, and follicular openings and ecrine sweat gland duct openings appear as white dots (WD) [7, 23].

2.2.2. Dots

Trichoscopy may distinguish whether hair follicle openings are normal, empty, fibrotic,or containing biological material, such as hyperkeratotic plugs or hair residues. "Dots" is a common term for small, round hair follicle openings seen by trichoscopy [5, 6, 24].

2.2.2.1. Yellow dots

Previous studies showed that yellow dots (YD) indicates dilated infundibula of follicles with remnants of hair [25–28, 41] and follicular openings filled with keratotic material and/or sebum [24, 29]. They vary in color, shape and size. Regularly distributed YD are present in 60% of patients with AA and are considered a marker of disease severity and less favorable prognosis [24] while there was no relation with disease severity according to our study [30]. Yellow dots are present in AA [24, 30] discoid lupus erythematosus (DLE), TE [28, 30], and AGA [19, 28]. Large, dark yellow to brownish YD (keratotic plugs) are characteristic of DLE and correspond to wide infundibula filled with keratotic material [31, 32] although we saw these brown dots in patients with AGA at the same time [28]. Yellow dots are also seen in patients with patterned hair loss, YD in the frontal area compared to the occipital area favors the diagnosis of female AGA [19], they differ from the YD observed in other diseases by their "oily" appearance that most probably results from the predominance of sebum over keratotic material [9].

Yellow dots imposed over dark hair shaft residues appearing as large "3D" soap bubbles have been described in dissecting cellulitis [31] and in trichotillomania [24]. According to some dermatologists [5], when there is no suspicion of AGA, if you see YD, the diagnosis of AA incognita is obvious to differ AA incognita from TE and trichotillomania. On the other hand, in addition to these diseases, YD may be seen in patients with TE, trichotillomania, psoriasis, and seborrheic dermatitis [28, 30].

2.2.2.2. Brown dots

Yellow dots are firstly described by Ross and colleagues [5] as uniform structures yellowish-pink in color, while some of these dots were found to be brown in color in our patients [28, 30]. Brown dots were found with a statistically higher frequency in patients with AGA [30]. Scattered brown areas are seen in actinic keratosis and DLE, and peripilar brown areas are seen in AGA, in TE and in healthy individuals, simply sometimes, we can see brown dots in a distribution similar to YD in dark-skinned patients [8, 28, 30], and therefore, I call them yellow-brown dots instead of YD as a separate category.

2.2.2.3. Black dots

Black dots (formerly "cadaverized hairs") are residues of pigmented hairs that have been broken or destroyed at the level of the scalp [33]. They are considered a marker of high disease activity while there was no relationship during our study [24, 30]. Black dots may be present in dissecting cellulitis, tinea capitis, chemotherapy-induced alopecia, trichotillomania, but may be incidentally observed also in other diseases and after laser depilation or trichogram [33, 34]. Black dots are not present in healthy individuals or in patients with patterned hair loss or TE [4, 28, 30, 35].

2.2.2.4. Black dotted pigmentation

Black dots sized smaller than declared black dots (cadaverized hairs) those are seen in AA previously [30] were named as black dotted pigmentation (BDP) by us, and they related positively with disease severity in AA. A biopsy from one of these areas in a patient with AA showed no cellular infiltration but revealed intense demodex colonization in follicular ostia, so it was thought that the trichoscopic appearance might be due to this infestation. In a study [36], dirty dots on scalp represented nonmicrobial environmental particles in healthy children.

2.2.2.5. Red dots

Red dots are widened follicles surrounded by dilated vessels and extravasated erythrocytes were described in DLE and are believed to be a positive prognostic factor [29]. Regularly distributed brown or brown-gray dots are a characteristic finding in the eyebrow area of patients with frontal fibrosing alopecia (FFA). This finding is a favorable prognostic factor for eyebrow regrowth [6]. Additionally, red dots have been described in individuals with vitiligo [37].

2.2.2.6. Grey dots

Pink-grey and grey dots have been observed in the eyebrow area of patients with FFA [9].

2.2.2.7. White dots

The classic, big, irregular WD represent areas of perifollicular fibrosis and are observed most commonly in lichen planopilaris (LPP) [6]. Another type of WD, the small, regular pinpoint WD are observed in the sun-exposed scalp of patients with skin phototypes III and IV and in the normal scalp of those with phototypes V and VI [6, 28, 30, 38]. They have been correlated with the acrosyringeal (ecrine sweat duct openings) and empty follicular openings [38–40]. According to us, another type of WD are cumulus like clustered WD that are intersecting WD in a nested form. We think in severe AA the classic, irregular WD is nested together with pinpoint WD, so we call them clustered WD similar to cumulus clouds [30]. In advanced stages of AGA, follicles can be replaced by connective tissues, afterwards causing atrophy. These empty follicular ostia are seen as WD [5, 19, 24, 28, 30, 31, 38, 39]. WD are more common in the late stages of AGA [5, 28]. Kossard and Zagarella [42] observed WD in scarring alopecia and considered these WD as being the melanin pour places in fibrous tracts of scar tissue.

2.2.3. Hair shafts

Abnormalities in hair shaft structure may provide diagnostic clues for multiple acquired and inherited causes of hair loss. Rudnicka et al. recently proposed a classification of hair shaft abnormalities observed by trichoscopy [18, 43–45]. The features of hair shafts include exclamation mark hair in AA, trichotillomania, and chemotherapy-induced alopecia (also called "tapering hairs ": 1- to 2-mm-long fractured hairs, whose tips are wider than the proximal portion of the shaft), broken hairs (fractured hairs with uniform shaft diameter), vellus hairs in patterned hair loss and in long-lasting AA (less than 0.03 mm in thickness and less than 3-mm long, representing miniaturized hairs or regrowing hairs can be differentiated from short, healthy regrowing hairs, which are darkly pigmented and straight with pointed ends), coiled hairs in trichotillomania (broken hairs that curl back), comma hairs (short, c-shaped hairs), and cork screw hairs in tinea capitis (short hairs, spiral in shape), Pohle Pinkus constrictions in AA, chemotherapy-induced alopecia, blood loss, malnutrition, and chronic intoxication, flame hairs (semitransparent, wavy, and cone-shaped highly specific hair residues, resembling a fire flame that remain attached to the scalp after anagen hairs have been pulled out), V-signs (two or more hairs emerging from one follicular unit and broken at the same length),and sprinkled hairs (only a sprinkled "hair powder", resulting from hair damage, is visible) in trichotillomania, and tulip hairs (diagonally fractured short hair shafts with a tulip leaf-like hyperpigmentation at the distal end] in trichotillomania and AA [43, 44]. Trichoscopy has also been successfully used to diagnose many genetic hair shaft disorders [45].

2.2.4. *Perifollicular and interfollicular epidermis*

According to the color and structure (scaling, discharge, and surface structure) of the areas, the classification of perifollicular and interfollicular skin surface abnormalities in trichoscopy can be classified as; perifollicular discoloration (hyperpigmentation), predominant in androgenetic alopecia,and perifollicular fibrosis, characteristic for some form of fibrosing alopecia [8, 46].

Due to epidermal and perifollicular inflammation in seborrheic dermatitis and psoriasis [47, 48], proximal hair shaft with macropits [49] may look relatively hidden under a white-grey epidermal diffuse proliferation that we called as hidden hair [50] that differs from perifollicular scaling observed in LPP and in folliculitis decalvans [6, 31].

During our knowledge, honeycomb hyperpigmentation is a normal finding in sun-exposed areas (chronic sun exposure) and in patients with Fitzpatrick skin phototypes IV, V, and VI [5–7], but in our study, when this pattern is observed trichoscopically, the estimated alopecia risk was 3.2 times higher regardless of age that is why, we do not think it is the characteristic of normal aging scalp [28]. Perifollicular brown coloration ("peripilar sign") is believed to correspond to the perifollicular presence of lymphocytic infiltrates [51] and is common in patients with patterned hair loss [2]; however, the peripilar sign may be observed in up to10% of hair follicles in healthy individuals [21]. Scattered brown discoloration is characteristic of DLE [31].

2.2.5. *Blood vessels*

Appearance of cutaneous microvessels in trichoscopy may vary in type and number depending on disease and activity of the process. The significance of blood vessel abnormalities observed on trichoscopy has not been explored in detail thus far. Common types of vessels in alopecia includes elongated vessels in LPP, thick arborizing vessels in DLE and seborrheic dermatitis, twisted red loops and comma vessels in seborrheic dermatitis, atypical red vessels, structureless red areas, signet ring vessel, twisted red loops and glomerular or coiled vessels in linear or circular alignment in psoriasis [9, 19, 31, 50, 52].

2.2.6. Other structures

Other common trichoscopy signs include yellow or yellow-red discharge (e.g., folliculitis decalvans, bacterial infections, dissecting cellulitis, and tinea capitis) and structural changes in the skin surface (e.g., starburst pattern hyperplasia in folliculitis decalvans) [9, 31].

2.3. Alopecia areata

The most characteristic trichoscopic findings include the following: black dots, exclamation mark hairs, tapered hairs, broken hairs, coudability hairs (hairs of normal length with a narrowed proximal shaft and are mostly found in the scalp surrounding the alopecic patch), coiled hairs, YD, hypopigmented vellus hairs, trichorrhexis nodosa, monilethrix-like hairs (constrictions in the hair shaft),and Pohle Pinkus constrictions [4–9, 24, 30, 53–57]. Broken hairs are not exclusive to AA, as they may also be observed in trichotillomania [7]. Exclamation mark hairs represent the most specific signs of acute AA [17]; however, they are also observed in chemotherapy alopecia. Black dots may also be observed in trichotillomania, cicatritial alopecia, and tinea capitis. Yellow dots may be observed both in acute and in chronic forms of AA and generally have a regular distribution and in severe forms have a nested formation [5, 7, 24, 30]. Yellow dots are highly sensitive but have low specificity for AA, as they may be seen in other hair disorders, including AGA, congenital hypotrichoses, and DLE [7, 28]. Short, hypopigmented vellus hairs are a common finding in AA and are usually indicative of remitting disease [4, 7].

In our study [30], major risk factors for AA were determined to be black dots, WD, and YD (risk ratios were estimated as 170-fold, 5.9-fold,and 5.3-fold, respectively).

Active (acute) AA can be distinguished from nonactive AA using trichoscopy. Features of disease activity include black dots, exclamation marks, broken hairs, trichoptilosis, pig tail, short vellus hairs,and upright regrowing hair whereas YD, WD, clustered WD, honeycomb pigmentation, black dotted pigmentation, and vellus hairs are markers of disease severity and inactive late stage disease [4, 12, 20, 24, 30, 55, 58]. In addition to this, disease activity showed negative relation with atypical red vessels in our study, we believed that these atypical red vessels indicated rejuvenation after the catabolic process in progressive AA [30]. Early features of hair regrowth include the presence of pigmented, upright, regrowing hairs [24], and pigtail hairs [23]. Recent data show that trichoscopy may also be applied in the evaluation of treatment response in AA patients [59].

2.4. Androgenetic alopecia

Male and female pattern hair loss share similar trichoscopic features. These include hair shaft thickness heterogeneity (anisotrichosis, hair diameter diversity), YD, pinpoint WD, honeycomb pigmentation, focal atrichia, epidermal scaling, arborizing red lines, perifollicular brown,and white discoloration (peripilar sign), an increased proportion of vellus hairs, and an increased proportion of follicular units with only 1 emerging hair shaft instead of 2–4 hair shafts [4, 5, 9, 11, 19, 28, 43, 60–63]. On the other hand, in early AGA, we saw multihair follicular unit more than follicular units with only 1 emerging hair shaft [28].

Trichoscopy was demonstrated to be superior to the classical trichogram for the evaluation of early female AGA [64], showing 75% sensitivity and 61.54% specificity in a recent study [65].

All of the trichoscopic features appear most prominently in the frontal scalp area [19, 21]. An increased ratio of vellus hairs to all hairs in androgen dependent scalp regions is characteristic of AGA [6, 7, 19, 28]. The most important finding of AGA is the hair diameter variability, which reflects hair miniaturization [44]. Hair miniaturization does not equally affect all hair follicles of the same area, resulting in the simultaneous presence of terminal, intermediate, and vellus hairs. When the hair diameter variability of more than 20%, which means that vellus hairs account for more than 20% of all the hairs in the same view, was regarded as a hallmark of AGA in previous reports [6, 7, 60]. In addition to this, three major diagnostic criteria for female AGA have been suggested: more than four yellow dots in four images (70-fold magnification) of the frontal area, a lower than average hair thickness in the frontal area compared to the occipital area, and vellus hairs (below 0.03 mm) comprising more than 10% of hairs in the frontal area [19]. Recently, some authors have suggested that the presence of more than six vellus hairs in the frontal scalp may be indicative of initial female AGA [66].

In more advanced and severe stages of AGA, trichoscopy shows the presence of empty follicular ostia, YD, brown dots,and a honeycomb-like pigmented network in bald, sun-exposed areas [5, 7, 28, 63].

In our study, PFP was detected to be a characteristic trichoscopic finding of AGA that was described as a normal feature of the scalp in healthy persons younger than 25 years [21, 28].

2.4.1. Telogen effluvium

Although no specific trichoscopic criteria of TE have been recognized, the diagnosis may be suspected when empty hair follicles (sometimes appearing as YD), a high percentage of follicular units with only 1 hair, brown perifollicular discoloration (the peripilar sign), and short, dark, multiple upright regrowing hairs of normal thickness are present in the absence of the characteristic features of other scalp disorders [7, 19, 40, 67, 68]. In TE patients, no significant differences are observed in the trichoscopic findings between the frontal and occipital areas; this differentiates TE from patterned hair loss [9].

2.5. Trichotillomania

Trichoscopy shows the presence of broken hair shafts of different lengths with no significant changes in the perifollicular area. The extremities of the hairs have a typical frayed aspect (split ends) [69]. Trichoscopy is also useful to demonstrate the signs of plucking to the parents [70]. Recently, a number of other signs, all variants of broken hairs, have been described, including coiled hairs, flame hairs (semitransparent, wavy, and cone-shaped highly specific hair residues, resembling a fire flame that remain attached to the scalp after anagen hairs have been pulled out), V-signs (2 or more hairs emerging from one follicular unit and broken at the same length), tulip hairs (diagonally fractured short hair shafts with a tulip leaf-like hyperpigmentation at the distal end), and sprinkled hairs (only a sprinkled "hair powder", resulting from hair damage, is visible) [68]. Black dots and exclamation mark hairs may be sometimes observed [6, 57, 68], and it can be very difficult to distinguish these cases from AA.

2.6. Congenital triangular alopecia

Trichoscopy shows normal follicular openings, highlights the clinical presence of long, thin vellus hairs that are surrounded by normal terminal hairs in the adjacent scalp and allows for differential diagnosis with AA and cicatritial alopecia [7, 71, 72].

2.7. Tinea capitis

Comma hairs are comma-like structures that are associated with both ectothrix and endothrix types of fungal invasion [73–76]. In some patients, hairs are more intensely coiled than typical comma hairs. These hairs have been called "corkscrew hairs" [73, 75, 76]. Corkscrew hairs are also observed in patients of African descent who are infected by *Trichophyton soudanense* [75], *Trichophyton tonsurans* [76], *Trichophyton violaceum* [77], and *Trichophyton verrucosum* [78]. Other less common findings include Morse code hairs (interrupted hairs), bent hairs, zigzag hairs, broken hairs, and black dots [6, 18, 68, 73, 79].

2.8. Anagen effluvium

Trichoscopic images of anagen effluvium are characterized by the presence of black dots, monilethrix-like hairs, and exclamation mark hairs [33, 34].

2.9. Psoriasis and seborrheic dermatitis

Kim et al. reported that red dots and globules, twisted red loops,and glomerular vessels were mostly seen in psoriasis while atypical red vessels, arborizing red lines,and structureless red areas were seen in seborrheic dermatitis [52]. On the other hand, in our study we observed red dots and globules, atypical red vessels, structureless red areas, hidden hair and signet ring vessel mostly in psoriasis while twisted red loops and comma vessels mostly in seborrheic dermatitis [50]. Twisted red loops are thought to be the characteristic videodermatoscopic figure of scalp psoriasis in comparison with seborrheic dermatitis [5]. On the other hand, we considered red dot and globules as the characteristic videodermatoscopic figure of psoriasis and arborizing red lines for seborrheic dermatitis according to our study [50].

2.10. Common cicatricial alopecias

2.10.1. Discoid lupus erythematosus

One of the most typical trichoscopic features of active DLE is the presence of large YD that differ from the YD observed in AA by their larger size and darker, yellow-brownish color [31, 32, 80]. Occasionally, in long-lasting DLE, thin and radial arborizing vessels are observed to emerge from these dots ("red spider in YD" appearance) which some authors consider a characteristic of DLE [6, 31]. Thick arborizing vessels are commonly present at the periphery of the lesion. Trichoscopic findings for long-lasting, inactive DLE lesions do not differ from those for other types of cicatricial alopecia and are characterized by structureless milky-red or white areas lacking follicular openings [31]. When present, red dots, which are regularly distributed around follicular openings, indicate the expression of active disease and are related to a good prognosis with possible hair regrowth upon prompt treatment [29, 31].

2.10.2. *Lichen planopilaris*

Trichoscopy reveals the absence of follicular openings and the presence of whitish perifollicular casts that surround the hair shafts at their emergence as the most characteristic feature [4–7, 31, 81, 82]. Scales migrate along the hair shafts and form tubular structures that cover the proximal portions of the emerging hair shafts. This phenomenon is called tubular perifollicular scaling [31]. Some authors have described the presence of blue-gray dots arranged in a target pattern around the hair follicles (due to the presence of melanophages) [80]. In dark-skinned subjects affected by LPP the persistence of a normal pigmented network inside the plaques of hair loss is typical, as the interfollicular epidermis is commonly unaffected by the inflammatory process [83].

Milky-red areas are characteristic for inflammation-mediated fibrosis of recent onset [31]. Small hair tufts, of 5–9 hairs, may be present in late LPP [31]. To sum up, possible differences between DLE and LPP are the presence of blue-gray dots with a diffuse distribution along the patch "speckled" pattern, resulting from interface dermatitis and the subsequent pigment incontinence [80] and the loss of the normal pigmented network in dark-skinned patients due to the involvement of the interfollicular epidermis.

2.10.3. *Frontal fibrosing alopecia*

Trichoscopic findings in FFA include the lack of follicular openings and minor perifollicular scaling is lower than that of LPP [84–87]. A characteristic finding of FFA is the abrupt interruption of the hairline, with the absence of the vellus hairs that are typically observed in normal scalp. The background in patients with FFA is usually ivory-white to ivory-beige [86, 87]. Pink-grey and grey dots are commonly observed in the lateral eyebrow area of patients with FFA [9]. To sum up, lonely hairs, surrounded by areas of fibrosis [84], and the absence of vellus hairs in the frontal hairline [85] have been discussed as possible clues for the diagnosis of FFA.

Trichoscopy is very helpful in the differential diagnosis with other types of alopecia involving the scalp margin in female patients; in AGA, it shows an increased presence of vellus hairs at the hairline, in FFA, the absence of vellus hairs represented the predominant trichoscopic pattern, followed by perifollicular scaling, and the absence of follicular openings, in ophiasic AA, it shows the typical signs of the disease, while in traction alopecia vellus hairs are preserved [85].

2.10.4. *Folliculitis decalvans*

Trichoscopy shows severe pustulation, scaling,and crusting that are generally prominent around follicular units. When cicatritial alopecia occurs, trichoscopy shows the absence of follicular openings and, in cases of tufted folliculitis, the outgrowth of several hairs (hair tufts) from single and dilated residual follicular openings [5, 88, 89] that is the most characteristic trichoscopic feature [82, 90]. Some authors have described the presence of a perifollicular hyperplasia with a typical starburst pattern in such cases. A perifollicular concentration of blood vessels may also be present. In long-standing disease, white and milky red areas lacking follicular openings are predominant [31].

2.10.5. Dissecting cellulitis

In early stages, dissecting cellulitis shows trichoscopic features that may be similar to those observed in AA [39]. In a study [54] including 11 patients with dissecting cellulitis, trichoscopy showed the presence of YD, red dots, empty follicular openings,and black dots and may mimic AA [33, 54]. As the diseases progresses, other trichoscopic features become more prominent, including yellow structureless areas and YD with "3-dimensional" structure imposed over dystrophic hair shafts [31]. Some authors describe these yellow dots with "3D" structure that are imposed over dystrophic hair shafts as the most characteristic feature of dissecting cellulitis [6, 31]. End-stage fibrotic lesions are characterized by confluent ivory-white or white areas lacking follicular openings [31, 91].

2.10.6. Central centrifugal alopecia

One article described the trichoscopic aspect of the disease as reduced hair density with hair shaft variability, pinpoint WD, and peripilar white halos. Moreover, pigmented, asterisk-like macules with sparse terminal and vellus-like hairs may be present. The residual terminal hairs may emerge as a single hair or as a group of two hairs and are generally surrounded by a characteristic, peripilar gray-white halo [7].

2.11. Hair shaft disorders

When using light microscopy, multiple samples may be needed before an abnormal hair shaft is identified therefore trichoscopy may replace light microscopy in the evaluation of genetic hair shaft defects, such as monilethrix [92, 93], trichorrhexis invaginata [94, 95], trichorrhexis nodosa [45], pili annulati [45, 96], pili torti [5, 96], and others [17, 18]. On the other hand, in trichothiodystrophy, the characteristic tiger tail pattern is not visible on trichoscopy, and polarized microscopy remains the criterion standard for diagnosing this condition [9, 45]. When using trichoscopy, different features may be observed in the following disorders:

2.11.1. Monilethrix

Elliptical nodes of normal hair thickness that are regularly separated by dystrophic constrictions in which the hairs have no medulla and that are the sites of fracture; this finding has also been described as the "regularly bended ribbon sign" [10, 45, 92, 93, 96, 97].

2.11.2. Pili torti

Flattened hair shafts with regular twists at irregular intervals along the long axis [10, 92, 96].

2.11.3. Pili trianguli and canaliculi (uncombable hair)

Triangular-shaped shafts with longitudinal grooving or flattening [9].

2.11.4. Pili annulati

Alternating light and dark bands, light bands corresponding to air-filled cavities within the hair shaft [6, 17, 45, 96].

2.11.5. Trichorrexis nodosa

White knots along the distal shafts and brush-pattern fractured ends [17].

2.11.6. Trichorrexis invaginata (bamboo hair)

Multiple ball-shaped nodes along hairs that resemble the ball-in-cup rings of bamboo and are due to invagination of the distal portion of the hair shaft into its proximal portion; the fragile node breaking off results in ragged, cupped proximal hair (golf-tee hairs) [17, 95, 96].

2.11.7. Woolly hair

Hair shafts resembling a crawling snake with short wave cycles [45].

2.11.8. Trichothiodystrophy

Nonhomogeneous structure resembling grains of sand and having a wavy contour [45].

3. Trichogram

In this procedure, 60–80 hairs are plucked with a rubber-armed forceps from a 5-day unwashed hair. Hair bulbs are immediately placed with their roots on a glass slide in an embedding medium, which allows information about the state of the proximal end of the hair shaft (the root), the distal end (the tip) and hair root is necessary [98].

The trichogram is a useful complementary tool for clinical evaluation, diagnosis, and the monitoring of treatment response [99].

It should be noted that the trichogram simply provides a snapshot of the hair follicle at the time of examination and that the condition of follicles can vary within the same patient depending on numerous factors, such as sampling site, previous washing or brushing of the hair, and time of the year [100].

3.1. Trichogram equipment

Appropriate sampling site for male pattern hair loss should be taken from the central interparietal area, while the second sample, if needed, should be taken from the temporal or occipital area. In female pattern hair loss, samples should be taken from the center and the vertex of the scalp. The sites for telogen hair loss and scarring alopecia are, respectively, the central interparietal area and the advancing border of the alopecic patch. Using a rubber-sheathed Kocher forceps, a tuft of 15–20 hairs must be removed. To do this, you have to place the forceps 1–2 cm from the scalp and pluck out the hairs rapidly and firmly in the direction of the natural growth of the hair. If the hairs are not plucked out firmly, they may appear as pseudo-dystrophic hairs under the microscope, or exhibit frayed or broken roots [99].

The next step is to prepare the hairs for examination under the microscope. They should be parallel to each other and that the roots are aligned. Next, they are covered with clear adhesive tape. To avoid artifacts and obtain a sharper, cleaner image, you may apply several drops of balsam (such as that used to mount histological slides) and cover the hairs with a cover slip. The use of polarized light improves image quality [99].

3.2. Hair examination

The sample is examined using a 4× objective, although a 10× or 40× objective can be used if higher magnification is needed. A higher-quality image can be obtained by fitting 2 polarizers to the microscope: 1 between the condenser and the sample and the other between the sample and the observer [99].

3.2.1. The proximal end

Anagen hair shafts are longer, have a uniform diameter, a rectangular shape, and a slight distal angle. Pigmentation is intense in the bulb area and there are sheaths and membranes.

Telogen hair shafts are shorter and appear higher up in the trichogram, above the roots of anagen hairs; the root is thick and club shaped and there are no distal angles.

Pigmentation is weak or absent; the sheath is also absent or found only at the distal end.

Very few hairs in the catagen phase are observed in the trichogram as they account for a very small percentage of all hair.

The anagen to telogen ratio varies, mainly according to age and sex. Children have the highest percentage of anagen hair (95% anagen vs. 5% telogen), and the ratio decreases with age. The anagen to telogen ratio is 86:11 in women and 83:15 in men. In a normal trichogram, an average of 89% of hairs are in anagen, 10% in telogen, and 1% in catagen. A diagnosis of telogen effluvium is established when over 20% of the hairs examined are in telogen phase.

Dystrophic hairs have a decreased proximal diameter, an irregular contour, no epithelial sheaths, and an angle of over 20. They are common in AGA or in hair that has not been removed correctly from the scalp. Keratotic material may be observed on the tip of the hair in conditions such as seborrheic dermatitis, psoriasis, and folliculitis. A common finding in patients with demodicosis is the presence of Demodicosis folliculorum in contact with the root of the hair, although this condition is usually diagnosed by superficial skin biopsy [99].

3.2.2. The hair shaft

Normal hair is uniform in appearance and structure along the entire length of the hair shaft; this uniformity is also observed between the different hairs in a sample. Hair dysplasias are

http://dx.doi.org/10.5772/66836

malformations of the hair shaft. Although scanning electron microscopy is the diagnostic tool of choice in such cases, certain signs may be observed in the trichogram [101]:

3.2.2.1. *Monilethrix (beaded hair)*

Alternating segments of narrowings and nodosities, giving a characteristic beaded appearance.

3.2.2.2. *Pseudomonilethrix*

Round hairs with irregular, sporadic rounded nodosities. There are no narrowings.

3.2.2.3. *Pili torti*

Twists of hairs with bending at different angles and regular intervals.

3.2.2.4. *Trichorrhexis invaginata (bamboo hair)*

Ball-shaped deformity with cupping at the proximal end of the hair shaft.

3.2.2.5. *Trichothiodystrophic hair*

Patients with trichothiodystrophy may have hair with ribbon-like flattening, characteristic trichoschisis-like fractures (clean transverse breaks), with an irregular surface, and tiger-tail banding.

3.2.2.6. *Trichonodosis*

Single or double knots on the hair shaft. Tie knots and other more complex knots are also observed.

3.2.2.7. *Trichorrhexis nodosa*

Bulging hair characterized by fracture nodes with open splitting of the cortex on both sides of the node. If the hair eventually splits, it will leave a brush-like appearance at both ends.

3.2.2.8. *Bubble hair*

Short, broken hairs with a wavy surface,and bubbles inside the shaft.

3.2.2.9. *Loose anagen hair*

Twisted anagen hairs with a ruffled cuticle at the proximal end. Long, pili canaliculi type canals on the shaft are a common finding [102].

3.2.2.10. *Pili annulati*

Hair shafts with alternating light and dark bands.

3.2.2.11. *Woolly hair*

Thin curly hair forming small woolly balls.

3.2.2.12. Uncombable hair (pili canaliculi)

Canalicular formation along the entire length of the hair shaft. This formation can be difficult to spot under a microscope but the micrometer can be moved if pili canaliculi is suspected.

3.2.3. The distal end

Three types of hair shaft tips can be observed:

Javelin tip: A very sharp, spear-like tip is seen in hair that is growing well and has never been cut, paintbrush tip: Fractures in the hair shaft (trichoschisis) give the tip a paintbrush-like appearance, seen in hair shaft anomalies such as monilethrix, alopecia areata, or in hair fragility induced by cosmetic products an clean-cut tip: The distal end has been cut and ends in a perfectly straight line. It is typically seen in hair that has been cut and in cases of trichotillomania [99].

3.3. Common alopecia in trichogram

In alopecia areata, hair shaft is with alternating narrow and normal sections. Pseudomonilethrix and/or trichoschisis may be observed in some hairs. Hair shaft diameter variability has been demonstrated in women, with larger diameters seen in higher stages of the Ludwig Scale [103]; the differences were minimal at stage I and maximal at stage III. In TE, the hairs are shorter than normal, have a uniform diameter, a rounded proximal end (club-like appearance) and a lack of pigment and membranes. In anagen effluvium normal anagen hairs that are longer than telogen hairs, pigmented, and having sheaths and membranes whose distal end is angled like a golf club are seen in the trichogram. Nits or lice may be seen in patients with pediculosis capitis [99].

Abbreviations

AA	alopecia areata
AGA	androgenetic alopecia
DLE	discoid lupus erythematosus
FFA	frontal fibrosing alopecia
LPP	lichen planopilaris
TE	telogen effluvium
WD	white dots
YD	yellow dots

Author details

Melike Kibar

Address all correspondence to: kibarmelike@hotmail.com

Department of Dermatology, Kecioren Training and Research Hospital, Turkey

References

[1] Olszewska M, Rudnicka L, Rakowska A, Kowalska-Oledzka E, Slowinska M. Trichoscopy. Arch Dermatol 2008; 144: 1007.

[2] Inui S. Trichoscopy for common hair loss diseases: algorithmic method for diagnosis. J Dermatol 2011; 38: 71–5.

[3] Lacarrubba F, Misciali C, Gibilisco R, Micali G. Circle Hairs: clinical, trichoscopic and histopathologic findings. Int J Trichology 2013; 5: 211–3.

[4] Lacarrubba F, Dall'Oglio F, Nasca MR, Micali G. Videodermatoscopy enhances diagnostic capability in some forms of hair loss. Am J Clin Dermatol 2004; 5: 205–8.

[5] Ross EK, Vincenzi C, Tosti A. Videodermoscopy in the evaluation of hair and scalp disorders. J Am Acad Dermatol 2006; 55: 799–806.

[6] Rudnicka L, Olszewska M, Rakowska A, Slowinska M. Trichoscopy update 2011. J Dermatol Case Rep 2011; 4: 82–8.

[7] Miteva M, Tosti A. Hair and scalp dermatoscopy. J Am Acad Dermatol 2012; 67: 1040–8.

[8] Rudnicka L, Rakowska A, Olszewska M. Trichoscopy: how it may help the clinician. Dermatol Clin 2013; 31: 29–41.

[9] Rudnicka L, Olszewska M, Rakowska A. Atlas of trichoscopy: Dermoscopy in hair and scalp disease. London: Springer; 2012.

[10] Micali G, Lacarrubba F, Massimino D, Schwartz RA. Dermatoscopy: alternative uses in daily clinical practice. J Am Acad Dermatol 2011; 64: 1135–46.

[11] Rudnicka L, Olszewska M, Rakowska A, Oledzka E, Slowinsja M. Trichoscopy: a new method for diagnosing hair loss. J Drugs Dermtol 2008; 7(7): 651–4.

[12] Lee BS, Chan JY, Monselise A, McElwee K, Shapiro J. Assessment of hair density and caliber in Caucasian and Asian female subjects with female pattern hair loss by using the Folliscope. J Am Acad Dermatol 2012; 66: 166–7.

[13] Hoffmann R. TrichoScan: a novel tool for the analysis of hair growth in vivo. J Investig Dermatol Symp Proc 2003; 8: 109–15.

[14] Saraogi PP, Dhurat RS. Automated digital image analysis [TrichoScan[R]] for human hair growth analysis: ease versus errors. Int J Trichology 2010; 2: 5–13.

[15] Guarrera M, Fiorucci MC, Rebora A. Methods of hair loss evaluation: a comparison of TrichoScan[[R]] with the modified wash test. Exp Dermatol 2013; 22: 482–4.

[16] Miteva M, Tosti A. Dermoscopy guided scalp biopsy in cicatricial alopecia. J Eur Acad Dermatol Venereol 2013; 27: 1299–303.

[17] Miteva M, Tosti A. Dermatoscopy of hair shaft disorders. J Am Acad Dermatol 2013; 68: 473–81.

[18] Rudnicka L, Rakowska A, Kerzeja M, Olszewska M. Hair shafts in trichoscopy: clues for diagnosis of hair and scalp diseases. Dermatol Clin 2013; 31: 695–708.

[19] Rakowska A, Slowinska M, Kowalska-Oledzka E, Olszewska M, Rudnicka L. Dermoscopy in female androgenic alopecia: method standardization and diagnostic criteria. Int J Trichology 2009; 1: 123–30.

[20] Jain N, Doshi B, Khopkar U. Trichoscopy in alopecias: diagnosis simplified. Int J Trichology 2013; 5(4): 170–8. doi:10.4103/0974-7753.130385

[21] Rakowska A. Trichoscopy [hair and scalp videodermoscopy] in the healthy female. Method standardization and norms for measurable parameters. J Dermatol Case Rep 2009; 3: 14–9.

[22] Vogt A, McElwee KJ, Blume-Peytavi U. Biology of the hair follicle. In: Blume-Peytavi U, Tosti A, Whiting D, Trüeb R, editors. Hair; From Basic Science to Clinical Application. Berlin: Springer-Verlag; 2008. pp. 1–22.

[23] Torres F, Tosti A. Trichoscopy: an update. G Ital Dermatol Venereol 2014; 149: 83–91.

[24] Inui S, Nakajima T, Nakagawa K, Itami S. Clinical significance of dermoscopy in alopecia areata: analysis of 300 cases. Int J Dermatol2008; 47: 688–93. PMID: 18613874

[25] Ardigò M, Tosti A, Cameli N et al. Reflectance confocal microscopy of the yellow dot pattern in alopecia areata. Arch Dermatol 2011; 147: 61–4.

[26] Lee WS. Ultrastructural and immunohistological changes of the follicular keratinocytes in alopecia areata: comparison from active lesion, stable lesion and non-lesional scalp. In: van Neste D, Randall V, editors. Hair Research for the Next Millennium. Amsterdam: Elsevier, 1996. pp. 203–7.

[27] McElwee KJ, Silva K, Boggess D et al. Alopecia areata in C3H/HeJ mice involves leukocyte-mediated root sheath disruption in advance of overt hair loss. Vet Pathol 2003; 40: 643–50.

[28] Kibar M, Aktan S, Bilgin M. Scalp dermatoscopic findings in androgenetic alopecia and their relations with disease severity. Ann Dermatol 2014; 26(4): 478–84. doi:10.5021/ad.2014.26.4.478. Epub 2014 Jul 31

[29] Tosti A, Torres F, Misciali C, Vincenzi C, Starace M, Miteva M, Romanelli P. Follicular red dots: a novel dermoscopic pattern observed in scalp discoid lupus erythematosus. Arch Dermatol 2009; 145: 1406–9. PMID: 20026850

[30] Kibar M, Aktan S, Lebe B, Bilgin M. Trichoscopic findings in alopecia areata and their relation to disease activity, severity and clinical subtype in Turkish patients. Australas J Dermatol 2015; 56(1): e1–6. doi:10.1111/ajd.12102. Epub 2013 Aug 29.

[31] Rakowska A, Slowinska M, Kowalska-Oledzka E, Warszawik O, Czuwara J, Olszewska M, et al. Trichoscopy of cicatricial alopecia. J Drugs Dermatol 2012; 11: 753–8.

[32] Lanuti E, Miteva M, Romanelli P, Tosti A. Trichoscopy and histopathology of follicular keratotic plugs in scalp discoid lupus erythematosus. Int J Trichology 2012; 4: 36–8.

[33] Kowalska-Oledzka E, Slowinska M, Rakowska A, Czuwara J, Sicinska J, Olszewska M, et al. 'Black dots' seen under trichoscopy are not specific for alopecia areata. Clin Exp Dermatol 2012; 37: 615–9.

[34] Pirmez R, Piñeiro-Maceira J, Sodré CT. Exclamation marks and other trichoscopic signs of chemotherapy-induced alopecia. Australas J Dermatol 2013; 54: 129–32.

[35] Amer M, Helmy A, Amer A. Trichoscopyas a useful method to differentiate tinea capitis from alopecia areata in children at Zagazig University Hospitals. Int J Dermatol 2016. doi:10.1111/ijd.13217. [Epub ahead of print]

[36] Fu JM, Starace M, Tosti A. A new dermoscopic finding in healthy children. Arch Dermatol 2009; 145: 596–7.

[37] Pirmez R, Piñeiro-Maceira J, de Almeida BC, Sodré CT. Follicular red dots: a normal trichoscopy feature in patients with pigmentary disorders? An Bras Dermatol 2013; 88: 459–61.

[38] Abraham LS, Pineiro-Maceira J, Duque-Estrada B, Barcaui CB, Sodre CT. Pinpoint white dots in the scalp: dermoscopic and histopathologic correlation. J Am Acad Dermatol 2010; 63: 721–2. PMID: 20846575.

[39] De Moura LH, Duque-Estrada B, Abraham LS, Barcaui CB, Sodre CT. Dermoscopy findings of alopecia areata in an African-American patient. J Dermatol Case Rep 2008; 2: 52–54. PMID: 21886714.

[40] Chiramel MJ, Sharma VK, Khandpur S, Sreenivas V. Relevance of trichoscopy in the differential diagnosis of alopecia: A cross-sectional study from North India. Indian J Dermatol Venereol Leprol 2016. doi:10.4103/0378-6323.183636. [Epub ahead of print]

[41] Ihm CW, Hong SS, Mun JH, et al. Histopathological pictures of the initial changes of the hair bulbs in alopecia areata. Am J Dermatopathol 2004; 26: 249–53.

[42] Kossard S, Zagarella S. Spotted cicatricial alopecia in dark skin. A dermoscopic clue to fibrous tracts. Australas J Dermatol 1993; 34: 49–51.

[43] Mubki T,Rudnicka L,Olszewska M,Shapiro J. Evaluation and diagnosis of the hair loss patient: part II. Trichoscopic and laboratory evaluations. J Am Acad Dermatol 2014; 71(3): 431.e1–431.e11. doi:10.1016/j.jaad.2014.05.008

[44] Ioannides D, Tosti A (Eds.) Alopecias—Practical Evaluation and Management. Curr Probl Dermatol. Basel, Karger, 2015, vol. 47, pp. 21–32. doi:10.1159/000369402

[45] Rakowska A, Slowinska M, Kowalska-Oledzka E, Rudnicka L. Trichoscopy in genetic hair shaft abnormalities. J Dermatol Case Rep 2008; 2: 14–20.

[46] Van Neste D. Natural scalp hair regression in preclinical stages of male androgenetic alopecia and its reversal by finasteride. Skin Pharmacol Physiol 2006; 19: 168–76. PMID: 16679818.

[47] Braun-Falco O, Heilgemeir GP, Lincke-Plewig H. Histological differential diagnosis of psoriasis vulgaris and seborrheic eczema of the scalp. Hautarzt 1979; 30: 478–83.

[48] Murphy M, Kerr P, Grant-Kels JM. The histopathologic spectrum of psoriasis. Clin Dermatol 2007; 25: 524–8.

[49] Kim KS, Shin MK, Ahn JJ, Haw CR, Park HK. A comparative study of hair shafts in scalp psoriasis and seborrheic dermatitis using atomic force microscopy. Skin Res Technol 2013; 19: e60–4.

[50] Kibar M, Aktan S, Bilgin M. Dermoscopic findings in scalp psoriasis and seborrheic dermatitis; two new signs; signet ring vessel and hidden hair. Indian J Dermatol 2015; 60(1): 41–5. doi:10.4103/0019-5154.147786

[51] Deloche C, de Lacharriere O, Misciali C, Piraccini BM, Vincenzi C, Bastien P, et al. Histological features of peripilar signs associated with androgenetic alopecia. Arch Dermatol Res 2004; 295: 422–8.

[52] Kim GW, Jung HJ, Ko HC, Kim MB, Lee WJ, Lee SJ, et al. Dermoscopy can be useful in differentiating scalp psoriasis from seborrhoeic dermatitis. Br J Dermatol 2011; 164: 652–6.

[53] Errichetti E, Stinco G. Dermoscopy in General Dermatology: A Practical Overview. Dermatol Ther (Heidelb). 2016 Dec;6(4):471–507.

[54] Tosti A, Torres F, Miteva M. Dermoscopy of early dissecting cellulitis of the scalp simulates alopecia areata. Actas Dermosifiliogr 2013; 104: 92–3.

[55] Mane M, Nath AK, Thappa DM. Utility of dermoscopy in alopecia areata. Indian J Dermatol 2011; 56: 407–11.

[56] Inui S, Nakajima T, Itami S. Coudability hairs: a revisited sign of alopecia areata assessed by trichoscopy. Clin Exp Dermatol 2010; 35: 361–5.

[57] Abraham LS, Torres FN, Azulay-Abulafia L.Dermoscopic clues to distinguish trichotillomania from patchy alopecia areata. An Bras Dermatol 2010; 85: 723–6.

[58] Thakur BK, Verma S, Raphael V, Khonglah Y. Extensive tonsure pattern trichotillomania-trichoscopy and histopathology aid to the diagnosis. Int J Trichol 2013; 5(4): 196–8.

[59] Trink A, Sorbellini E, Bezzola P, Rodella L, Rezzani R, Ramot Y, et al. A randomized, double-blind, placebo and activecontrolled, half-head study to evaluate the effects of platelet rich plasma on alopecia areata. Br J Dermatol 2013; 169: 690–4.

[60] Inui S, Nakajima T, Itami S. Scalp dermoscopy of androgenetic alopecia in Asian people. J Dermatol 2009; 36: 82–5.

[61] Sewell LD, Elston DM, Dorion RP. "Anisotrichosis": a novel term to describe pattern alopecia. J Am Acad Dermatol 2007; 56: 856.

[62] Zhang X, Caulloo S, Zhao Y, Zhang B, Cai Z, Yang J. Female pattern hair loss: clinico-laboratory findings and trichoscopy depending on disease severity. Int J Trichology 2012; 4: 23–8.

[63] Hu R, Xu F, Han Y, Sheng Y, Qi S, Miao Y, Yang Q. Trichoscopic findings of androgenetic alopecia and their association with disease severity. J Dermatol 2015; 42(6): 602–7. doi:10.1111/1346-8138.12857. Epub 2015 Mar 26

[64] Galliker NA, Trueb RM. Value of trichoscopy versus trichogram for diagnosis of female androgenetic alopecia. Int J Trichology 2012; 4: 19–22.

[65] Bhamla SA, Dhurat RS, Saraogi PP. Is trichoscopy a reliable tool to diagnose early female pattern hair loss? Int J Trichology 2013; 5: 121–5.

[66] Herskovitz I, de Sousa IC, Tosti A. Vellus hairs in the frontal scalp in early female pattern hair loss. Int J Trichology 2013; 5: 118–20.

[67] Olszewska M, Warszawik O, Rakowska A, Slowinska M, Rudnicka L. Methods of hair loss evaluation in patients with endocrine disorders. Endokrynol Pol 2010; 61: 406–11.

[68] Rakowska A, Slowinska M, Olszewska M, Rudnicka L. New trichoscopy findings in trichotillomania: flame hairs, v-sign, hook hairs, hair powder, tulip hairs. Acta Derm Venereol 2014; 94: 303–6.

[69] Micali G, Lacarrubba F. Possible applications of videodermatoscopy beyond pigmented lesions. Int J Dermatol 2003; 42: 430–3.

[70] Lee DY, Lee JH, Yang JM, Lee ES. The use of dermoscopy for the diagnosis of trichotillomania. J Eur Acad Dermatol Venereol 2009; 23: 731–2.

[71] Lacarrubba F, Micali G. Congenital triangular alopecia. BMJ Case Rep 2014 Jan 8;2014.

[72] Iorizzo M, Pazzaglia M, Starace M, Militello G, Tosti A. Videodermoscopy: a useful tool for diagnosing congenital triangular alopecia. Pediatr Dermatol 2008; 25: 652–4.

[73] Slowinska M, Rudnicka L, Schwartz RA, Kowalska-Oledzka E, Rakowska A, Sicinska J, et al. Comma hairs: a dermatoscopic marker for tinea capitis: a rapid diagnostic method. J Am Acad Dermatol 2008; 59(5 suppl):S77–9.

[74] Sandoval AB, Ortiz JA, Rodriguez JM, Vargas AG, Quintero DG. Dermoscopic pattern in tinea capitis. Rev Iberoam Micol 2010; 27: 151–2.

[75] Hughes R, Chiaverini C, Bahadoran P, Lacour JP. Corkscrew hair: a new dermoscopic sign for diagnosis of tinea capitis in black children. Arch Dermatol 2011; 147: 355–6.

[76] Neri I, Starace M, Patrizi A, Balestri R. Corkscrew hair: a trichoscopy marker of tinea capitis in an adult white patient. JAMA Dermatol 2013; 149: 990–1.

[77] Vazquez-Lopez F, Palacios-Garcia L, Argenziano G. Dermoscopic corkscrew hairs dissolve after successful therapy of *Trichophyton violaceum* tinea capitis: a case report. Australas J Dermatol 2012; 53: 118–9.

[78] Ekiz O, Sen BB, Rifaioğlu EN, Balta I. Trichoscopy in paediatric patients with tinea capitis: a useful method to differentiate from alopecia areata. J Eur Acad Dermatol Venereol 2014; 28: 1255–8.

[79] Lacarrubba F, Verzi AE, Micali G. Newly described features resulting from high-magnification dermoscopy of tinea capitis. JAMA Dermatol 2014, doi:10.1001/jamadermatol.2014.3313.[Epub ahead of print].

[80] Duque-Estrada B, Tamler C, Sodré CT, Barcaui CB, Pereira FB. Dermoscopy patterns of cicatricial alopecia resulting from discoid lupus erythematosus and lichen planopilaris. An Bras Dermatol 2010; 85: 179–83.

[81] Kang H, Alzolibani AA, Otberg N, Shapiro J. Lichen planopilaris. Dermatol Ther 2008; 21: 249–56.

[82] Otberg N. Primary cicatricial alopecias. Dermatol Clin 2013; 31: 155–66.

[83] Tosti A, Duque-Estrada B. Dermoscopy in hair disorders. J Egypt Women Dermatol Soc 2010; 7: 1–4.

[84] Tosti A, Miteva M, Torres F. Lonely hair: a clue to the diagnosis of frontal fibrosing alopecia. Arch Dermatol 2011; 147: 1240.

[85] Lacarrubba F, Micali G, Tosti A. Absence of vellus hair in the hairline: a videodermatoscopic feature of frontal fibrosing alopecia. Br J Dermatol 2013; 169: 473–4.

[86] Inui S, Nakajima T, Shono F, Itami S. Dermoscopic findings in frontal fibrosing alopecia: report of four cases. Int J Dermatol 2008; 47: 796–9.

[87] Rubegni P, Mandato F, Fimiani M. Frontal fibrosing alopecia: role of dermoscopy in differential diagnosis. Case Rep Dermatol 2010; 2: 40–5.

[88] Lacarrubba F, Dall'Oglio F, Micali G. Massive tufted hair folliculitis associated with chronic use of systemic corticosteroids. G Ital Dermatol Venereol 2011; 146: 164–65.

[89] Braun RP, Oliviero M, Kolm I, French LE, Marghoob AA, Rabinovitz H. Dermoscopy: what's new? Clin Dermatol 2009; 27: 26–34.

[90] Otberg N, Kang H, Alzolibani AA, Shapiro J. Folliculitis decalvans. Dermatol Ther 2008; 21: 238–44.

[91] Mundi JP, Marmon S, Fischer M, Kamino H, Patel R, Shapiro J. Dissecting cellulitis of the scalp. Dermatol Online J 2012; 18: 8.

[92] Rakowska A, Slowinska M, Czuwara J, Olszewska M, Rudnicka L. Dermoscopy as a tool for rapid diagnosis of monilethrix. J Drugs Dermatol 2007; 6: 222–4.

[93] Jain N, Khopkar U. Monilethrix in pattern distribution in siblings: diagnosis by trichoscopy. Int J Trichology 2010; 2: 56–9.

[94] Rakowska A, Kowalska-Oledzka E, Slowinska M, Rosinska D, Rudnicka L. Hair shaft videodermoscopy in netherton syndrome. Pediatr Dermatol 2009; 26: 320–2.

[95] Burk C, Hu S, Lee C, Connelly EA. Netherton syndrome and trichorrhexis invaginata—a novel diagnostic approach. Pediatr Dermatol 2008; 25: 287–8.

[96] Wallace MP, de Berker DA. Hair diagnoses and signs: the use of dermatoscopy. Clin Exp Dermatol 2010; 35: 41–6.

[97] Liu CI, Hsu CH. Rapid diagnosis of monilethrix using dermoscopy. Br J Dermatol 2008; 159: 741–743.

[98] Blume-Peytavi U, Orfanos CE. Microscopy of the hair—The trichogram, In Serup J, Jemec GBE, Grove GL, (Eds.) Handbook of Non-Invasive Methods and the Skin [ed 2]. Boca Raton, FL, CRC Press Taylor & Francis Group, 2006, pp. 875–88.

[99] Serrano-Falcón C, Fernández-Pugnaire MA, Serrano-Ortega S. Hair and scalp evaluation: the trichogram. Actas Dermosifiliogr 2013; 104(10): 867–76. doi:10.1016/j.ad.2013.03.004. Epub 2013 Jul 18. English, Spanish.

[100] Kahn CM, Guerrero AR, Césped MC. Seasonal variation of trichogram in Chilean subjects. Rev Med Chil 2009; 137: 1437–40.

[101] Ferrando J, Moreno-Arias G. Displasias pilosas. [cited 2013 June 8]. Available from: http://antoniorondonlugo.com/blog/wp-content/uploads/2010/05/104-Displasias-Pilosas4.pdf

[102] Agusti-Mejias A, López-Davia J, García R, Febrer I, Alegre de Miquel V. Loose anagen hair syndrome. Diagnostic use of the trichogram. An Pediatr 2010; 73: 293–5.

[103] Serrano Ortega S, Dulanto Campos MC, Simón F, Saucedo. Value of the hair shaft diameter in female androgenetic allopecia. Actas Dermosifiliogr 1994; 85: 474–6.

Section 4

Diffuse Hair Loss

Chapter 7

Alopecia Areata

Burhan Engin, Muazzez Çiğdem Oba and
Yalçın Tüzün

Additional information is available at the end of the chapter

http://dx.doi.org/10.5772/66594

Abstract

Alopecia areata is an organ-specific autoimmune disease targeting hair follicles. It causes nonscarring hair loss. The prevalence rate of the disease is approximately 1 in 1000 people worldwide. The condition is most commonly seen as circular areas of hair loss, but it may sometimes be as extensive as to involve the whole scalp or whole body. The complex pathophysiology of alopecia areata involves an autoimmune basis. Association of alopecia areata with other autoimmune diseases, such as thyroiditis and vitiligo, and the good response of patients to immunosuppressive treatment support an autoimmune etiology. Although some poor prognostic signs are defined, the course of the disease is unpredictable and the response to treatment can be variable. To date, there are neither preventive nor curative measures to deal with the condition. First-line therapy for patchy disease is topical and intralesional steroids, whereas extensive disease is conventionally managed with immunotherapy. New treatment agents, such as excimer laser, low-dose recombinant interleukin 2, Janus kinase inhibitors, and simvastatin/ezetimibe, are promising.

Keywords: alopecia areata, pathogenesis, autoimmunity, squaric acid dibutylester (SADBE), diphenylcyclopropenone (DPCP)

1. Introduction

Alopecia areata is an organ-specific autoimmune disease targeting hair follicles. It causes nonscarring hair loss. The condition is most commonly seen as circular areas of hair loss, but may sometimes be as extensive as to involve the whole scalp or whole body [1]. Although some poor prognostic signs are defined, the course of the disease is unpredictable and the response to treatment can be variable [2]. To date, there are neither preventive nor curative measures to deal with the condition [3].

2. Epidemiology

Alopecia areata is the most prevalent autoimmune disorder and the second most frequent disease causing hair loss after androgenetic alopecia [3]. The prevalence rate of the disease is approximately 1 in 1000 people worldwide; in the United States, the lifetime risk is estimated to be 1.7% [2, 4]. Alopecia areata is mainly a disease of young adults; as many as 60% of patients are under the age of 20 at first presentation. Pediatric cases constitute approximately 20% of alopecia areata patients [2]. However, patients of any age can be affected. There is no gender predilection [4]. Reported cases in elderly were of milder severity and had a better treatment response [5].

3. Pathogenesis

Alopecia areata is an organ-specific T cell mediated autoimmune disease targeting hair follicles. Peribulbar lymphocytic infiltration impairing the normal hair cycle is considered to be the main pathophysiologic mechanism responsible for the disease process. Normal hair cycle is disrupted in alopecia areata; dystrophic changes of anagen follicles along with rapid progression of hair follicles from anagen to catagen and telogen phases are observed. In alopecia areata, perifollicular inflammatory infiltrate spares the bulge region of the follicle where follicular epithelial stem cells reside. Thus, in contrast to cicatricial alopecias, the inflammation does not interfere with the hair follicle integrity [6].

The complex pathophysiology of alopecia areata involves an autoimmune basis. Association of alopecia areata with other autoimmune diseases such as thyroiditis and vitiligo is reported. Presence of lymphocytes around hair follicles and the good response of patients to immunosuppressive treatment also support autoimmune etiology [2].

Etiopathogenetic theories are based upon the loss of immune-privileged status of hair follicles leading to an immune response against follicular antigens. In fact, normal proximal epithelium of anagen hair follicles have a very low expression of MHC class I antigens and no MHC class II antigen expression, along with a potent expression of immunosuppressive cytokines, such as TGF-β1 and α-melanocyte–stimulating hormone (α-MSH) [6]. According to the recent evidence, mechanism leading to hair loss involves the following steps: firstly, hair follicles must enter an anagen phase without the immune privilege described above, making those vulnerable to immune reactions. Subsequently, perifollicular CD8+ T cell infiltration of the anagen hair bulb epithelium ensues, along with a significant increase in interferon-gamma (IFN-γ) and various other cytokines. This milieu further damages the immune-privileged status of hair follicles, autoreactive CD8+ T lymphocytes, and IFN-γ and causes hair follicle dystrophy and premature catagen induction, leading to clinical hair loss [7]. Patients with alopecia areata have also been found to have an increased frequency of hair follicle-specific autoantibodies [2].

Genetic basis is implicated in disease pathogenesis. Many patients report a family history of alopecia areata with a frequency ranging from 10% to 42% of cases [8]. Studies show a higher

http://dx.doi.org/10.5772/66594

concordance rate among monozygotic twins compared to dizygotic twins also supporting the role of genetics [9]. HLA-DRB1*1104 and DQB1*03 loci that have a role in regulating immunity is associated with susceptibility to alopecia areata [2].

Genome-wide association studies can recognize specific individual genes, which may represent an increased susceptibility to alopecia areata. Petukhova et al. surveyed the entire genome and identified 139 single nucleotide polymorphisms associated with alopecia areata. The study showed that genomic regions containing the CTLA4, IL2/IL21, IL-2RA and Eos genes regulating proliferation of inflammatory cells to be susceptibility loci for alopecia areata. Ligands for the NKG2D receptor were also found to be implicated in disease pathogenesis [10]. Mouse models for alopecia areata gave valuable information regarding the role of CD8+ NKG2D+ T lymphocytes in pathogenesis. Transfer of these cytotoxic cells from mice with alopecia areata induced alopecia areata in healthy mice; on the other hand, NKG2D+ T cell-depleted lymph node cells transferred from the diseased mice to the healthy mice did not cause any disease. Interferon produced by NKG2D+ T cell is thought to contribute to the loss of immune-privileged status of hair follicles [11].

4. Clinical features

Alopecia areata patches are mostly asymptomatic and are discovered incidentally. Rarely, patients may complain of burning or itching sensation preceding hair loss. Typically, hair loss presents as one or more well-demarcated round to oval skin-colored patches [1]. The affected skin has a normal appearance with visible follicular orifices. Rarely, a soft edematous infiltration can be felt upon palpation and a peachy or reddened coloration can be observed [12]. Any hair-bearing site may be affected [1]. The scalp is the most common site of involvement, with or without the involvement of other body sites, such as the eyebrows, eyelashes, and beard [3].

According to the extent of involvement, alopecia areata can be classified into alopecia circumscripta presenting with limited hair loss, alopecia totalis involving the entire scalp, and alopecia universalis involving whole body (**Figures 1** and **2**).

A clinical classification regarding the pattern of hair loss is also frequently used. Patchy alopecia is the most common type seen in up to 75% of patients. Reticular type has a net-like pattern with multiple active and regressing patches (**Figure 3**). A band-like pattern involving occipital scalp is called ophiasis type of alopecia areata. The very rare ophiasis inversus, also called sisaipho type, presents with hair loss in the central scalp, resembling androgenetic alopecia [12]. Another unusual variant, perinevoid alopecia, is reported as presenting with alopecia patches around the nevi [13]. Diffuse alopecia areata presents with widespread thinning of the scalp hair. A recently defined variant, acute diffuse and total alopecia is characterized with rapid progression, female preponderance, and a favorable prognosis [14].

Initially, white hairs may be spared in patients with graying hair. As disease progresses, the white hair will also be lost. Initial hair regrowth, spontaneous or therapy-induced may be depigmented or hypopigmented, but the color usually returns with time [2].

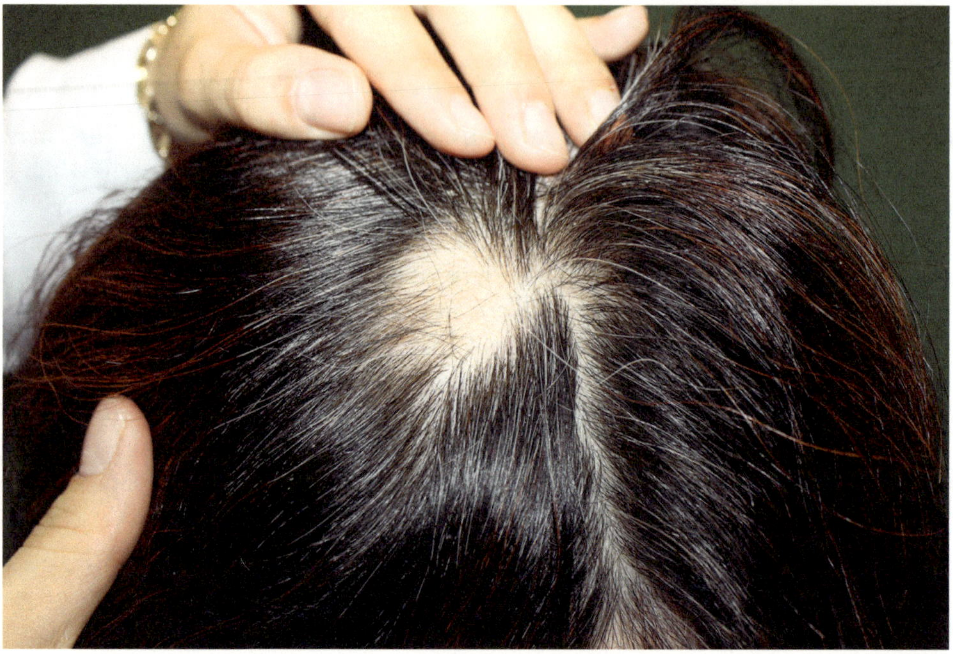

Figure 1. Circular area of nonscarring alopecia incidentally found in an adult patient.

Nail changes are observed in up to 7–66% of patients [15]. The nail matrix may be affected, resulting in pitting of the nail plate, which is the most common nail involvement in alopecia areata [6]. Other nail features found in alopecia areata are trachyonychia, Beau's line, onychorrhexis, onychomadesis, koilonychias, punctuate or transverse leukonychia, and red-spotted lunula [16]. Nail disease may precede, follow, or coexist with active hair loss [2].

5. Associated diseases

Alopecia areata is associated with many diseases, including other autoimmune diseases, atopy, ophthalmologic findings and psychiatric comorbidities.

Among autoimmune disorders, the two main associations are with thyroid disease and vitiligo [17]. Incidence of thyroid disease varies from 8% to 28% in patients with alopecia areata, compared with only 2% of the normal population. Among thyroid disorders, hypothyroidism is the most frequent association. [18] Prevalence of antithyroid antibodies is shown to be increased, but thyroid antibodies do not have any clinical correlation with disease severity [19]. Alopecia areata has also been shown to have a significant association with vitiligo; patients have a fourfold greater incidence of vitiligo compared with normal population. There are also reported associations of alopecia areata with pernicious anemia, lupus erythematosus, myasthenia gravis, rheumatoid arthritis, polymyalgia rheumatica, ulcerative colitis, and lichen planus [8]. A very strong disease association with the autosomal recessive disease autoimmune polyglandular syndrome type 1 (APS-1, chronic hypoparathyroidism-mucocutane-

http://dx.doi.org/10.5772/66594

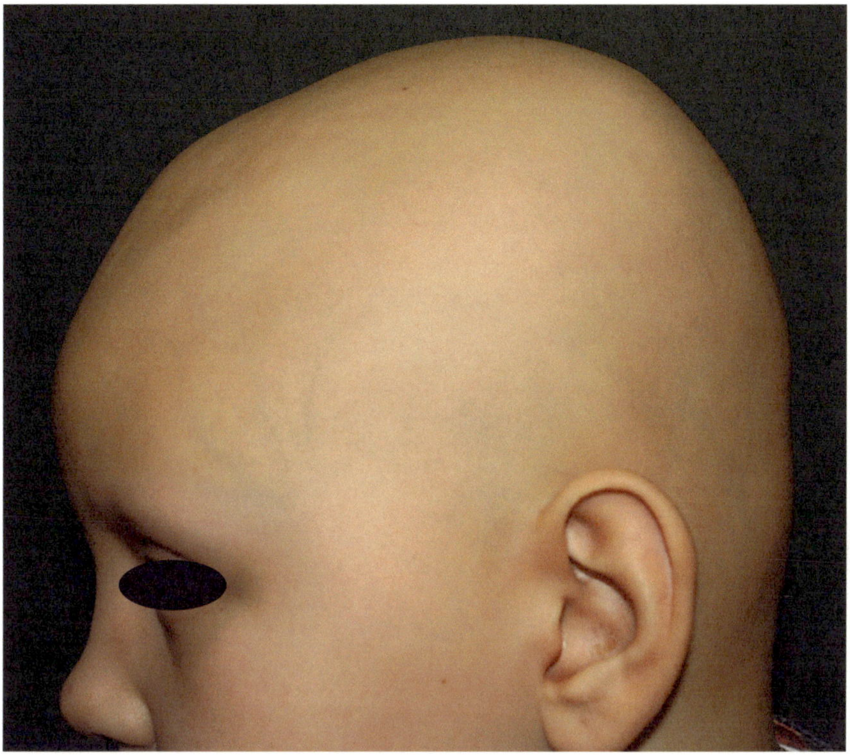

Figure 2. A patient with alopecia universalis having total loss of scalp hair and eyebrows.

ous candidiasis-autoimmune adrenal insufficiency) was recently reported [20]. Patients with Down's syndrome or Turner's syndrome also have increased risk of alopecia areata [17].

Atopic disorders, namely allergic rhinitis, asthma, and atopic dermatitis have been linked to alopecia areata. They have been found to occur in more than 40% of patients with alopecia areata, whereas their prevalence in the general population is estimated to be around 20% [17].

Interestingly, there is a decreased incidence of type 1 diabetes in alopecia areata patients and an increased incidence in their relatives. It was proposed that alopecia areata may have a protective effect against type 1 diabetes in predisposed individuals [21].

Ocular alterations, such as asymptomatic punctate lens opacities, and fundus changes can occur in up to 50% of patients with alopecia areata [22].

There may be a high psychiatric morbidity in alopecia areata patients. Depression, increased level of anxiety, generalized anxiety disorder, social phobia, posttraumatic stress disorder, and suicidal thoughts are among the reported psychiatric disturbances [23].

Incidence of nuchal nevus flammeus was reported to be increased in alopecia areata patients, especially in those showing a more severe course of the disease [24].

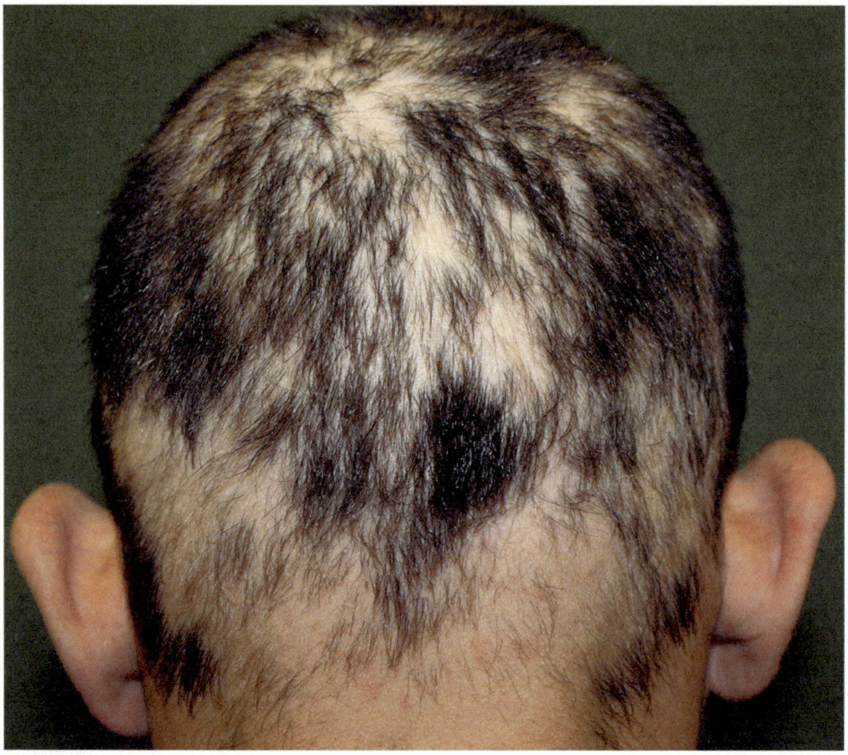

Figure 3. Reticular type alopecia areata with a net-like pattern.

6. Prognosis

The disease has an unpredictable course; spontaneous regrowth of hair is common as observed in about 80% of patients within one year [25]. However, patients usually present with several episodes of hair loss and hair regrowth during their lifetime [8]. Progression to alopecia totalis and universalis may occur in 5–10% of patients [3].

Extent of involvement (alopecia totalis/universalis)
Younger age of onset
Family history
Atopy
Ophiasis
Nail changes
Associated autoimmune disease

Table 1. Poor prognostic factors.

http://dx.doi.org/10.5772/66594

Some clinical factors that indicate a poor prognosis is defined (**Table 1**). The most important factor is the extent of the disease [1]. The chance of full recovery is less than 10% in alopecia totalis and universalis [12]. Acute diffuse and total alopecia variant constitutes an exception. As discussed earlier in this chapter, these patients have a favorable treatment response despite the substantial hair loss [15]. Other factors reported are young age at disease onset, a positive family history, atopy, ophiasis pattern of loss, nail changes, and associated autoimmune diseases [8, 15]. Positive family history is associated with the early age of onset. In fact, positive family history among first-degree relatives has been reported to be as high as 47% for patients with early onset, in contrast to 1.6% for all patients [6].

7. Diagnosis

Diagnosis of alopecia areata is made on clinical grounds. No routine laboratory investigations are needed. Routine thyroid screening is not indicated but screening may be performed in long-standing cases, females, patients with persistent patches, and patients with alopecia totalis and universalis [8].

Upon examination, exclamation mark hairs may be observed within or at the periphery of the lesions that are short hairs tapered towards their base [1]. Exclamation mark hairs occur only in acute forms of alopecia areata and are not seen in patients with long-standing areas of hair loss [15]. Pull test can be performed to assess disease activity; six hairs or more shed from the periphery of the lesion positively correlates with the disease activity [16].

Severity of the disease can be measured by SALT score, developed by the National Alopecia Areata Foundation working committee. The scalp is divided into 4 parts, the top constituting 40% of total surface, the posterior 24%, right side and left side of scalp 18% each. Percentage of hair loss in each area is determined and is multiplied by the percentage of scalp covered in that area of the scalp, and summing the products of each area will give the SALT score [26].

Several studies have shown that dermoscopy may be a useful tool to help in the diagnosis of alopecia areata. Dermatoscopic findings reported in the literature include: yellow dots, black dots, short vellus hairs, black dots, tapering hairs, and broken hairs [27].

In ambiguous cases, a scalp biopsy is required. Histopathological examination of 4 mm punch biopsy containing subcutaneous fat is necessary to establish correct diagnosis. Biopsy should be taken from the periphery of the lesion as this is the site where the disease activity is found [28]. Horizontal sections will give a better representation of the histopathology especially in bulb infiltration than vertical sections [29].

8. Histopathology

Histopathology depends on the stage of the disease [30]. In the acute stage, there is a dense inflammatory infiltrate surrounding the terminal anagen hair bulb situated in the deep subcutaneous tissue. Inflammatory infiltrate consists primarily of T lymphocytes and Langerhans cells, with occasional eosinophils, mast cells, and plasma cells [31, 32]. An early and typical feature is the presence of eosinophils in stellae and within hair bulbs [29]. Anagen hairs cycle through catagen then into telogen. A dense lymphocytic inflammation can cause breaking of the hair shaft with a trichorrhexis nodosa-like fracture. This is the exclamation point hair, which is in telogen phase and therefore shed [31, 32]. The horizontal section demonstrates a significant decrease in the anagen:telogen ratio. There is also a decrease in the number of terminal hairs with a slight increase in the number of vellus hairs [31].

In the subacute stage, the number of catagen hairs is markedly increased [30]. The number of telogen hairs also increases after a few weeks. The amount of terminal hairs decreases and the vellus hair increases [31, 32].

In the chronic stage, either no or a mild chronic peribulbar lymphocytic inflammation around the miniaturized hairs situated in the papillary dermis is observed [30, 31]. The terminal:vellus hair ratio decreases to 1.3:1 rather than 7:1, which is found in the normal population. Fibrosis is an uncommon finding. However, in approximately 10% of the patients with a long history of alopecia areata, fibrosis of the upper follicle can be detected [31].

Of note, diagnosis of alopecia areata does not depend on the presence of an inflammatory infiltrate. Histopathological examination reveals increased numbers of telogen hairs in the acute and chronic stages, increased miniaturized hairs in chronic stage, and markedly increased catagen hairs in the subacute stage, helping in the diagnosis of alopecia areata [30].

9. Differential diagnosis

Many other diseases may cause hair loss in a patchy or diffuse pattern [33, 34] (**Table 2**).

In children, tinea capitis, which is the most common dermatophyte infection seen in childhood and trichotillomania should be considered in differential diagnosis of alopecia areata. Clinically, patches of tinea capitis show scaling and signs of inflammation sometimes accompanied by cervical lymphadenopathy. Direct microscopic examination with potassium hydroxide, fungal culture, and trichoscopy can also help in the diagnosis [35]. In trichotillomania, diagnosis is straightforward when the patient or relatives accept the compulsive act of pulling. In dermatological examination, there are irregularly shaped patches and broken hairs of variable lengths. Residual hairs in patches of trichotillomania are anagen hairs firmly attached to the scalp; they are of normal texture and color, whereas residual hairs in alopecia areata are usually the exclamation mark hairs with their specific morphology, which are easily detached from the scalp. [33, 36] Rarely, alopecia areata and trichotillomania can coexist [37]. Histopathologically, there is an increase in catagen hairs, follicular hemorrhage, pigment casts, and trichomalacia, without the typical inflammatory infiltrate and miniaturization of hair follicles observed in alopecia areata [31, 36].

In adults, the differential diagnosis is usually between androgenetic alopecia and telogen effluvium. Patients with androgenetic alopecia usually demonstrate gradual loss of hair with

http://dx.doi.org/10.5772/66594

Tinea capitis
Trichotillomania
Androgenetic alopecia
Telogen effluvium
Cicatricial alopecia
Secondary syphilis
Loose anagen syndrome
Congenital triangular alopecia
Lupus erythematosus
Pressure alopecia
Traction alopecia

Table 2. Differential diagnosis of alopecia areata.

the typical distribution pattern. The pull test is usually negative in androgenetic alopecia [8]. In some cases, a scalp biopsy may be required to establish correct diagnosis. Many miniaturized hairs are found in both androgenetic alopecia and alopecia areata, but higher telogen hair counts and a decreased anagen to telogen ratio favors diagnosis of alopecia areata. Although a perifollicular lymphohistiocytic infiltrate may be observed in androgenetic alopecia, it is usually confined to the upper follicle [31]. Telogen effluvium may be difficult to differentiate from diffuse alopecia areata. In alopecia areata, hair pull test show either telogen or dystrophic anagen hairs, while they are purely telogen in telogen effluvium [2]. Upon histopathologic examination of horizontal sections of scalp biopsies, chronic telogen effluvium shows follicular counts that are similar to that of normal controls [31].

Cicatricial alopecia is characterized by patchy hair loss with loss of follicular orifices. Erythema, scaling, and pustulation may be observed in contrast to smooth, normal skin of alopecia areata patches [15]. Other forms of alopecia, such as syphilis, loose anagen syndrome, congenital triangular alopecia, and early lupus erythematosus, should also be considered [31]. Congenital triangular alopecia is a developmental abnormality of hair follicles that usually presents after 2 years of age as a triangular or round patch of hair loss near the frontotemporal hair line. Histopathological examination reveals vellus hairs [34]. Side pins used to keep the hair in place, may cause pressure alopecia, which presents with a patch of hair loss mimicking patches of alopecia areata [38]. Traction alopecia must be differentiated from alopecia areata, especially of ophiasis pattern [39].

10. Management

Currently, there is no curative or preventive treatment for alopecia areata. The main goal of therapy is to suppress the disease activity [16].

10.1. Intralesional corticosteroids

Intralesional corticosteroids have been used in treatment of alopecia areata, since 1958 [38]. Intralesional corticosteroids are considered as the first-line agents in limited alopecia areata. Injections are made every 4–6 weeks into the deep dermis using a 0.5-inch long 30-gauge needle. For lesions of the scalp, 0.1 mL of triamcinolone acetonide at concentration of 5 mg/mL is injected at 1-cm intervals. Intralesional corticosteroid application is also effective for beard and eyebrow alopecia areata at a concentration of 2.5 mg/mL. Maximum dose of triamcinolone acetonide should be limited to 3 mL for scalp, 0.5 mL for each eyebrow and 1 mL for beard [40]. Hair regrowth is usually observed within 4 weeks and intralesional corticosteroids should be discontinued, if there is no improvement in 6 months [28]. In some patients, resistance to steroid therapy can be explained by a decreased expression of thioredoxin reductase 1, an enzyme that activates the glucocorticoid receptor in the outer root sheath [41]. The most common side effect observed is atrophy, which may be prevented by avoiding superficial injections, and reducing the concentration and volume of injections [42]. Other side effects include hypopigmentation, depigmentation, and telangiectasias [40].

10.2. Topical corticosteroids

Midpotent and potent topical corticosteroids in forms of lotions, creams, and ointments are widely used in spite of the fact that evidence of their effectiveness is limited [42, 43]. In a double-blind placebo-controlled study, rate of complete hair growth was not statistically significant with 12 weeks use of 0.25% desoximetasone cream, twice daily, when compared with placebo [44]. A half-head comparison trial performed with 0.05% clobetasol propionate foam and vehicle found at least 50% regrowth of hair after 12 weeks of clobetasol treatment. Blood levels of cortisol and ACTH were not affected during the trial [45]. A recent study showed that twice daily treatment with clobetasol propionate 0.05% cream used in 2 cycles of 6 weeks on, 6 weeks off regimen for a total of 24 weeks was more effective than hydrocortisone 1% cream used in the same regime. Compared with only 33.3% of the children in the hydrocortisone group, 85% of the children in the clobetasol group had at least 50% reduction in the surface area with hair loss at 24 weeks [46]. Folliculitis is a common side effect; skin atrophy and telangiectasia can rarely be observed [47].

10.3. Topical immunotherapy

Topical immunotherapy is the most effective treatment option for patients with chronic severe alopecia areata, with greater than 50% scalp involvement [48].

Topical immunotherapy consists of applying a contact allergen to induce a low-grade chronic dermatitis. The mechanism of action is still unclear. Antigenic competition, induction of lymphocyte apoptosis, and diversion of the T cell response from the hair follicle to the epidermis are among the various suggested theories [49–60].

Dinitrochlorobenzene was the first topical sensitizer to be used in the treatment of extensive alopecia areata; however, it was abandoned because of its mutagenic effects [42, 51]. Squaric acid dibutylester (SADBE) and diphenylcyclopropenone (DPCP) are the two compounds still in use today. Although SADBE is an ideal immunogen that is not found in the natural environment and is not known to cross-react with other chemicals, DPCP is preferred because it is cheaper and is more stable in acetone for storage [42, 51]. DPCP is a very light sensitive compound and should be stored in amber bottles to protect it from exposure to ultraviolet and fluorescent lights [51].

Topical immunotherapy begins at first visit by the sensitization of the patient with 2% DPCP applied to a 5-cm circular area on the scalp. Two weeks later, a 0.001% DPCP solution is applied to the same half of the scalp. The concentration of DPCP is increased gradually each week to produce mild inflammation that manifests as pruritus and erythema lasting for 36–48 h. After establishing the appropriate concentration for the patient, subsequent therapy is continued once weekly with the same concentration [52]. DPCP should be left on the scalp for 48 h and the treated area must be protected from the sun during this time. Treatment of both sides is recommended only after achieving hair regrowth on the treated side. If there is no improvement in 6 months, DPCP is less likely to be successful; however, improvement in these "non-responder" patients with longer courses of DPCP therapy has been reported [42, 53]. If the patient does not develop an allergic reaction to 2% DPCP, SADBE can be tried [42]. The procedure with SADBE treatment is similar to DPCP.

The response rates of DPCP treatment in alopecia areata ranges from 5% to 85%. Patients with earlier onset of the disease or more extensive involvement were shown to be less likely to respond to diphenylcyclopropenone therapy [53].

Topical immunotherapy is generally well tolerated by most of the patients. The most commonly seen side effects are eczema, autoeczematization, blistering, and swelling of regional lymph nodes [54]. When a vesicular or bullous reaction develops, the patient should wash off the contact sensitizer and a topical corticosteroid should be applied to the affected area. Facial and scalp edema, contact urticaria, flu-like symptoms, erythema multiforme-like reactions, and pigmentary disturbances manifesting as hyperpigmentation, hypopigmentation, dyschromia in confetti, and vitiligo can also occur [42, 55, 56]. Patients may complain of burning sensation, after application of SADBE. Persistent allergic contact dermatitis of the primary site of sensitization, severe generalized dermatitis and systemic reactions characterized by fever, and arthalgias are among the rarely observed side effects [54].

10.4. Minoxidil

Topical minoxidil solution, approved by Food and Drug Administration and Health Canada for the treatment of androgenetic alopecia, can be used in alopecia areata. Evidence for the effectiveness of using 3% minoxidil, twice daily, was shown in a double-blind placebo controlled study [57]. A dose response effect exists, with the 5% solution being more effective than the 2% solution. However, few patients achieve cosmetically significant regrowth [58]. Minoxidil 5% solution, twice daily, is used in combination with topical or intralesional corticosteroids. Contact dermatitis and hypertrichosis are the most common side effects. Minoxidil foam, which does not contain propylene glycol, has less irritating effects than the solution [59].

10.5. Anthralin

Anthralin, 0.5–1%, short contact therapy is used as alternative treatment although evidence for its efficacy depends on case series without controls [47].

Anthralin 1% cream is applied daily for 15 or 20 min initially and then washed. The contact time is increased by 5 min weekly up to 1 h or to the time required to cause a low-grade dermatitis. Once the contact time sufficient to produce the mild dermatitis is found, subsequent therapy is continued daily for the established period of time. Anthralin should be applied at least 3 months before evaluating the response to treatment. Side effects include severe irritation, folliculitis, regional lymphadenopathy, and staining of skin, clothes and fair hair. Patients should avoid eye contact with this chemical, and the treated area should be protected from the sun [59].

10.6. Photochemotherapy

No controlled studies of oral or topical psoralen plus ultraviolet A (PUVA) therapy in alopecia areata have been reported [59]. The reports about the efficacy of PUVA therapy are conflicting. Several studies have shown low response rates of PUVA therapy [60, 61], while others have shown good response rates [62, 63]. PUVA therapy is thought to eradicate the mononuclear cell infiltrate, surrounding the hair follicle responsible for the disease [16]. Uncertainty about efficacy and concerns about PUVA-induced skin carcinogenesis make this therapy option a rarely chosen one [59].

10.7. Systemic glucocorticosteroids

Systemic corticosteroids have been used since 1952 in the treatment of alopecia areata; however, relapse rates are high upon dose reductions [64].

Long-term daily treatment with oral corticosteroids will produce favorable results in a part of the patients [33]. It was reported that 12–28% of patients with 1–99% scalp alopecia areata regrew 50% or more of their hair after a 6-week tapering course of prednisone therapy, starting at 40 mg daily. 2% minoxidil therapy may be useful for prolonging the response to the treatment after prednisone cessation [65]. However, oral corticosteroids are no longer used for chronic therapy of alopecia areata because of their side effects [33]. Side effects of oral steroids include avascular necrosis, weight gain, hypertension, diabetes, sleep alteration, mood changes, weakness, acneiform eruptions, irregular menses, and striae [52].

High-dose intravenous corticosteroid pulse therapy can be considered in patients with multifocal or ophiasis-type alopecia areata if treatment with topical sensitizers or highly potent topical corticosteroids during 6 months have failed. In more extensive involvement, such as alopecia totalis and universalis, treatment efficacy was shown to be diminished [64].

10.8. Immunosuppressive treatment

Immunosuppressive agents namely sulfasalazine, methotrexate, and cyclosporine can be used in the treatment of alopecia areata.

Sulfasalazine therapy can be an alternative treatment option in persistent alopecia areata cases. Studies have shown favorable treatment response, but a high relapse rate. The most common side effects include nausea, vomiting, headache, fever, and rash; less commonly hematologic abnormalities and hepatotoxicity can develop [66, 67].

http://dx.doi.org/10.5772/66594

Severe forms of alopecia areata resistant to conventional topical and/or systemic treatments may respond to methotrexate. In a retrospective study, weekly 15–25 mg methotrexate with or without 10–20 mg prednisolone daily was reported to be effective in 64% of cases [68].

Cyclosporine has been used alone or in conjunction with corticosteroids variable response rates [47]. Use of cyclosporine is limited because of side effects and high relapse rate. Side effects include nephrotoxicity, immune suppression, hypertension, and hypertrichosis of body hair [59].

10.9. Other therapies

10.9.1. Excimer laser

Mechanism of action of excimer laser in alopecia areata is thought to depend on induction of T cell apoptosis as proven in in vitro studies [69]. In a treatment of 18 patients with 42 alopecia areata patches with the 308 nm excimer laser, hair regrowth was observed in 41.5% of treated areas. Lesions on the extremities, patients with alopecia totalis, or alopecia universalis were resistant to the treatment [70].

10.9.2. Low-dose recombinant interleukin 2

Low-dose interleukin 2 (IL-2) is essential to proliferate Treg cells, which play a key role in alopecia areata [71]. A prospective study in 5 patients with extensive, treatment-resistant alopecia areata, 1.5 million IU/d subcutaneous interleukin 2 was administered during 5 days, followed by three 5-day courses of 3 million IU/d at weeks 3, 6, and 9. It was reported that 4 of the 5 patients attained considerable hair regrowth. Treatment adverse events were mild to moderate and included asthenia, arthralgia, urticaria, and injection site reactions [72].

10.9.3. Janus kinase inhibitors

Tofacitinib citrate is a small-molecule selective Janus kinase 1/3 (JAK 1/3) inhibitor that was approved by FDA, in late 2012, for the treatment of moderate-to-severe rheumatoid arthritis. A patient with longstanding alopecia universalis, treated with tofacitinib for psoriasis had hair regrowth, being the first documented case of alopecia areata responding to tofacitinib. After eight months of tofacitinib treatment (5 mg twice daily for 2 months followed by 10 mg in the morning and 5 mg at night thereafter), the patient had full regrowth of hair at all body sites [73]. There have been other case reports showing efficacy of tofacitinib treatment [74, 75]. Adverse effects of tofacitinib use include increased risk of severe infections including tuberculosis, anemia, neutropenia, headache, and mild nausea [74].

Another JAK inhibitor, ruxolitinib applied topically twice daily for 12 weeks in a patient with refractory alopecia universalis induced almost full eyebrow regrowth and approximately 10% regrowth of scalp hair [76].

10.9.4. Simvastatin/ezetimibe

Simvastatin 40 mg and ezetimibe 10 mg daily treatment for alopecia totalis and alopecia universalis was documented to have favorable responses in case reports [77]. In a prospective uncontrolled study, simvastatin/ezetimibe 40 mg/10 mg daily for 24 weeks was shown to be an effective treatment option for alopecia areata [78].

Author details

Burhan Engin*, Muazzez Çiğdem Oba and Yalçın Tüzün

*Address all correspondence to: burhanengin2000@yahoo.com

Dermatology Department, Cerrahpaşa Medical Faculty, Istanbul University, Istanbul, Turkey

References

[1] Alkhalifah A. Alopecia areata update. Dermatol Clin. 2013; **31**:93–108. doi: 10.1016/j.det.2012.08.010.

[2] Alkhalifah A, Alsantali A, Wang E, McElwee KJ, Shapiro J. Alopecia areata update: part I. Clinical picture, histopathology, and pathogenesis. J Am Acad Dermatol. 2010; **62**:177–188. doi: 10.1016/j.jaad.2009.10.032.

[3] Villasante Fricke AC, Miteva M. Epidemiology and burden of alopecia areata: a systematic review. Clin Cosmet Investig Dermatol. 2015; **8**:397–403. doi: 10.2147/CCID.S53985.

[4] Alzolibani AA. Epidemiologic and genetic characteristics of alopecia areata (part 1). Acta Dermatovenerol Alp Pannonica Adriat. 2011; **20**:191–198.

[5] Jang YH, Park KH, Kim SL, et al. Alopecia areata in the elderly: a 10-year retrospective study. Ann Dermatol. 2015; **27**:411–416. doi: 10.5021/ad.2015.27.4.411.

[6] Gilhar A, Paus R, Kalish RS. Lymphocytes, neuropeptides, and genes involved in alopecia areata. J Clin Invest. 2007; **117**:2019–2027.

[7] Gilhar A, Schrum AG, Etzioni A, Waldmann H, Paus R. Alopecia areata: animal models illuminate autoimmune pathogenesis and novel immunotherapeutic strategies. Autoimmun Rev. 2016; **15**:726–735. doi: 10.1016/j.autrev.2016.03.008.

[8] Madani S, Shapiro J. Alopecia areata update. J Am Acad Dermatol. 2000; **42**:549–566.

[9] Rodriguez TA, Fernandes KE, Dresser KL, Duvic M, National Alopecia Areata Registry. Concordance rate of alopecia areata in identical twins supports both genetic and environmental factors. J Am Acad Dermatol. 2010; **62**:525–527. doi: 10.1016/j.jaad.2009.02.006.

[10] Petukhova L, Duvic M, Hordinsky M, et al. Genome-wide association study in alopecia areata implicates both innate and adaptive immunity. Nature. 2010; **466**:113–117. doi: 10.1038/nature09114.

[11] Xing L, Dai Z, Jabbari A, et al. Alopecia areata is driven by cytotoxic T lymphocytes and is reversed by JAK inhibition. Nat Med. 2014; **20**:1043–1049. doi: 10.1038/nm.3645.

[12] Finner AM. Alopecia areata: clinical presentation, diagnosis, and unusual cases. Dermatol Ther. 2011; **24**:348–354. doi: 10.1111/j.1529-8019.2011.01413.x.

[13] Yesudian P, Thambiah AS. Perinevoid alopecia. An unusual variety of alopecia areata. Arch Dermatol. 1976; **112**:1432–1434.

[14] Sato-Kawamura M, Aiba S, Tagami H. Acute diffuse and total alopecia of the female scalp. A new subtype of diffuse alopecia areata that has a favorable prognosis. Dermatology. 2002; **205**:367–373.

[15] Spano F, Donovan JC. Alopecia areata: Part 1: pathogenesis, diagnosis, and prognosis. Can Fam Physician. 2015; **61**:751–755.

[16] Wasserman D, Guzman-Sanchez DA, Scott K, McMichael A. Alopecia areata. Int J Dermatol. 2007; **46**:121–131.

[17] Hordinsky M, Ericson M. Autoimmunity: alopecia areata. J Investig Dermatol Symp Proc. 2004; **9**:73–78.

[18] Thomas EA, Kadyan RS. Alopecia areata and autoimmunity: a clinical study. Indian J Dermatol. 2008; **53**:70–74. doi: 10.4103/0019-5154.41650.

[19] Kasumagić-Halilović E. Thyroid autoimmunity in patients with alopecia areata. Acta Dermatovenerol Croat. 2008; **16**:123–125.

[20] Collins SM, Dominguez M, Ilmarinen T, Costigan C, Irvine AD. Dermatological manifestations of autoimmune polyendocrinopathy-candidiasis-ectodermal dystrophy syndrome. Br J Dermatol. 2006; **154**:1088–1093.

[21] Wang SJ, Shohat T, Vadheim C, Shellow W, Edwards J, Rotter JI. Increased risk for type I (insulin-dependent) diabetes in relatives of patients with alopecia areata (AA). Am J Med Genet. 1994; **51**:234–239.

[22] Recupero SM, Abdolrahimzadeh S, De Dominicis M, et al. Ocular alterations in alopecia areata. Eye (Lond). 1999; **13**:643–646.

[23] Kuty-Pachecka M. Psychological and psychopathological factors in alopecia areata. Psychiatr Pol. 2015; **49**:955–964. doi: 10.12740/PP/39064.

[24] Hatzis J, Kostakis P, Tosca A, et al. Nuchal nevus flammeus as a skin marker of prognosis in alopecia areata. Dermatologica. 1988; **177**:149–151.

[25] MacLean KJ, Tidman MJ. Alopecia areata: more than skin deep. Practitioner. 2013; **257**:29–33.

[26] Olsen EA, Hordinsky MK, Price VH, et al, National Alopecia Areata Foundation. Alopecia areata investigational assessment guidelines—Part II. National Alopecia Areata Foundation. J Am Acad Dermatol. 2004; **51**:440–447.

[27] Inui S, Nakajima T, Nakagawa K, Itami S. Clinical significance of dermoscopy in alopecia areata: analysis of 300 cases. Int J Dermatol. 2008; **47**:688–693. doi: 10.1111/j.1365-4632.2008.03692.x.

[28] Stengel FM. Indications and technique of biopsy for diseases of the scalp. J Dermatol Surg Oncol. 1978; **4**:170–171.

[29] Restrepo R, McKee PH, Calonje E. Diseases of the hair. In: McKee PH, Calonje E, Granter SR, editors. Pathology of the Skin. 3rd ed. Philadelphia: Elsevier Mosby; 2005. pp.1073–1079.

[30] Ahmed Z, Banik RL, Paul HK, Jaigirdar QH, Begum F, Chowdhury SA. Histopathological changes in different stages of alopecia areata. Mymensingh Med J. 2010; **19**:100–105.

[31] Dy LC, Whiting DA. Histopathology of alopecia areata, acute and chronic: why is it important to the clinician? Dermatol Ther. 2011; **24**:369–374. doi: 10.1111/j.1529-8019.2011.01414.x.

[32] Whiting DA. Histopathologic features of alopecia areata: a new look. Arch Dermatol. 2003; **139**:1555–1559.

[33] Messenger AG, McKillop J, Farrant P, McDonagh AJ, Sladden M. British Association of Dermatologists' guidelines for the management of alopecia areata 2012. Br J Dermatol. 2012; **166**:916–926.

[34] Gupta LK, Khare A, Garg A, Mittal A. Congenital triangular alopecia: a close mimicker of alopecia areata. Int J Trichol. 2011; **3**:40–41. doi :10.4103/0974-7753.82135.

[35] Ekiz O, Sen BB, Rifaioğlu EN, Balta I. Trichoscopy in paediatric patients with tinea capitis: a useful method to differentiate from alopecia areata. J Eur Acad Dermatol Venereol. 2014; **28**:1255–1258. doi: 10.1111/jdv.12246.

[36] Shelleh HH, Khan SA, Al-Hatiti HS. Trichotillomania or alopecia areata? Int J Dermatol. 2006; **45**:1196–1198.

[37] Brzezinski P, Cywinska E, Chiriac A. Report of a rare case of alopecia areata coexisting with Trichotillomania. Int J Trichology. 2016; **8**:32–34. doi: 10.4103/0974-7753.179388.

[38] Seetharam KA. Alopecia areata: an update. Indian J Dermatol Venereol Leprol. 2013; **79**:563–575. doi: 10.4103/0378-6323.116725.

[39] Heath CR, Taylor SC. Alopecia in an ophiasis pattern: traction alopecia versus alopecia areata. Cutis. 2012; **89**: 213–216.

[40] Ross EK, Shapiro J. Management of hair loss. Dermatol Clin. 2005; **23**:227–243.

[41] Sohn KC, Jang S, Choi DK, et al. Effect of thioredoxin reductase 1 on glucocorticoid receptor activity in human outer root sheath cells. Biochem Biophys Res Commun. 2007; **356**:810–815.

[42] Alkhalifah A. Topical and intralesional therapies for alopecia areata. Dermatol Ther. 2011; **24**:355–363. doi: 10.1111/j.1529-8019.2011.01419.x.

[43] Delamere FM, Sladden MM, Dobbins HM, Leonardi-Bee J. Interventions for alopecia areata. Cochrane Database Syst Rev. 2008; CD004413. doi: 10.1002/14651858.CD004413.pub2.

[44] Charuwichitratana S, Wattanakrai P, Tanrattanakorn S. Randomized double-blind placebo-controlled trial in the treatment of alopecia areata with 0.25% desoximetasone cream. Arch Dermatol. 2000;**136**:1276–1277.

[45] Tosti A, Iorizzo M, Botta GL, Milani M. Efficacy and safety of a new clobetasol propionate 0.05% foam in alopecia areata: a randomized, double-blind placebo-controlled trial. J Eur Acad Dermatol Venereol. 2006; **20**:1243–1247.

[46] Lenane P, Macarthur C, Parkin PC, et al. Clobetasol propionate, 0.05%, vs hydrocortisone, 1%, for alopecia areata in children: a randomized clinical trial. JAMA Dermatol. 2014; **150**:47–50. doi: 10.1001/jamadermatol.2013.5764.

[47] Alkhalifah A, Alsantali A, Wang E, McElwee KJ, Shapiro J. Alopecia areata update: part II. Treatment.. J Am Acad Dermatol. 2010; **62**:191–202. doi: 10.1016/j.jaad.2009.10.031.

[48] Sutherland L, Laschinger M, Syed ZU, Gaspari A. Treatment of alopecia areata with topical sensitizers. Dermatitis. 2015; **26**:26–31. doi: 10.1097/DER.0000000000000094.

[49] Happle R. Antigenic competition as a therapeutic concept for alopecia areata. Arch Dermatol Res. 1980; **267**:109–114.

[50] Herbst V, Zöller M, Kissling S, Wenzel E, Stutz N, Freyschmidt-Paul P. Diphenylcyclopropenone treatment of alopecia areata induces apoptosis of perifollicular lymphocytes. Eur J Dermatol. 2006; **16**:537–542.

[51] Rokhsar CK, Shupack JL, Vafai JJ, Washenik K. Efficacy of topical sensitizers in the treatment of alopecia areata. J Am Acad Dermatol. 1998; **39**:751–761.

[52] Spano F, Donovan JC. Alopecia areata: part 2: treatment. Can Fam Physician. 2015; **61**:757–761.

[53] Wiseman MC, Shapiro J, MacDonald N, Lui H. Predictive model for immunotherapy of alopecia areata with diphencyprone. Arch Dermatol. 2001; **137**:1063–1068.

[54] Hill ND, Bunata K, Hebert AA. Treatment of alopecia areata with squaric acid dibutylester. Clin Dermatol. 2015; **33**:300–304. doi: 10.1016/j.clindermatol.2014.12.001.

[55] Perret CM, Steijlen PM, Zaun H, Happle R. Erythema multiforme-like eruptions: a rare side effect of topical immunotherapy with diphenylcyclopropenone. Dermatologica. 1990; **180**:5–7.

[56] Nilforoushzadeh MA, Keshtmand G, Jaffary F, Kheirkhah A. Diphencyprone induced vitiligo: a case report. Case Rep Med. 2012; **2012**:356236. doi: 10.1155/2012/356236.

[57] Price VH. Double-blind, placebo-controlled evaluation of topical minoxidil in extensive alopecia areata. J Am Acad Dermatol. 1987; **16**:730–736.

[58] Fiedler-Weiss VC. Topical minoxidil solution (1% and 5%) in the treatment of alopecia areata. J Am Acad Dermatol. 1987; **16**:745–748.

[59] Shapiro J. Current treatment of alopecia areata. J Investig Dermatol Symp Proc. 2013; **16**:42–44. doi: 10.1038/jidsymp.2013.14.

[60] Healy E, Rogers S. PUVA treatment for alopecia areata—does it work? A retrospective review of 102 cases. Br J Dermatol. 1993; **129**:42–44.

[61] Taylor CR, Hawk JL. PUVA treatment of alopecia areata partialis, totalis and universalis: audit of 10 years' experience at St John's Institute of Dermatology. Br J Dermatol. 1995; **133**:914–918.

[62] Mitchell AJ, Douglass MC. Topical photochemotherapy for alopecia areata. J Am Acad Dermatol. 1985; **12**:644–649.

[63] Claudy AL, Gagnaire D. PUVA treatment of alopecia areata. Arch Dermatol. 1983; **119**:975–978.

[64] Luggen P, Hunziker T. High-dose intravenous corticosteroid pulse therapy in alopecia areata: own experience compared with the literature. J Dtsch Dermatol Ges. 2008; **6**:375–378. doi: 10.1111/j.1610-0387.2007.06608.x.

[65] Olsen EA, Carson SC, Turney EA. Systemic steroids with or without 2% topical minoxidil in the treatment of alopecia areata. Arch Dermatol. 1992; **128**: 1467–1473.

[66] Aghaei S. An uncontrolled, open label study of sulfasalazine in severe alopecia areata. Indian J Dermatol Venereol Leprol. 2008; **74**:611–613.

[67] Rashidi T, Mahd AA. Treatment of persistent alopecia areata with sulfasalazine. Int J Dermatol. 2008; **47**:850–852. doi: 10.1111/j.1365-4632.2008.03700.x.

[68] Joly P. The use of methotrexate alone or in combination with low doses of oral corticosteroids in the treatment of alopecia totalis or universalis. J Am Acad Dermatol. 2006; **55**:632–636.

[69] Zakaria W, Passeron T, Ostovari N, Lacour JP, Ortonne JP. 308-nm excimer laser therapy in alopecia areata. J Am Acad Dermatol. 2004; **51**:837–838.

[70] Al-Mutairi N. 308-nm excimer laser for the treatment of alopecia areata. Dermatol Surg. 2007; **33**:1483–1487.

[71] Hordinsky M, Kaplan DH. Low-dose interleukin 2 to reverse alopecia areata. JAMA Dermatol. 2014; **150**:696–697. doi: 10.1001/jamadermatol.2014.510.

[72] Castela E, Le Duff F, Butori C, et al. Effects of low-dose recombinant interleukin 2 to promote T-regulatory cells in alopecia areata. JAMA Dermatol. 2014; **150**:748–751. doi: 10.1001/jamadermatol.2014.504.

[73] Craiglow BG, King BA. Killing two birds with one stone: oral tofacitinib reverses alopecia universalis in a patient with plaque psoriasis. J Invest Dermatol. 2014; **134**:2988–2990. doi: 10.1038/jid.2014.260.

[74] Gupta AK, Carviel JL, Abramovits W. Efficacy of tofacitinib in treatment of alopecia universalis in two patients. J Eur Acad Dermatol Venereol. 2016; **30**:1373–1378. doi: 10.1111/jdv.13598.

[75] Jabbari A, Nguyen N, Cerise JE, et al. Treatment of an alopecia areata patient with tofacitinib results in regrowth of hair and changes in serum and skin biomarkers. Exp Dermatol. 2016; **25**:642–643. doi: 10.1111/exd.13060.

[76] Craiglow BG, Tavares D, King BA. Topical ruxolitinib for the treatment of alopecia universalis. JAMA Dermatol. 2016; **152**:490–491. doi: 10.1001/jamadermatol.2015.4445.

[77] Robins DN. Case reports: alopecia universalis: hair growth following initiation of simvastatin and ezetimibe therapy. J Drugs Dermatol. 2007; **6**:946–947.

[78] Lattouf C, Jimenez JJ, Tosti A, et al. Treatment of alopecia areata with simvastatin/ezetimibe. J Am Acad Dermatol. 2015; **72**:359–361. doi: 10.1016/j.jaad.2014.11.006.

Chapter 8

Telogen Effluvium

Emin Ozlu and Ayse Serap Karadag

Additional information is available at the end of the chapter

http://dx.doi.org/10.5772/66975

Abstract

Telogen effluvium (TE) is a noninflammatory disease characterized by diffuse loss of telogen hair. It is the most frequent cause of diffuse hair loss and the actual incidence of the disease is not known. According to the underlying etiology, TE could be physiologically and pathologically classified. The evaluation of a patient with TE includes a detailed history, physical examination, and laboratory tests. The patients should be questioned in terms of TE subtype, duration, and clinical course of hair loss. The most important point in the treatment of TE is to consult about the natural course of the disease.

Keywords: hair loss, iron deficiency, management, treatment, telogen hair

1. Introduction

Hair is important for social communication and healthy appearance, and acts as marker for identity of one's personal image. It can be, indeed, directly related to a feminine appearance, sexuality, attractiveness, and the concept of personality in females. In addition, hair is the second fastest growing tissue of the body, followed by bone marrow. Therefore, many metabolic derangements can be manifested with alopecia, and hair loss may be the initial clinical sign of a systemic disease [1]. Although hair loss may cause anxiety in individuals, irrespective of age and sex, and results in reduced quality of life and restriction of social relations in females, more than males. As a result, hair loss is the most frequent cause of admission to dermatology clinics [2].

2. Definition

Telogen effluvium (TE) was first termed by Kligman to define an increased shedding of normal club hairs based on the hypothesis that, irrespective of the cause, the follicle tends to act in a similar manner undergoing a premature termination of anagen and precipitating telogen [3].

Telogen effluvium is a noninflammatory disease characterized by diffuse loss of telogen hair, caused by any disruption of hair cycle which leads to increased and synchronized telogen shedding [4]. It is the leading cause of diffuse hair loss. However, the actual incidence of the disease remains unknown [2]. It has been suggested to result from an abrupt shift of large numbers of anagen hairs to telogen hairs on the scalp with altered ratio of anagen hair to telogen hair from the normal ratio of 90:10–70:30 [1]. The degree of telogen effluvium depends on the severity and duration of exposure, but not the type of the agent [5].

Although the effect of age also remains unclear; elderly women are reported to be more vulnerable to acute TE following high fever, surgical trauma, severe hemorrhage, or immense psychological stress. In children, TE is responsible for only a minority of cases with hair loss [6, 7].

Telogen effluvium can be classified into two groups, according to the duration of disease, as acute and chronic. The duration of disease is shorter than 6 months in acute TE, while it takes more than 6 months in chronic state. In acute TE, hair loss typically begins 2–3 months later than the triggering event, although the triggering factor is unknown in 33% of the cases. However, chronic TE is frequent in healthy females in the fourth to fifth decades [7]. In addition, telogen gravidarum is a variant of TE which follows childbirth. Significant telogen gravidarum can affect a third to a half of all women following childbirth [8]. In postpartum TE, follicles remain in a prolonged anagen phase, rather than cycling into the telogen phase. Once released from anagen, an increased shedding of telogen hair is one of the clinical signs of the disease [9].

3. Epidemiology

The majority of TE is subclinical; however, its actual incidence or prevalence still remains unclear. It has no predilection for particular racial or ethnic groups. Although it affects both sexes, women are more likely to present for the evaluation of acute TE than men [10]. A higher number of women also suffer from chronic TE than men. Chronic TE, which is less common than the acute variant, mostly affects women between the ages of 30 and 60 years [11, 12].

4. Etiology and pathogenesis

The cycle of hair follicle includes anagen, catagen, and telogen phases. In a normal scalp, about 90–95% of the hair follicles are in the anagen phase, 5–10% are in the telogen phase, and a loss of 100–150 hairs per day is accepted as normal. Telogen effluvium is an abnormality of hair cycling during which a higher percentage of the scalp hairs are in the telogen phase. In TE, the number and ratio of hair follicles in the telogen phase increase. The physiological daily shedding of about 100–150 telogen club hair from the scalp is a usual nature of the hair cycle. In addition, follicles normally retain telogen hair, until the reentry to the anagen phase. Eventually, a new anagen hair pushes the old telogen hair out. It is unlikely to result in visible alopecia and to alter the trichogram [13]. Temporary alopecia may develop, since the shorter telogon hair is replaced by the long telogen hair. When the new anagen hair grows within 3–6 months, alopecia resolves [7]. In addition, no genetic cause for TE has been proposed to date [2, 9].

http://dx.doi.org/10.5772/66975

According to the underlying etiology, TE can be physiologically and pathologically categorized. Physiological causes include neonatal and physiological TE. However, pathological causes of TE include inflammatory diseases, stress, drugs, endocrine disorders, organ dysfunctions, nutritional causes, exogenous factors, syphilis, and systemic lupus erythematous [2]. The main causes of TE are shown in **Table 1** [2, 10].

Acute telogen effluvium
Acute or chronic major illness
Collagen vascular disease
Febrile illness:
• HIV infection
• Malaria
• Tuberculosis
• Typhoid
Major surgery
Endocrine disorders:
• Hypothyroidism
• Hyperthyroidism
Nutritional:
• Protein or caloric dietary restriction
• Nutritional deficiencies
• Iron deficiency anemia
• Congenital or acquired zinc deficiency
• Rapid weight loss
Drugs, supplements, or toxins
Physiological:
• Telogen gravidarum
• Physciological effluvium of newborn
Significant emotional stress
Inflammatory conditions of the scalp (e.g., seborrheic dermatitis)
Infectious conditions that affect the scalp (e.g., fungal, bacterial, or spirochetal)
Chronic telogen effluvium
Shortened anagen
May follow acute TE or telogen gravidarum
Chronic diffuse telogen hair loss
Thyroid disorders
Iron deficiency anemia
Acrodermatitis enteropathica
Crash dieting
Chronic starvation
Hypoproteinaemia
Metabolic disturbances
Advanced malignancy
Senility
Systemic lupus erythematosus
Dermatomyositis
Syphilis
Drugs
HIV infection
Anorexia nervosa
HIV: human immunodeficiency virus, TE: telogen effluvium

Table 1. Causes of telogen effluvium [2, 10].

5. Functional types of telogen effluvium

Headington defined five types of functional TE, according to the different follicular cycles. These include the immediate anagen release, delayed anagen release, immediate telogen release, delayed telogen release, and short anagen phase [2].

5.1. Immediate anagen release

It is a common form of TE which is related to physiological stress, severe illness, and drug use. During stress, the cytokines induce apoptosis of hair follicle keratinocytes, first with catagen, followed by telogen [2]. Therefore, follicles, which are induced to leave the anagen, enter telogen early [14].

5.2. Delayed anagen release

It typically occurs in women with postpartum hair loss, and when the oral contraceptives are discontinued. It is also known as telogen gravidarum. It is caused by high levels of circulating placental estrogen, which prolongs the anagen phase, result in a full head of hair during pregnancy. The withdrawal of these hormones during delivery stimulates the overdue anagen hair to enter into the catagen phase simultaneously. As a result, an increased shedding of telogen hair can be seen after a couple of months of delivery [2, 15].

5.3. Immediate telogen release

Drug-induced shortening of telogen results in follicles with the reentry of the anagen prematurely [14]. Hair follicles typically release the club hair 100 days later. It is caused by a shortened normal telogen cycle. This type of hair shedding usually occurs 2–8 weeks, following therapy with topical minoxidil [16]. As the exogen hair at resting is released, this paradoxical phenomenon occurs, by stimulated anagen phase [2].

5.4. Delayed telogen release

Hair follicles do not shed or recycle into anagen, but remain in prolonged telogen. When teloptosis defined as the termination of telogen phase with hair shedding occurs, the main clinical manifestion of increased shedding of the club hair presents. In such cases, the major cause is seasonal hair loss [2, 16].

5.5. Short anagen phase

Idiopathic shortening of anagen duration results in persistent telogen shedding. The condition is not associated with the hair shaft fragility or hair unruliness. It leads to resistant and chronic TE. It is common in hereditary hypotrichosis and ectodermal dysplasia and as an isolated disorder in otherwise healthy children [2, 16].

http://dx.doi.org/10.5772/66975

6. Clinical findings

6.1. Acute telogen effluvium

Women with acute TE are usually admitted with complaints of increased hair loss while washing hair and combing or brushing hair. These patients often have a concern of baldness. Despite excessive hair shedding, the density of the hair is visible [14]. If the main triggering cause of TE is eliminated, hair loss lasts for up to 6 months [1].

In the absence of a concomitant hair or scalp disorder, the scalp and hair shafts seem normal without any symptoms. In TE, the distribution of the scalp hair loss is diffuse; however, the bitemporal area may be the most affected area [10, 11]. In general, patients do not relate these events to their recent illness and have a concern of baldness [7]. In addition, no scarring or inflammation is present [2, 13].

To date, several factors have been suggested to be associated with the induction of TE, depending on clinical observations. However, there is no data to confirm and define the level of risk for TE related to these factors. It is estimated that an inciting factor is unable to be detected in about one-third of patients with acute TE [10].

In postpartum TE, time to hair loss often takes 2 or 3 months after delivery, although it can be delayed up to 6 months, depending on the length of the telogen phase. More interestingly, TE can be more pronounced, if delivery occurs in the fall, as the time of postpartum TE coincides with an increased seasonal hair shedding during the winter. In addition, breastfeeding may partially reduce TE with the effects of prolactin, since lactating women have an increased anagen-to-telogen ratio at 4 months in the postpartum period, compared to the nonlactating women. The condition often resolves by 12 months after delivery, even if breastfeeding continues [14, 17].

6.2. Chronic telogen effluvium

Women with chronic TE usually suffer from a prolonged, fluctuating course of TE for more than 6 months. In general, there is no trigger factor; however, some patients may have a continuation of acute TE with a shortened anagen phase, underlying a complaint of shortened hair as well as hair shedding seen in all patients with TE [13, 14].

In some cases, this type of hair loss may last for several years. Prolonged TE may be caused by multiple sequential triggers, although no trigger is identified in certain cases [1, 12].

In primary chronic TE, there is no specific triggering agent. Chronic TE can be induced by an acute TE [16]. Both hypothyroidism and hyperthyroidism are associated with chronic diffuse telogen hair loss (CDTHL). This is usually reversible upon reestablishment of the euthyroid state, although at times, longstanding hypothyroidism may cause hair follicle atrophy [18].

Iron deficiency anemia is also a causative factor of CDTHL, since follicles need iron to stimulate the anagen phase of the hair cycle [19]. The hair loss can be reversed with the iron supplementation. Iron deficiency without anemia is more controversial, as it has a potential relationship with CDTHL [20]. In the majority of cases, drug-induced CDTHL occurs mechanistically via the immediate anagen release [19]. It typically occurs within 6–12 weeks of treatment and progresses while on the medication. It, then, begins to resolve after the discontinuation of the drug [21]. To the best of our knowledge, no controlled trials showing a causal relationship for specific medications have been conducted; however, if a medication is suspected, it should be discontinued for a period of at least 3 months to examine its possible link to the hair loss [4, 14].

Moreover, diet is associated with the hair condition. Therefore, each patient should be questioned for the protein intake. Eating disorders can also lead to hair loss. In a study, 67% of the patients with TE had bulimia, while 61% had anorexia nervosa [22].

7. Diagnosis

In the presence of hair loss, the key step is taking a thorough history of the patient. In addition, the affected areas of the scalp should be examined to determine the presence or absence of follicular orifices. It helps to distinguish the scarring and nonscarring alopecia [23]. In the presence of follicular orifices, nonscarring alopecia can be suspected, although further history findings are useful to unveil the main cause [14].

The diagnosis of TE is usually based on the patient's history, physical examination findings, and hair pull test results (**Table 2**) [10]. The recognition of diffuse, noninflammatory, nonscarring hair loss should raise the clinical suspicion for TE, when it occurs acutely and is preceded by a physiological or psychological stressor, in particular. In the majority of cases, scalp biopsy is not required [10].

Anamnesis, clinical diagnosis
Hair pull test
Trichogram
Light microscoby
Biopsy
Laboratory evaluation
Wash test

Table 2. Diagnosis of telogen effluvium [10].

http://dx.doi.org/10.5772/66975

8. Histopathology

With the exception of TE induced by inflammatory disorders affecting the scalp, scalp biopsies of TE not show an inflammation. On the other hand, increased telogen follicles are the main histopathological finding [24]. Unlike androgenetic alopecia, the rate of vellus hair follicles does not increase [12].

9. Evaluation

Patients with TE should be evaluated with a detailed history, physical examination, and laboratory tests (**Table 3**) [1]. In addition, TE subtype, duration, and clinical course of hair loss should be also questioned. In particular, possible triggering factors within 2–5 months before hair loss begins should be addressed [7]. In the absence of no causative factor, a complete blood count, serum ferritin, biochemical markers, and thyroid function tests should be performed [2].

In addition, hair-care practices of patients which may damage hair such as braiding leading to traction alopecia, and the loss of eyelashes, eyebrows, and axillary, pubic, or body hair should be questioned, as alopecia areata or trichotillomania may affect any hair-bearing area. A detailed history, childbirth, prior surgeries, and psychosocial stress should be also assessed. Furthermore, drugs that may cause TE should be examined (**Table 4**) [1, 2]. Additionally, acne, irregular menstrual cycles, or hirsutism may indicate androgen excess, which contributes to female pattern hair loss. Symptoms of hyperthyroidism or hypothyroidism should be also evaluated and current and previous medications should be carefully reviewed. A history of following a strict vegetarian diet or heavy menses may suggest iron deficiency anemia [1].

Duration
Thinning, shedding
Localization: localized diffuse
Associated symptoms: itching, pain, burning
Systemic symptoms, personal history
Nutritional history
Drug history
Psychosocial history
Hair care products-cosmetics history
Family history

Table 3. History of hair loss checklist [1].

More than 5%:	1–5%:	Less than 1%
Mood stabilizers (lithium and valproic acid): *the most common*	Oral contraceptives	Amiodarone
Antidepresants (fluoxetine)	Acyclovir	Amitriptyline
Oral retinoids (acitretin, isotretinoin)	Allopurinol	Azathioprine
Anticoagulant (heparin,enoxaparine, warfarin)	Buspirone	Dopamine
Antimicrobial (isoniazid)	Captopril	Naproxen
Antiviral (indinavir)	Carbamazepine	Omeprazole
Interferon alpha	Cyclosporine	Paroxetine
Terbinafine	Lamotrigine	Sertraline
Beta-blockers (metaprolol, propronolol)	Nifedipine	Verapamile
	Hypolipidemic drugs	Venlafaxine
	Cetirizine	Vinblastine
	Gold	Vincristine

Table 4. Drugs associated with telogen effluvium [1, 2].

10. Laboratory

Although the majority of female patients with hair loss have normal laboratory test results, a complete blood count, ferritin, thyroid-stimulating hormone, antinuclear antibody titer, and vitamin D level can be studied, as abnormal levels of these parameters are likely to be associated with distinct forms of alopecia. In addition, serum and free testosterone, dehydroepiandrosterone sulfate, and prolactin should be analyzed, in the presence of any signs of potential endocrine abnormalities including severe acne, hirsutism, virilization, galactorrhea, menstrual irregularities, or infertility [14]. In case of any risk factors for syphilis, the venereal disease research laboratory test is recommended [1].

The link between serum levels of ferritin or vitamin D and TE is controversial. To date, studies investigating the relationship between serum ferritin levels and TE have shown controversial results [20, 25–27].

Iron deficiency anemia and thyroid disorders are the common conditions associated with TE. However, in the majority of cases, no apparent clinical features suggesting these conditions are observed [2].

A strict vegetarian diet or heavy menses may be suggestive for iron-deficiency anemia. Iron supplementation is recommended for TE patients who have had a serum ferritin level less than 70 ng per milliliter [20]. However, the effects of iron supplementation for TE have not been extensively investigated in controlled trials. The efficacy data are limited to case series, indicating cessation of hair loss and new hair growth with iron supplementation in women with low ferritin levels. On the other hand, the beneficiary effect of iron supplementation has not been established in all cases [27, 28].

Furthermore, perimenopausal symptoms such as hot flashes and irregular bleeding should be evaluated in older women. In this age group, starting or interrupting hormonal replacement therapies should be ruled out as a possible cause of TE [29].

11. Physical examination

The scalp hair and scalp skin should be carefully examined in all patients. Scale, inflammation, pustules, and scarring or abnormalities of the hair shaft should not be evaluated as the manifestations of an isolated TE. On physical examination, the entire skin surface should be examined to identify the extent of hair loss and to detect the main features of other hair or scalp disorders [10].

11.1. Hair pull test

A hair pull test should be performed as part of the physical examination in patients with suspected TE. The test is helpful to detect active hair shedding. About 50–60 hair fibers close to the skin surface are grasped and the hairs from the proximal to distal ends are tugged. Normally, only two or three hairs are pulled out by this method. In the presence of abnormal shedding, more than 10% hair (6–10 hair) can be easily pulled out from any part of the scalp, if the patient has not shampooed for more than 24 h [2, 30]. The test should be performed in four regions of the scalp: the frontal, occipital, and both temporal regions. The hair should not be shampooed for at least a day [29]. Light microscope is used to examine the hair shafts and to confirm that the loose hairs are telogen hairs [10].

Of note, the hair pull test may produce a false-negative result, if the patient has shampooed or vigorously groomed the hair on admission. In addition, if the patient has not shampooed or combed the hair for several days, the test may yield false positivity [10].

11.2. Trichogram (hair pluck test)

From a hair pluck, sample is abnormal, which indicates higher than 25% telogen hair [13]. Since telogen rate in this test is not associated with the severity of the hair loss, the sensitivity of the hair pull test is low [2].

11.3. Wash test

As daily hair count is troublesome, the wash test has been proposed. In wash test, the patient is instructed to wash hair after 5 days of last shampoo in a sink with its drain covered by gauze. The hair entrapped in the gauze is, then, counted [2].

11.4. Dermoscopy

Data relating to the dermoscopic findings of TE are limited. Acute TE may indicate empty follicles and regrowing hairs of normal thickness (>0.03 mm). Dermoscopic findings are useful to distinguish chronic TE from female pattern hair loss (female androgenetic alopecia). The latter variably exhibits a greater hair diameter [31].

11.5. Wood's light examination

TE can be due to seborrheic dermatitis of the scalp. On physical examination, a greasy scale and erythema on the scalp can be seen with a characteristic distribution. In addition, examination with a Wood's lamp (a source of ultraviolet A light) can be useful for the definite diagnosis of seborrheic dermatitis, which unveils the scale [32].

11.6. Procedures

In the majority of cases, further investigation is not required, beyond the clinical history and physical examination. However, additional diagnostic tools can be useful in patients in whom the diagnosis remains unclear [10].

11.7. Scalp biopsy

In most cases, scalp biopsies are not required and are only reserved for certain patients with an obscure diagnosis. Although scalp biopsy is not mandatory, it helps to exclude female pattern hair loss and alopecia areata. In general, biopsy results are normal, except increased telogen follicles (normal telogen counts vary between 6 and 13%). The rate of telogen follicles more than 15% indicates TE, while more than 25% is the major manifestation of TE [2, 30].

A 4-mm punch biopsy is sectioned horizontally for each specimen, and a second specimen is sectioned vertically. In general, we perform biopsy in an area outside of predilection for androgenetic alopecia to reduce the possibility of diagnostic uncertainty; therefore, we avoid bitemporal, frontal, and vertex areas of the scalp, if applicable. We usually select the leading edge of the alopecic area and avoid completely bald areas [10].

11.8. Trichograms and phototrichograms

Although these techniques are less common, they may be helpful to confirm the diagnosis of TE. With the use of these techniques, the rate of telogen and anagen hair follicles on the scalp can be evaluated. Currently, trichograms and phototrichograms are mostly used in specialized clinical hair centers and research studies. These procedures are described in detail in a separate section [10].

12. Differential diagnosis

The pattern of hair thinning or shedding can be helpful in the differential diagnosis. Diffuse thinning of the scalp hair in both temporal regions is highly suggestive of TE [33]. Frontal fibrosing alopecia almost particularly affects the frontal and frontotemporal hairlines. In case of traction alopecia, the periphery of the scalp is usually affected. Central centrifugal cicatricial alopecia (CCCA) typically begins at the vertex of the scalp, expanding centrifugally [34]. Alopecia areata may present in varying patterns. The patchy type is usually localized, whereas a more diffuse pattern has also been described [29, 35].

13. Treatment

Consulting on the natural course of the disease is the mainstay of the treatment of TE. A detailed evaluation should be performed to identify the underlying cause. In general, hair loss halts within 3–6 months in patients in whom a triggering factor is identified and eliminated [2].

Although spontaneous improvement is expected for patients with TE related to an isolated event such as childbirth, those related to a persisting insult should have the cause eliminated or treated, if applicable. In case of drug-induced TE, the suspected drug should be discontinued for at least 3 months to identify whether hair loss improves with the discontinuation of therapy. In addition, concomitant hair or scalp disorders such as seborrheic dermatitis should be simultaneously treated [10].

Furthermore, hair loss may profoundly affect the psychosocial status of the patient, irrespective of the degree of hair loss. Therefore, emotional well-being of the patient is critical in the management. All concerns of the patient should be sensitively addressed by the clinician. In addition, patients should be educated on the hair growth cycle and the expected course of TE, including an explanation that complete hair loss is not expected to occur, to reassure patients. Follow-up is also helpful both to encourage the patient and to identify those requiring further evaluation for persistent TE [10].

Moreover, the diagnosis and treatment of TE should be briefly discussed with the patient. Potential therapeutic options include the followings, based on the pathogenesis of TE:

1. Inhibition of catagen.
2. Induction of anagen in telogen follicles.
3. Inhibition of exogen.

Currently, no potent, FDA-approved catagen inhibitors or anagen inducers are commercially available. However, catagen-inducing drugs such as beta-blockers, retinoids, anticoagulants, or antithyroid drugs should be avoided and catagen-inducing endocrine disorders including thyroid dysfunction, hyperandrogenism, or hyperprolactinaemia should be simultaneously treated. Replacement therapy for catagen-promoting deficiencies such as iron, zinc, estradiol, or proteins can be also prescribed [2].

Today, no proven vitamins or supplements for any form of hair loss are commercially available. In case of a measurable deficiency such as iron-deficiency anemia, replacement therapy may be initiated. However, a balanced diet and stable body weight are the critical measures. In the literature, biotin supplementation has been shown no effect on TE [36]. Despite their claimed benefits, there are no controlled studies investigating the efficacy of iron or thyroxine replacement on TE [4]. In addition, maintaining serum ferritin above 40 ng/dL has been suggested to reverse hair loss [26]. In case of poor response, possible factors such as poor compliance, misdiagnosis, malabsorption, coexisting anemia, or persistent blood loss should be considered. Iron supplementation should be continued for 3–6 months, until the iron stores are replenished [37].

Of note, unnecessary long-term iron supplementation may result in iron overload [38]. On the other hand, there is no proven effect of antioxidants or other supplements on TE [39].

14. Conclusion

In conclusion, TE is a common disease that causes diffuse hair loss. The diagnosis of acute TE is based on patient's history and examination findings. Since acute TE is self-limiting, the clinician should monitor the patient, until spontaneous resolution. However, in case of severe or prolonged shedding, further investigations are warranted. On the other hand, chronic TE can be only diagnosed, after other causes of chronic diffuse telogen hair loss are ruled out. There is no specific treatment for TE. In the management of TE, the major aspect is to educate the patient relating to the natural history of the condition.

Author details

Emin Ozlu[1] and Ayse Serap Karadag[2]*

*Address all correspondence to: karadagaserap@gmail.com

1 Duzce University, School of Medicine, Department of dermatology, Bolu, Turkey

2 Istanbul Medeniyet University, School of Medicine, Department of Dermatology, Istanbul, Turkey

References

[1] Shapiro J. Clinical practice. Hair loss in women. N Engl J Med. 2007 Oct 18;357(16):1620–30. DOI: 10.1056/NEJMcp072110

[2] Malkud S. Telogen effluvium: A review. J Clin Diagn Res. 2015;9:WE01-3. DOI: 10.7860/JCDR/2015/15219.6492.

[3] Kligman AM. The human hair cycle. J Invest Dermatol. 1959 Dec;33:307–16. PMID: 14409844

[4] Harrison S, Sinclair R. Telogen effluvium. Clin Exp Dermatol. 2002 Jul;27(5):389–5. PMID: 12190639

[5] Tosi A, Misciali C, Piraccini BM, Peluso AM, Bardazzi F. Drug-induced hair loss and hair growth. Incidence, management and avoidance. Drug Saf. 1994 Apr;10(4):310–7. Review. PMID: 8018303

[6] Nnoruka EN, Obiagboso I, Maduechesi C. Hair loss in children in South-East Nigeria: Common and uncommon cases. Int J Dermatol. 2007 Oct;46 Suppl 1:18–22. DOI: 10.1111/j.1365-4632.2007.03457.x

[7] Grover C, Khurana A. Telogen effluvium. Indian J Dermatol Venereol Leprol. 2013 Sep–Oct;79(5):591–603. DOI: 10.4103/0378-6323.116731. Review.

[8] Dawber RP, Connor BL. Pregnancy, hair loss, and the pill. Br Med J. 1971 Oct 23;4(5781):234. PMID: 5115836

[9] Chartier MB, Hoss DM, Grant-Kels JM. Approach to the adult female patient with diffuse nonscarring alopecia. J Am Acad Dermatol. 2002 Dec;47(6):809–18; quiz 818-20. Review. DOI: 10.1067/mjd.2002.128771

[10] Bergfeld W. Telogen effluvium. http://www.uptodate.com/contents/telogen-effluvium. Literature review current through: Jul 2016.

[11] Trüeb RM. Systematic approach to hair loss in women. J Dtsch Dermatol Ges. 2010 Apr;8(4):284–97, 284–98. DOI: 10.1111/j.1610-0387.2010.07261.x.

[12] Whiting DA. Chronic telogen effluvium: increased scalp hair shedding in middle-aged women. J Am Acad Dermatol. 1996 Dec;35(6):899–906. PMID: 8959948

[13] Sinclair R. Diffuse hair loss. Int J Dermatol. 1999 May;38 Suppl 1:8–18. Review. PMID: 10369535

[14] Harfmann KL, Bechtel MA. Hair loss in women. Clin Obstet Gynecol. 2015 Mar;58(1):185–99. doi: 10.1097/GRF.0000000000000081.

[15] Courtois M, Loussouarn G, Hourseau C, Grollier JF. Ageing and hair cycles. Br J Dermatol. 1995 Jan;132(1):86–93. PMID: 7756156

[16] Trueb RM. Diffuse hair loss. In: Blume-Peytavi U, Tosti A, Whiting DA, Trueb R, editors. Hair growth and disorders, 1st edn. Berlin: Springer; 2008. pp. 259–272.

[17] Gizlenti S, Ekmekci TR. The changes in the hair cycle during gestation and the post-partum period. J Eur Acad Dermatol Venereol. 2014 Jul;28(7):878–81. DOI: 10.1111/jdv.12188. Epub 2013 May 20.

[18] Church RE. Hypothyroid hair loss. Br J Dermatol. 1965;77:661–2.

[19] Headington JT. Telogen effluvium. New concepts and review. Arch Dermatol. 1993 Mar;129(3):356–63. Review. PMID: 8447677

[20] Trost LB, Bergfeld WF, Calogeras E. The diagnosis and treatment of iron deficiency and its potential relationship to hair loss. J Am Acad Dermatol. 2006 May;54(5):824–44. Review. DOI: 10.1016/j.jaad.2005.11.1104

[21] Brodin MB. Drug-related alopecia. Dermatol Clin. 1987 Jul;5(3):571–9. Review. PMID: 3301114

[22] Glorio R, Allevato M, De Pablo A, Abbruzzese M, Carmona L, Savarin M, Ibarra M, Busso C, Mordoh A, Llopis C, Haas R, Bello M, Woscoff A. Prevalence of cutaneous manifestations in 200 patients with eating disorders. Int J Dermatol. 2000 May;39(5):348–53. PMID: 10849124

[23] Jackson AJ, Price VH. How to diagnose hair loss. Dermatol Clin. 2013 Jan;31(1):21–8. DOI: 10.1016/j.det.2012.08.007. Epub 2012 Sep 29.

[24] Weedon D. Diseases of cutaneous appendages. In: Weedon's Skin Pathology, 3rd ed, Elsevier Limited, Edinburgh. 2010. p.397

[25] Olsen EA, Reed KB, Cacchio PB, Caudill L. Iron deficiency in female pattern hair loss, chronic telogen effluvium, and control groups. J Am Acad Dermatol. 2010 Dec;63(6):991–9. DOI: 10.1016/j.jaad.2009.12.006. Epub 2010 Oct 13.

[26] Karadag AS, Ertugrul DT, Tutal E, Akın KO. The role of anemia and vitamin D levels in acute and chronic telogen effluvium. Turk J Med Sci 2011;41(5):827–833.

[27] Sinclair R. There is no clear association between low serum ferritin and chronic diffuse telogen hair loss. Br J Dermatol. 2002 Nov;147(5):982–4. PMID: 12410711

[28] Hard S. Non-anaemic iron deficiency as an etiologic factor in diffuse loss of hair of the scalp in women. Acta Derm Venereol. 1963;43:562–9.

[29] Mubki T, Rudnicka L, Olszewska M, Shapiro J. Evaluation and diagnosis of the hair loss patient: part II. Trichoscopic and laboratory evaluations. J Am Acad Dermatol. 2014 Sep;71(3):431.e1–431.e11. DOI: 10.1016/j.jaad.2014.05.008. Review.

[30] Shrivastava SB. Diffuse hair loss in an adult female: approach to diagnosis and management. Indian J Dermatol Venereol Leprol. 2009 Jan–Feb;75(1):20–7; quiz 27–8. Review. PMID: 19172026

[31] Miteva M, Tosti A. Hair and scalp dermatoscopy. J Am Acad Dermatol. 2012 Nov;67(5):1040–8. DOI: 10.1016/j.jaad.2012.02.013. Epub 2012 Mar 8. Review.

[32] Mayser P, Stapelkamp H, Krämer HJ, Podobinska M, Wallbott W, Irlinger B, Steglich W. Pityrialactone – a new fluorochrome from the tryptophan metabolism of Malassezia furfur. Antonie Van Leeuwenhoek. 2003;84(3):185–91. PMID: 14574113

[33] Rudnicka L, Olszewska M, Rakowska A, Kowalska-Oledzka E, Slowinska M. Trichoscopy: a new method for diagnosing hair loss.J Drugs Dermatol. 2008 Jul;7(7):651–4. Review. PMID: 18664157

[34] Rakowska A, Slowinska M, Kowalska-Oledzka E, Warszawik O, Czuwara J, Olszewska M, Rudnicka L. Trichoscopy of cicatricial alopecia. J Drugs Dermatol. 2012 Jun;11(6):753–8. PMID: 22648224

[35] Lacarrubba F, Dall'Oglio F, Rita Nasca M, Micali G. Videodermatoscopy enhances diagnostic capability in some forms of hair loss. Am J Clin Dermatol. 2004;5(3):205–8. PMID: 15186200

[36] McMichael A. Approach to office visits for hair loss in women. Cutis 2011;87:8–9. PMID: 21323092

[37] Goddard AF, McIntyre AS, Scott BB. Guidelines for the management of iron deficiency anaemia. British Society of Gastroenterology. Gut 2000;46:1–5.

[38] Bottomley SS. Secondary iron overload disorders. Semin Hematol 1998;35:77–86.

[39] Esfandiari A, Kelly AP. The effects of tea polyphenolic compounds on hair loss among rodents. J Natl Med Assoc 2005;97:1165–9.

Chapter 9

Androgenic Alopecia: Cross-Talk Between Cell Signal Transduction Pathways

Anastasia Nesterova and Anton Yuryev

Additional information is available at the end of the chapter

http://dx.doi.org/10.5772/67845

Abstract

Signaling pathways that control coordination of hair follicle cells genetic program are the convenient model for explaining the hierarchy of intercellular interactions governing cyclic growth of hair. This chapter describes models of molecular signaling pathways specific to dermal papilla cells from balding human scalp in hair follicle cycle. These models include already published data, as well as information inferred from pathway analysis of microarray data and protein-protein interaction database. Interplay of androgenic-alopecia-related signaling pathways FGF, TGFB, BMP, and WNT, as well as cyclin-dependent kinases signaling, is shown.

Keywords: hair follicle, dermal papilla, catagen, androgen receptor, alopecia, microarray, pathway analysis, SNEA

1. Introduction

Androgenetic alopecia (AGA) is the state of progressive cessation of hair growth on the human frontal area of the scalp, most likely inherited and androgen-dependent (OMIM locus numbers are 109200, 612421, 300710). In women, as well as in men with androgenic alopecia, the growth of frontal scalp hairs slows down, and the transition occurs from terminal (pigmented and thick) hair type to vellus (nonpigmented and thin) hair type. The duration of fast growth periods (anagen) gradually reduces with each hair cycle, hair follicles become narrower and shorter, and progressively miniaturized [1]. Peak of the disease in most male patients occurs at the age of 40–50 years. Male pattern hair loss ultimately leaves narrow bands of hair on temples and occiput, where hair never fall off during AGA [2, 3].

It was thought that AGA is associated with high levels of androgens circulating in blood. However, currently prevalent firm opinion is that it is not increased levels of androgens cause this disease, but rather altered androgen cell sensitivity [4]. There is evidence that in AGA, in dermal papilla cells of hair follicles from the frontal and parietal scalp skin, 5a-reductase-driven synthesis of topical androgens is increased just as well as activation of androgen receptor complex [5]. The paradoxical situation occurs with accepting the androgen-dependent paradigm of AGA: when the activity of androgen-related signaling stimulates beard growth, while the same signaling arrests hair growth from frontal area of the scalp [5–8].

Nevertheless, failures in treatment of AGA using anti-androgens or 5a-reductase blockers suggest that additional causative factors do take part in the development of the disease. Present day search for beginnings of AGA is in fact search for answers to the following questions: (a) To which extent do cell-specific signaling pathways contribute to the initiation and maintenance of hair growth cessation in a frontal scalp skin? (b) What are the features of hair follicles from a beard or an occipital scalp and from a frontal scalp that manage baldness in first two cases and hair growth in another? One of the accepted answers is that despite great variety of causes, the basic mechanism of hair growth pathologies consists in discoordination of cross-talk between canonical signaling pathways within hair follicle dermal papilla and hair follicle outer root sheath stem cells [9, 10].

Signaling pathways are the convenient model for explaining the hierarchy of intercellular proteins interactions, which control the hair follicle cells genetic destiny. The pathway models described in the chapter include specific to cells of hair follicle already published data, as well as information inferred from publicly available results of microarray essays and ResNet® Mammalian database [11].

2. Hair follicle-related signaling pathways in androgenic alopecia

Pathway is the term from molecular biology which denotes the way or the mechanism by which a cell reacts to stimuli. In general, pathway is a simplified model of any process in a cell. More accurate scientific definition of the pathway could be as follows: Pathway is a biological process, which initiates when extracellular signaling molecule activates a specific receptor located on the cell surface or inside the cell. In turn, this receptor triggers a chain of events inside the cell, creating a response. Usually, a pathway is visualized as a graphical map. Besides graphical information, a signaling pathway model also includes annotations and references about entities and relations between entities from curated database. There are software applications that allow a researcher to use such signaling pathway models in microarray data analysis and for dynamic simulation of signal propagation [12, 13].

Hair follicle is a multicellular organ that has strictly organized structure and that follows distinct patterns in its development [14, 15]. As opposed to other human organs that grow constantly, hair growth occurs in a cyclic manner. A normal hair cycle of scalp hair includes a fast growing period (anagen phase, 2–6 years), regression period (catagen phase, 2–3 weeks), and resting period (telogen phase, 10–12 weeks). The duration of the anagen phase defines hair length and pigmentation. Normally, 80–90% of hairs in hairy part of scalp are in active growth phase—anagen [1]. Numerous reviews are focused on cyclic growth of hair follicles [15–19].

The earliest sign of AGA is increased amount of frontal scalp area skin hair follicles at telogen phase [20]. Developing the alopecia is a long-term process. There is progressive reduction of the duration of anagen phase of hair follicles on the frontal scalp area with each passage through the hair cycle. Other discovered physiological changes in AGA: dermal papilla cell reduction; thinning of the dermis; the sebaceous glands enlargement; connective tissue streamers presence; number of mast cells increased; and T-cell infiltration of follicular stem cell epithelium [21–23]. There are strong evidences that AGA is androgen signaling-dependent disease. Pattern of AGA inheritance is related with an autosomal dominant trait. Castration in men stops progression of hair loss while administration of testosterone restores balding [2]. Men with type 2 5a-reductase deficiency syndrome do not develop AGA balding phenotype [24]. Finasteride (type 2 5a-reductase inhibitor) reduces dihydrotestosterone (DHT) level in scalp skin and increases hair growth in more than 60% of men with AGA [25]. Androgen receptor (AR) gene is the only risk gene for AGA phenotype confirmed in gene association studies [26]. Androgen receptors level was higher in cultured dermal papilla cells derived from balding scalp hair follicles, compared to dermal cell from nonbalding follicles [5, 8]. The concentration of DHT has been shown to be higher in the balding scalp than in the nonbalding scalp [27]. Both type 1 and type 2 5a-reductase have higher level in frontal than occipital follicles from AGA scalp [5]. Expression of enzymes involved in DHT synthesis (STAR and HSD3B1) was enhanced in the bald frontal area, in comparison with occipital areas of AGA patients [28].

Another layer in research of androgen-dependent hair growth covers seeking differences in androgen sensitivity of distinct areas of skin. Follicles from frontal and parietal areas of the human scalp are considered to be androgen-sensitive. There are also two more types of hair follicles: androgen-independent hair follicles, such as eyelashes, and androgen-dependent pigmented terminal hair follicles, such as beard [26, 29, 30]. Why do hair follicles have different sensitivity to androgens is still open question. There are few studies towards difference between androgen-dependent and androgen-independent hair follicles [8, 30–35].

Thus, from the point of view of signaling pathways research, studying AGA mainly focuses on DHT synthesis in the skin and AR signaling affecting cell processes that cause arrest of anagen phase in frontal scalp. Precisely, these include diminishing of dermal papilla cell proliferation and hair bulge stem cell inactivation. Also, there are important pathways of sebocyte and melanocyte maintenance, keratinocytes apoptosis, and macrophages migration.

2.1. Dermal papilla-specific signaling pathways

The entire hair develops from the niche of activated dermal papilla (DP) cells—group of mesenchymal cells in lower part of hair follicle adjacent to dermis, which provide the regulation of hair keratinocyte differentiation [36]. The changes in molecular signaling which follow the dermal papillae burst in balding scalp of a person with AGA result in suppressed growth of hair keratinocytes derived from DP cells [29]. Dermal papilla in developed hair follicle in anagen is surrounded by a proliferative zone within the hair bulb named matrix. Dermal papilla and matrix include heterogenic cell populations with even multi-lineage potential [37, 38]. For example, adult DP cells were induced to differentiate into adipogenic and osteogenic lineages, as well as in pluripotent stem (iPS) cells [39]. The activity of alkaline phosphatase (ALP) can be used both in mice and human hair follicles as a marker for detecting DP activity [40].

Androgen synthesis is the first fragment of AGA-related signaling pathway in DP cells (**Figure 1**). DP cells can synthesize androgens themselves to stimulate androgenic receptor. All types of hair follicle DPs (beard, pubic, and scalp) have testosterone and androstenedione. But normally, only beard cells produce more potent androgen 5-alpha-dihydrotestosterone produced by SRD5A2. In AGA, DP cells from androgen-sensitive frontal scalp contain more SRD5A2 than those from androgen-insensitive occipital scalp [5]. Steroid sulfatase (STS) in the dermal papillae of human terminal hair follicles hydrolyzes dehydroepiandrosterone sulfate (DHEAS) to dehydroepiandrosterone (DHEA). In healthy human occipital scalp, as well as in the beard, STS activity was significantly higher in the hair dermal papillae than in the outer root sheaths [41].

AR signaling is the key fragment of AGA-related signaling pathway in DP cells. Dermal papilla appears to be the site of androgen action in hair follicle, as androgen receptors are only found in DP cells. In AGA, dermal papilla cells from balding scalp express higher levels of androgen receptors than nonbalding scalp cells [5, 35]. *AR* gene isoforms or functional mutation near the androgen receptor gene may explain the aberrant expression of the AR protein in the balding scalp of AGA patients. Of the many *AR* gene polymorphisms known, G allele of StuI and polyQ polymorphisms has the most significant association with AGA, especially in white populations [42]. DNA methylation of the *AR* promoter is increased in hair follicles from

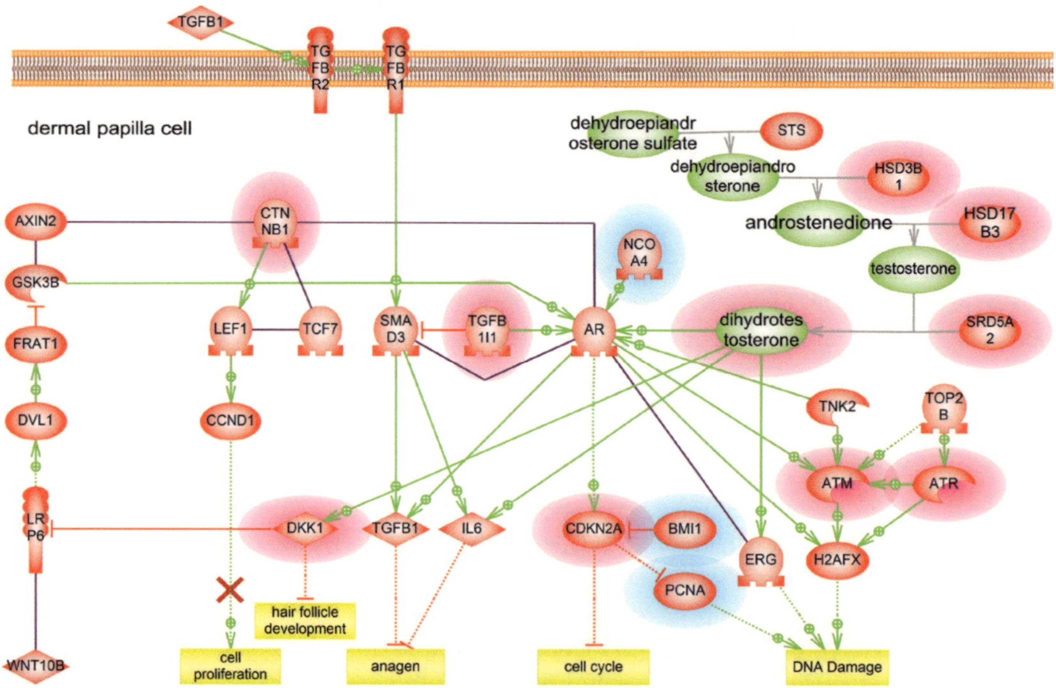

Figure 1. Androgens promote scalp dermal papilla cells dysfunction in AGA. Highlighted entities are underexpressed genes (blue) or overexpressed genes (red) in AGA, according to previous studies. Pathway was built in Pathway Studio environment. The legend for the pathway is provided in Methods section (**Figure 7**).

http://dx.doi.org/10.5772/67845

occipital scalp compared with those from vertex AGA scalp, indicating efficacy of the DNA methylation for protecting occipital hair follicles against AR expression [43]. Human DP cells from AGA express dihydrotestosterone-driven TGFB1, DKK1, and IL6 proteins. TGFB1, DKK1, and IL6 were able to promote apoptosis in outer root sheath keratinocytes derived from dermal papilla cells, which results in hair growth arrest [44–46].

Intersections between WNT, TGF, and AR signaling comprise the next important fragment of AGA-related signaling pathway in DP cells. DHT suppresses WNT signaling (LEF/TCF-mediated transcriptional activity) in DP cells from bald scalp. However, these phenomena could not be observed in DP cells of non-AGA males. It was shown that AR and beta-catenin 1 (CTNNB1) interact with each other [47]. In response to DHT, high expression level of dickkopf 1 (DKK1) was shown in balding dermal papilla cells in AGA [48]. DKK1 acts as inhibitor of canonical WNT/CTNNB1 signaling and hair follicle growth in mice [49]. In mice, in cells of outer root sheath layer of hair follicle, recombinant human DKK1 as inhibitor of WNT induced the pro-apoptotic protein BAX, resulting in apoptosis [45].

TGFB1 can enhance androgens sensitivity in balding dermal papilla cells through SMAD3 signaling, in cooperation with TGFB1I1 as a coactivator of the androgen receptor [50]. In beard and bald frontal scalp dermal papilla cells, expression of *TGFB1I1* mRNA was higher than in cells from the occipital scalp [39]. Also the common fact is that increased expression of cytokines (TGFB1, IL6) promotes apoptosis [44].

IL6 is expressed in DP cell, whereas its receptors IL11RA and IL6ST are expressed in the inner and outer root sheaths of human hair follicles [46]. It was shown that DHT induces IL6 expression in the balding DP of human cells compared with nonbalding DP cells. This results in anagen-to-catagen transition in hair follicle and hair growth arrest [51]. Direction of the IL6 expression change by androgens is cell-specific. In several studies, testosterone and DHT were found to inhibit production of IL6 by human peripheral blood monocytes and osteoblasts. In study of acute wound healing, DHT reduced the expression and secretion of *Il6* (and *Tgfb1*) in mice dermal fibroblasts [52].

Expression of NCOA4, AR coactivator, and a cell growth promoter was found to be reduced in dermal papilla of balding areas [53]. The dermal papilla and hair bulb expressed only the short (beta) but not the long (alpha) form of NCOA4. NCOA4 is capable to enhance AR transactivation induced by ligands such as estradiol, androstenediol, and the phytoestrogen daidzein. Studies indicate that AR competes with VDR and PPARG/RXR for NCOA4 availability [54].

Finally, PTGDS (prostaglandin D2 synthase) is elevated at the mRNA and protein levels in bald scalp, compared to haired scalp of men with AGA. Prostaglandin D2 (PGD2) is similarly elevated in bald scalp. PGD2 is a potent vessel contractor and may contribute to AGA development throughout deterioration of blood supply of hair follicle. PGD2 inhibits hair follicle regeneration through the PTGDR2 receptor [55].

Induction of androgen-accelerated premature senescence (loss of proliferative capacity) in bald scalp dermal papilla cells of AGA patients is one more fragment of the pathway. Loss of proliferative capacity of balding DPC was associated with higher expression of CDKN2A and lower expression of BMI1 and PCNA. CDKN2A protein levels were upregulated in response to androgen, and knockdown of the AR diminished the effects of androgen [56]. This suggests that balding DP cells are sensitive to environmental stress. Three important DNA damage sensors, H2AX, ATM, and ATR, were detected only in balding DP cells. Expression levels of H2AX protein were further increased with AR overexpression [57].

In general, the hypothesis of the pathway is that increase in AR signaling promotes regression of dermal papilla in AGA scalp, and the phase of hair follicle degeneration (catagen) gets initiated earlier than it normally should. AR signaling stimulates catagen likely through (a) TGFB1/HIC5/ARA55 cross-talk [57]; (b) increased level of DNA damage and loss of proliferative capacity induction, which is associated with higher expression of CDKN2A [56]; (c) DKK1 expression, which inhibits cell growth and WNT signaling [47]. However, none of these mechanisms alone is sufficient for the development of AGA, highlighting the combinatorial causes in the disease progression (**Figure 1**).

2.2. Bulge stem cells renewal pathway

Defect in differentiation of hair follicle stem cells (keratinocyte stem cells) could play a key role in the pathogenesis of AGA. New anagen phase and hair follicle arise due to activity of stem and stem-like cells of hair follicle which activate and fill the dermal papilla slow-cycling stem cells (pluripotent/multipotent cells) locate in outer root sheath of hair follicle (bulge region). Other pool of cells with features of "stemness" (secondary germ cells or hair germ cells) becomes morphologically defined between dermal papilla and bulge area in the end of telogen phase [58]. Moreover, in mice, mesenchymal self-renewing cell populations (hair follicle dermal stem cells) were found within the surrounding of DP dermal sheath [59].

Different molecular markers were suggested for distinguishing populations of hair follicle stem cells [58, 60]. Mice cells from bulge area express such specific marker as CD34. Human bulge cells could be found with CD34 as negative marker and CD200 as best positive marker [60, 61]. Mouse bulge cells distinct from secondary germ cells with expression of markers S100A6 and S100A4. Human hair follicle stem cells were categorized into nine subpopulations in Ref. [62] according to different expression of cell-specific markers. CD34 and CD271 expression in human hair follicle is confined to stem cells from sub-bulge area in outer root sheath of the hair follicle [63]. The sub-bulge area is the area between the bulge and dermal papilla, which become distinct in the telogen phase [64]. Stem cells in bulge (and sub-bulge) areas and secondary germ cells are considered to be functionally related cell populations. The CD34+ cells from sub-bulge area are considered to be a reservoir to the secondary hair germ cells upon the end of anagen. Also, secondary germ cells appeared to transform back (or send proliferative signals) into bulge cells in the telogen phase in mice [58, 64].

In bald areas in patients with androgenic alopecia, K15+ITGA6+ cells were present, but CD200+ITGA6+ cells and CD34+ cells were greatly diminished. The authors remarked that AGA likely results from diminished conversion of hair follicle stem cells in outer root sheath to progenitor secondary germ cells [65]. A decrease in second germ generation progenitor cells population attached to dermal papilla in telogen, possibly due to a lack of replenishment from sub-bulge cells, could potentially lead to AGA phenotype, when the each next anagen phase is characterized by new hair follicle smaller than its predecessor. Although these results can

http://dx.doi.org/10.5772/67845

explain decrease in amount of hair follicles in anagen phase in balding scalp in AGA, they do not point at what causes the hair fallout, since human cells from the outer root sheath of hair follicles display CD34 only during anagen phase [63]. To address this question, the detailed research of stem cells maintenance in hair follicle cycle in AGA involving modern techniques is required. The paper that summarizes the data on human hair follicle cycle and proposes standardized approach in this field was recently published [1].

Signaling pathways in stem cells during hair follicle cycle currently lack human-specific information and are mostly based on data from animal models. According to "bulge activation hypothesis," stem cells in bulge area are activated through interactions with the adjacent dermal papilla before the anagen phase [66]. Activation of new anagen and new hair growth can be described in two steps [64]. First, secondary germ cells become activated at the end of telogen. This activation characterized by WNT signaling and subsequent stabilization of beta-catenin. Second, secondary germ cells stimulate activation of stem cells in bulge area of outer root sheath, which in turn maintain the pool of matrix and dermal papilla cells. The initial pre-first step of anagen phase activation is depended on inductive signal coming from DP. It is supposed that the close proximity of the secondary germ cells to the DP in telogen results in their prior than bulge area activation [64, 67].

In AGA, anagen activation appears to fail, and telogen phase lasts longer [23]. In the next cycle, anagen phase onset is often absent at all [29].

Telogen is the resting phase for the cells and major proliferative signaling pathways within. In healthy mouse, bulge area cells WNT signaling is silent in catagen and telogen [68]. Microarray data suggest that mice bulge cells overexpress inhibitory factors for WNT signaling (*sFRP1, Dkk3, Wif*) [69]. In human bulge cells, increased expression of the WNT inhibitors *WIF1* and *DKK3* was also shown [60]. In patients with AGA, dermal papilla cells were shown to produce excessive amounts of factors inhibiting WNT signaling (for instance, DKK1) [45].

Balance between BMP and WNT signaling was discovered to be important in regulating the transition between quiescence and activation state of murine bulge stem cells [70]. High levels of BMP signaling during early (refractory) telogen are considered the cause of bulge stem cells retention in the quiescent state. In contrast, bulge stem cells activation in the late telogen is thought to require inhibition of BMP signaling. Both BMP and WNT signaling can regulate each other. Quiescence happens due to reciprocal negative feedback loops in these signaling pathways [71, 72]. In mice, *Bmp2* and *Bmp4* gene expression as well as expression of *Dkk1* and *Sfrb4* genes inhibit the expression of WNT family genes and thus limit hair follicle development to the stage of refractory telogen [70]. BMP signaling pathway suppresses itself by triggering the expression of *Noggin* [73, 74].

In human bulge stem cells, the BMP signaling antagonist FST was found overrepresented in the bulge in outer root sheath (ORS) [60]. Also, TGFb2 counteracted BMP signaling in mice bulge stem cells by enhancing the expression of *Tmeff1*, another antagonist of the BMP pathway. TGFB signaling needs to be activated for the hair cycle renewal [75].

Normally, telogen ends and anagen begins when the balance shifts towards WNT signaling is activated [70]. What signaling pathways normally initiate stem cells proliferation and subsequent anagen, and whether such signals are missed in case of AGA remains unknown. Perhaps, the external signals from adipocytes or fibroblasts in sebaceous gland surrounding hair follicle could be the origin of this initial stimulus [19].

3. Pathway analysis of microarray experimental data in AGA

Microarray technology allows detecting simultaneously the expression of thousands of genes in cells. Data acquired using microarray technology expose differences in gene expression between samples, such as cells from balding and nonbalding human scalp skin.

There are a lot of statistical and bioinformatics methods that can be used to identify cellular processes and signaling pathways with high activity in various cell types in hair bulge. Pathway analysis is the common term for these methods [12, 76]. We used sub-network enrichment analysis (SNEA) method [77] for pathway analysis of AGA hair follicle-related public microarray data. SNEA is based on the Gene Set Enrichment Analysis algorithm [78]. It uses a variation of a nonparametric statistic tests and considers "sub-network" as gene sets. SNEA uses Mann-Whitney statistic enrichment test to find sub-networks statistically enriched with nearest neighbors of the testing entity ("seed") that are most differentially expressed in the microarray experiment. In context of Pathway Studio data model, a seed can be a protein, complex, protein functional class, metabolite or drug, cellular process, disease, or a cell type. SNEA algorithm uses existing relationships in Pathway Studio ResNet® database to build "sub-networks" based on user-specified criteria. Significant seeds calculated by SNEA can be further used to identify the pathways or gene ontology groups that are significantly enriched with seeds. This analysis can point on pathways activated or repressed in different cell types or diseases. SNEA algorithm implemented in Pathway Studio® software iterates through the database of six million relations between proteins, molecules, cell processes, and diseases extracted from biomedical research literature by natural language processing technology. SNEA implementation in Pathway Studio allows to determine major transcription factors, receptors, and hormone upstream of differentially expressed genes in an experiment and identify small molecules that are associated with the diseases through changes in the proteins activity.

There are several public microarray datasets measuring expression of genes in the bald scalp of patients with AGA. Datasets with accession numbers GSE6664 [31] and GSE36169 [55] [65] could be uploaded from Gene Expression Omnibus (GEO) database [79]. Two more experiments were described by Midorikawa et al. [34] and Kwack et al. [48]. Besides oligonucleotide microarray experiments, microRNAs differential expression analysis was conducted in balding and nonbalding dermal papilla cells [32]; the expression of sex-determining genes in bald frontal scalp area was examined by real-time RT-PCR [80]. Also, microarray analysis to find differences in expression between beard and scalp dermal papilla cells is available [30].

The results of gene expression studies conducted for bald scalp in AGA patients are often controversial. For example, two gene microarray analyses with DP cells from AGA frontal and occipital scalp areas reveal either high level of DKK1 expression in DP cells from bald frontal scalp [48] or diminished DKK1 expression [31]. Most probably, this mismatch is due to differences in methods for DP cells isolation and culture or different levels of DHT treatment between experiments. It is also not clear from the corresponding articles if the DP cell donors were taking hair loss medications at the time of biopsy. In one more microarray experiment [81], higher levels of DKK1 were shown in human palmoplantar fibroblasts (human skin area without hair follicles) compared to nonpalmoplantar fibroblasts. So, one more putative cause of the mismatch could be the presence of mRNA from other cell type in the sample.

Nevertheless, some genes still have similar differential expression trends in DP cells from balding scalp in several experiments. The following genes were found to be overexpressed: TGFb2, ODC1, RYBP, FGF7, and CDKN2B/A. Genes BMI1, MCL1, SERPINE2, NCOA4, and others were found to be underexpressed. All results from human balding scalp from patients with AGA are summarized in **Table 1**.

Gene	Level	Source	Method	Treatment	Pathway	References
ARA70b (NCOA4b)	Down	DP cells	Hybridization		AR signaling	[55]
BMI1	Down	DP cells	ELISA		Cell senescence	[86]
CLDN11, CDKN1A, POSTN, KBTBD11, PSG5	Down	DP cells	cDNA array	1–10 nM DHT		[87]
SCF	Down	DP cells	ELISA		Impeding bulbar melanocyte pigmentation	[4]
SERPINE2	Down	DP cells	PCR	10 nM DHT	Extracellular matrix turnover	[88]
TIMP2, MCL1, IL6, TYRO3, RHOB	Down	DP cells	cDNA array			[36]
ACTG2, DNER, NPTX2, BEX1, GDF15	Up	DP cells	cDNA array	1–10 nM DHT		[87]
AR	Up	Early-passage DP cells			Induces apoptosis in ORS cells	[50]
ARA55 (TGFB1I1)	Up	DP cells	PCR		AR signaling	[89]
CDKN2A, SOD1, CAT, ATRIP	Up	DP cells	ELISA		Cell senescence	[86]
DAX1 (NR0B1), SRY, WT1, SOX9	Up	Scalp	RT-PCR, Western blotting			[84]
DKK1	Up	DP cells, scalp	cDNA array, immunoblotting	50–100 nM DHT	Induces apoptosis in ORS cells	[50]
DNPH1, CASP4, MOG, CDKN2B, ICAM1	Up	DP cells	cDNA array			[36]
IL6	Up	DP cells	ELISA	10–100 nM DHT		[53]
MIR221, MIR125b, MIR106a and MIR410	Up	DP cells	microRNA APM			[33]
PTGDS	Up	Scalp, HF in catagen	cDNA array		Inhibit hair growth	[82]

Gene	Level	Source	Method	Treatment	Pathway	References
StAR, HSD3B1	Up	Scalp	RT-PCR			[90]
TGFB1	Up	DP, keratinocytes	ELISA	Androgen	Induces apoptosis in ORS cells	[91]
TGFB2	Up	DP cells	Protein level	10 nM DHT	Induces apoptosis in ORS cells	[92]
YARS, SGK, ADAMTS5, SLC19A2, SLC2A3	Up	DP cells	cDNA array, immunoblotting	50–100 nM DHT		[50]
SRD5A1, SRD5A2	Up	HF in anagen	Northern blotting			[5]
H2AX						[58]
SOX9						[84]

For cDNA arrays, only top five significant genes ranked by fold change are shown.

Table 1. Genes with altered levels of mRNA expression in bald scalp from patients with AGA.

3.1. In silico analysis of microarray experimental data on dermal papilla cells

Dermal papilla (DP) is the key part of hair follicle that defines growth rate, thickness, and shape of hair shaft. GEO microarray dataset with accession number GSE66664 [31] compared gene expression in cultured immortalized human DP cells from balding (frontal) and nonbalding (occipital) scalps in response to DHT treatment. DP immortalized cell lines were obtained from two white 26-year-old men with Hamilton–Norwood grade IV AGA. The authors reported underexpression of vasculature-related genes in DP cells of balding hair follicles. Overexpressed genes were mostly enriched by genes from gene ontology groups related to cell cycle and mitosis. DP cells from both bald and nonbald scalp samples included classical DP signature genes, such as ALPL, WIF1, LEF1, and VCAN, expression of which correlated with inductive role of DP cells in hair morphogenesis [40].

Using gene array downloaded from GEO GSE66664 dataset, we found overexpressed and underexpressed genes in balding versus nonbalding immortalized dermal papilla cells cultured with 1 and 10 nM DHT. We also found differentially expressed (DE) genes in balding versus nonbalding dermal papilla cells cultured without DHT treatment. These genes were chosen with 0.05 p-value and twofold change of the expression cutoff. Both lists of differentially expressed (DE) genes were used for further pathway analysis as datasets 1 and 2, respectively.

The differential expression between genes in balding DP cell samples cultured with DHT versus balding DP cell samples cultured without DHT has founded to limit the number of external factors affecting the experiment. As result, we obtained 2 datasets with DE genes in bald DP cells—one for 1 nmol/L and the second for 10 nmol/L (nM) of DHT treatment's level. Each dataset contains 11 DE genes lists with values as results of calculation the ratio between values of genes in sample without DHT treatment (0 min) and 11 samples with DHT treatment periods from 15 min to 48 h. Two equivalent datasets for nonbald DP cell samples were also calculated. Lists of DE genes from all datasets were used for further pathway analysis (**Table 2**).

http://dx.doi.org/10.5772/67845

Dataset	Samples	DHT treatment	DE ratio[3]
Dataset 3	bDP[1]	1 nM	0 h vs 15 min—48 h
Dataset 4	bDP[1]	10 nM	0 h vs 15 min—48 h
Dataset 5	nbDP[2]	1 nM	0 h vs 15 min—48 h
Dataset 6	nbDP[2]	10 nM	0 h vs 15 min—48 h
Dataset 1	bDP, nbDP (15 min—48 h)	1 and 10 nM	bDP vs nbDP
dataset 2	bDP, nbDP (15min—48 h)	-	bDP vs nbD P

[1]Bald dermal papilla cells sample.
[2]Nonbald dermal papilla cells sample.
[3]Two samples between which differential expressions of genes were calculated.

Table 2. Datasets with differentially expressed genes were used in current analysis based on gene array GSE66664.

3.2. AR-related differentially expressed genes in microarray with AGA DP cells

In response to DHT, AR completely translocates to the nucleus after 30 min [82]. Considering additional 30–50 min for transcription, we concluded that the optimal time to find AR-related targets in studied microarray data is 1 h after of DHT treatment. All changes in expression after 1 h are likely related with paracrine signaling pathways following AR activation.

Total number of AR neighbors in ResNet13® database is 4931 genes. Among DE genes in bald compared to nonbald scalp DP cells samples with DHT treatment (dataset 1), we found 114 DE genes—neighbors of AR. We also found 126 DE genes—neighbors of AR in DP cells samples without DHT treatment (dataset 2) (**S. Table 1**). Out of them, only five genes (NOS3, EGR1, SMAD6, BTG2, and LATS2) were underexpressed in bald DP cells samples more in presence of DHT (dataset 1) while less in absent of DHT. Relations between these genes and AR are not specific for DP cell and were discovered mostly in cancer cells. However, reconstruction of the pathway model based on data from other tissues is routine practice in pathway analysis (**Table 3**).

BTG2 controls G1/S phase transition negatively by direct inhibition of cyclin D1 (CCND1) transcription in human cancer cells [83]. Inhibition of BTG2 (B-cell translocation gene 2) expression by DHT/TNF axis was shown in human keratinocytes [84]. LATS2 is also involved in the regulation of the G1/S transition of the cell cycle and degrades cyclin-dependent kinase inhibitor 1A (CDKN1A) by phosphorylation [85]. LATS2 was shown to modulate expression of AR target genes in cancer cells [86]. In rat immortalized dermal papilla cells, DHT also increased cell cycle arrest, increased *Cdkn1b* level, and decreased *cyclin E* (*Ccne1*), *cyclin D1* (*Ccnd1*), and *cyclin-dependent kinase* 2 (*Cdk2*) levels [87].

There evidences that AR-related SMAD6, EGR1, and NOS3 genes founded in dataset 1 may play role in hair follicle functioning. SMAD complex is regulated by TGFB signaling was shown to induce the catagen phase of the hair cycle in mammals [87].

Early growth response-1 (EGR1) is induced by various stressor factors. EGR1 had found functionally interacting with the androgen receptor and promoting androgen receptor nuclear

Name	Log change (d. 1)	p-value (d. 1)	Log change (d. 2)	p-value (d. 2)	Relation with AR	Localization
NOS3	−1.0376	5.175E-78	−0.935	2.25E-07	Regulation, PMID: 20416296	Vessel endothelial cell
EGR1	−2.096	1.45E-36	−0.947	8.47E-04	Binding, PMID: 12890669	Prostate carcinoma cell
SMAD6	−1.0187	9.55E-34	−0.9821	2.77E-07	Binding, PMID: 16249187	Colon carcinoma cell
BTG2	−1.0740	6.587e-07	−0.8412	0.0003658	Binding, PMID: 21172304	Prostate cancer cell
LATS2	−1.2569	7.83E-39	−0.8982	0.01183	Binding, PMID: 20935475	Breast cell

Lowering of activity of AR target genes in bald DP cells after DHT treatment that we found in datasets 1 could be related with cell cycle dysregulation.

Table 3. AR neighbors underexpressed in bald DP cells samples (datasets 1–2).

translocation in prostate cancer cells [88]. EGR1 has been also reported to be involved with apoptosis and cell migration in several cell types [89, 90]. The lower EGR1 expression in the dataset 1 (bald DP cells samples) may perhaps be result of competing of EGR1 and AR coactivators and corepressors. SHP inhibits both androgen receptor and EGR1 by competing coactivators and inhibitory proteins [91]. In mice embryonic fibroblasts, TP53 was shown to inhibit Egr1 through angiogenesis-associated gene Elk3 [92]. Egr1 inhibition also may be modulated in part via the binding to mesenchymal-specific corepressors NAB1 and NAB2 [93].

NOS3 does not have direct connection with AR, but its expression in epithelial cells is shown to be regulated through AR signaling, as well as its phosphorylation [94]. NOS3 causes the NO-induced vascular relaxation and may trigger angiogenesis in bald scalp. NR0B1, PTGDS, and SGK1 were among other DE genes in dataset 1 that has relations with AR. These genes had been reported previously to play important role in scalp hair follicle development in AGA (**Table 1, S. Table 1**).

The examination of datasets 3–6 (in view of time impact and DHT level impact on the differential expression) reveals more genes with expression correlated with DHT/AR signaling in bald DP cells (**Figure 2**).

Among genes with highest differential expression values (±2-fold change values) in datasets 3–6, we found 32 genes neighbors of AR or DHT in ResNet12® database (**S. Table 1**). Several AR neighbors differ in expression by more than 20% between bald and nonbald DP cell samples (**Figure 2**). Differential expression of genes such as CYB1P1 or CTGF had positively increased in bald samples versus nonbald, whereas SPRY1 and CEPBD genes had negatively deepened expression trend in bald samples. A lot of genes reduced their expression in bald samples compare with nonbald. For example, EGR1 and EGR2 genes reduced their expression by more than 70% in balding versus nonbalding scalp. We noticed also that EGR1 is responsible gene to 1 nM level of DHT treatment in bald DP cells samples, while EGR2 (and S100A14)

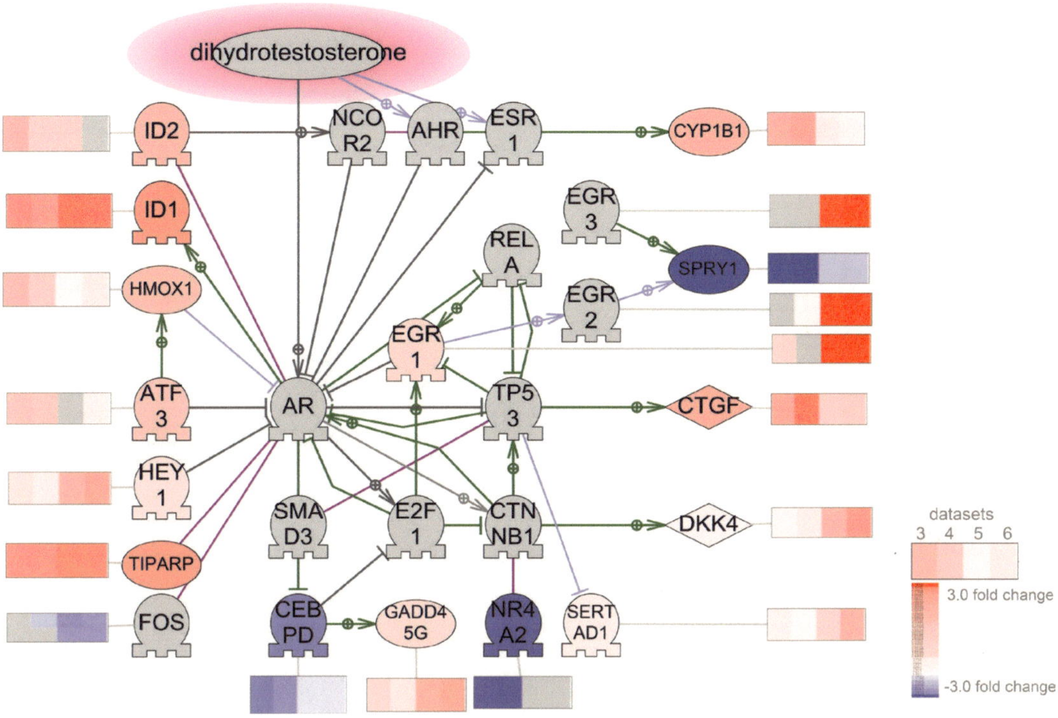

Figure 2. The impact of DHT and AR on DE genes with notably variances between bald versus nonbald dermal papilla cell samples after 1 h of 1–10 nM of DHT treatment. Highlighted proteins are corresponded to DE values in bald DP cell sample after 1 h of 1 nM DHT treatment (dataset 3). SPRY1, NR4A2 and CEBPD are underexpressed genes. ID1-2, CYP1B1, TIPARP and CTGF are overexpressed genes. Changing in DE values is represented by heat maps (rectangles near proteins).

are responsible genes to higher (10 nM) level of DHT. The 1 h of higher (10 nM) DHT level treatment correlated also with the lowering of SPRY1 differential expression in bald DP cells. The same conditions in nonbald DP cell samples correlated with slightly increasing of DKK4 and SERTAD1 differential expression (**Figure 3**).

Dickkopf WNT signaling pathway inhibitor 1 (DKK1) is a familiar target in AGA research. DKK4 also was shown to be able to inhibit WNT signaling in mice hair follicle [95]. AR could trigger DKK4 expression due to CTNNB1 activation [96]. Beta-catenin (CTNNB1) the central protein in WNT signaling in negative feedback loops manner activates DKK4 expression [97]. One more possible option how AR may impact on DKK4 expression in bald DP cells is through TRPS1. In the rat vibrissa follicles, AR could repress TRPS1, which in turn upregulates the expression of the Dkk4 [98, 99].

EGR1, EGR2, and EGR3 are early stress response transcriptional factors. In bald DP cell samples in dataset 1, EGR1 underexpressed severely. In datasets 3–6, EGRs rather downregulated expression in bald cell samples than higher differential expression in nonbald cell samples. Growth factors induce Egr2 and its target Igfbp5 expression, which are important for mice zigzag hair development [100]. Also Smad3 is involved in regulation of Egfr2 and Egr3 activation in mice skin [101]. The low expression of SPRY1 in datasets 3–4 could be associated with insufficient

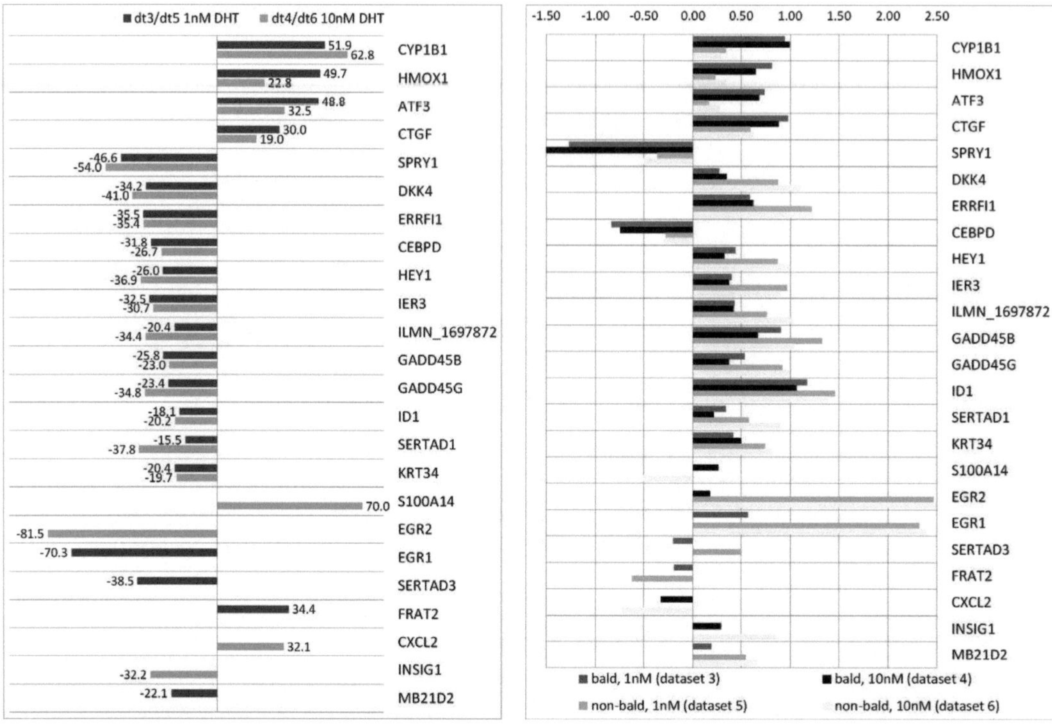

Figure 3. Genes with more than 20% distinguish in differential expression values between bald versus nonbald dermal papilla cell samples after 1 h of 1–10 nM of DHT treatment. The percent of ratio between DE values of genes in bald and nonbald samples (on the left). The comparison of DE values (log fold changes) of genes in datasets 3–6 (on the right).

EGR3 expression as Spry1 is expression target of Egr3 in mice T-cell [102]. In its turn, SPRY1 may inhibit EGR1 by disrupting the GRB2-SOS interaction in FGF or CTGF signaling [103]. SPRY1 also was shown to be down-regulated by androgens in prostate cancer cells [104].

CYP1B1 is necessary for metabolizing intracellular oxidative stress molecules. In addition, CYP1B1 catalyzes the generation 4-hydroxy estradiol which causes DNA damage in ovarian cancer [105]. CYP1B1 contains an estrogen response element and addition to aryl hydrocarbon receptor response elements in its promoter [106]. SERTAD1 expression level was significantly increased in conditions with low levels of nutrients [107]. Relation of this protein with AR signaling is unclear. ID1 and ID2 are key BMP signaling target transcriptional factors, and their important role was shown in mice hair follicle as well as in other organs [71]. Most probably, ID1 and ID2 overexpression marked the BMP signaling activation in DP cell samples at the time point 1 h after DHT treatment. AR-related activation of ID1 was shown in cancer [108]. ID2 was shown to interact with AR though NCOR2 [109]. CEBPD and NR4A2 both were underexpressed in bald DP cell samples, in datasets 3 and 4. NR4A2 is required for neuronal differentiation and is also induced as an immediate early gene in dermal endothelial cells and melanocytes [110]. NR4A2 binding to CTNNB disrupts co-repressor complexes, allowing co-activators to bind and activate NR4A2 [111]. There is some evidence that androgens may participate in NR4A2 activation [112]. Hypothetically, AR may be involved in NR4A2 inhibition

http://dx.doi.org/10.5772/67845

with NR0B1 (nuclear receptor DAX-1) partnership. CEBPD is important for differentiation, survival, and cell death in many cell types including adipocytes and fibroblasts. The most important transcription factors regulating CEBPD transcription are CREB, SP1, and STAT3 [113].

There is an important note that, among others, such genes as HEY1, SPRY1, PTGS1, EGR3 are considered to be DP signatures genes [31].

3.3. Pathway and ontology analysis of AGA DP cells microarray data

3.3.1. Regulators and ontology analysis

SNEA processing of DE genes from GSE6664 array in Pathway Studio application revealed top 100 significant regulators of differentially expressed genes in datasets 1–6 (see Section 5). Regulators themselves are not genes with DE in the bald versus haired scalp, but the ones that have genes from DE list as expression targets (connected with them with expression or promoter binding relation types). SNEA regulators help to reveal activated signaling pathways that include genes with altered expression.

TGFB1I1, TGFB2, CDKN2A, ATM/ATR, and MAP2K3 appeared in the list of regulators from dataset 1, which support previous data about their pivotal role in AGA development (**S. Tables 2** and **1**). TGFB1I1, TGFB2, ATM/ATR, and MAP2K3 are found to be the regulators of underexpressed genes in bald DP cells. CDKN2A was found to be the regulator of overexpressed genes.

Anaphase-promoting complex (APC), AURKA, E2F2, and E2F7 are also found as regulators of overexpressed genes in bald DP cells. E2F transcription factors are well-known transcription factors in the cell cycle. Anaphase-promoting complex (APC/C) allows the sister chromatids at the metaphase plate to separate and move to the poles. AURKA (aurora kinase A) is required for spindle pole formation during chromosome segregation in mitosis [114].

Moreover, using SNEA, we found that MIR106A (median change −1.10844, p-value 2.02e-03) to be the first significant miRNA regulator of DE genes in balding DP cells. Overexpression of MIR106A was shown in DP cells from patient with AGA in [32]. Among genes that MIR106 could regulate, there are such specific for hair follicle development genes as VIM, SPP1, and IL6. SPP1 (osteopontin) is expressed only during catagen but not in anagen or telogen in cultured rat vibrissae dermal papilla cells [115]. IL6 (interleukin 6) gene is a thoughtful candidate for DHT inducible catagen phase and regression of human hair shafts [51]. BMP2 is also a direct target of MIR106A [116].

The most number of genes with differential expression more than 2-fold change values in datasets 3–6 come about 6–12 h' time point transition after DHT treatment compared to absent of DHT (data not shown). We are presume that genes with extremes of expression of these time points point to paracrine signaling pathways initiated afterward DHT/AR signaling. SNEA regulators of DE genes in 6/12 time point are representing AR signaling follow-on cell processes and pathways.

RUNX1, CRTC1, FGF8, and others appeared in the list of regulators of expression which were common for bald DP cells samples (dataset 3 and 4) at 12 h after DHT treatment (**S. Table 2**).

Inductors of mesenchymal cell differentiation were the notable group in the regulator's list. A lot of detected regulators are important for mesenchymal cell differentiation in brain, bone, and hematopoietic cell lineage. For example, CREB-regulated transcription coactivator 1 (CRTC1) is a coactivator of NOTCH and mesenchymal cell differentiation and also regulates the expression of KISS1 in normal melanocytes [117]. RUNX1 is the well-known transcriptional factor that drives the development of skin appendages as well as hematopoietic cell lineage [118]. In hair follicle stem cells, RUNX1 promotes proliferation and simultaneously represses cell-cycle-related p21, p27, p57, and p15 transcription. Expression targets of RUNX1 and CRTC1 SNEA regulators include top DE genes in 6/12 h after DHT treatment in datasets 3–6 (**Figure 4**). The relations between regulators and their targets are not specific to dermal papilla cells (described for different cell models).

AR-related proteins, such as PIAS2, LATS2, and URI1, were found as regulators in dataset 4. PIAS2 binds to the androgen receptor and inhibits in a testosterone-dependent manner AR transcription activity in testis [119]. PIAS2 decreases N-cadherin protein expression during the neural crest development [120]. We found that at 12-h time point, N-cadherin expressed more intensively only in nonbald DP cell samples (dataset 5 and 6) versus bald DP cell samples. During epithelial-mesenchymal transition, ID1 and ID2 also repress E-cadherin promoter expression [121]. URI1 (prefoldin RPB5 interactor) was revealed as repressor regulator of AR transcription in human cancer prostate cell lines [122]. LATS2 already has been noticed as underexpressed DE gene in the dataset 1.

DP signature genes, such as MYLIP, SPRY1, FABP5, and GPM6B, were found to be underexpressed after 12 h of DHT treatment in bald DP cell samples.

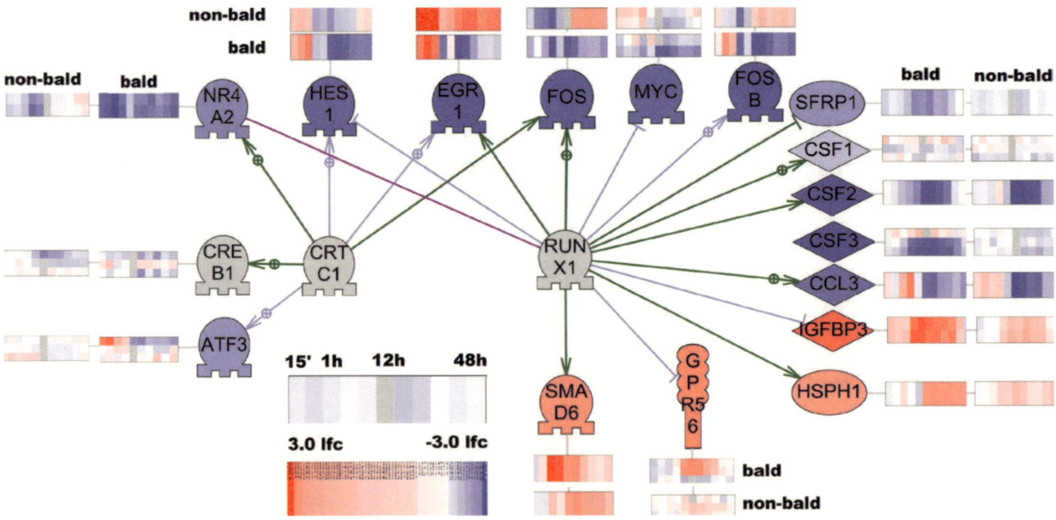

Figure 4. Expression targets of SNEA regulators RUNX1 and CRTC1 associated with DE genes in bald and nonbald DP AQ15 cell samples after 12 h of 1–10 nM DHT treatment. Highlighted proteins are corresponded to DE values in bald DP cellsample after 12 h of 1 nM DHT treatment (dataset 3). CREB1, CRC1 and RUNX1—genes without significantly DE in the dataset 3 (12 h'time point). ATF3, NR4A2, HES1, EGR1, FOS, MYC, FOSB, SFRP1, SCF1-3 and CCL3—underexpressed in bald DP cell sample genes. IGFBP3, HSPH1, GPR56 and SMAD6—overexpressed genes. Changing in DE values is represented by heat maps (rectangles near proteins). Chemokines, cytokines, and proteins involved in hematopoietic cell differentiation are widely presented in the list of regulators in datasets 3–6 (CSF1, TYROBP, L6ST, and others).

Statistical methods in the gene expression analysis such as Fisher's exact test and SGEA help to quickly reveal general picture of actual genes group, cell processes, and signaling pathways preceded the experiment. Several GO (Gene Ontology) groups and cell processes enriched with top DE genes from datasets 1–6 have revealed with GSEA. Specific biological cell processes such as cytokine-mediated immune response, regulation of apoptotic process, angiogenesis, and other similar to those in original research [31] were associated with underexpressed DE in bald frontal DP cells in dataset 1. Cellular response processes related to overexpressed DE genes were also similar to results in [31] and included DNA damage, collagen fibril organization, mitotic spindle organization, telomere maintenance, skin development, and others. Regulators of overexpressed DE genes from dataset 1 were significantly associated with "cell cycle," "response to DNA damage," and "apoptosis" cell processes. Regulators of underexpressed DE genes were associated with "apoptosis," "cell adhesion and migration," and "angiogenesis" (**S. Table 2**). Several ligands (TGFB2, THBS1, PTHLH, and ANGPT2) associated with cell process "catagen progression" also have been found to be regulators of underexpressed genes in bald DP cells from dataset 1.

We found stem cell and endothelial cells differentiation cell processes associated the list of regulators of DE genes after 12 h of DHT treatment for the datasets 3–6. Other types of GO and cell processes associated with regulators were "response to DNA damage stimulus," "induction of positive chemotaxis," and "angiogenesis." "Estrogen metabolic process" was found in the top of GO groups enriched with regulators for the datasets 3–6 in 12-h time point.

DE genes after 12 h of DHT treatment from datasets 3–6 associated themselves with "negative regulation of pathway-restricted SMAD protein phosphorylation," "regulation of WNT signaling pathway," "positive regulation of epithelial to mesenchymal transition" cell processes. DE genes after 12 h of DHT treatment characterized with "positive regulation of BMP signaling pathway," "regulation of angiogenesis," and other cell processes. (**S. Table 2**).

3.3.2. *Pathways analysis*

Pathway analysis with the lists of DE gene regulators from the dataset 1 on Elsevier PS Pathway Collection (PS Collection) reveals activation of cell cycle-related pathways. Pathways related to chromatin remodeling were most significantly enriched with DE genes in bald DP cells. G2/M and G2/S cell cycle phase transition pathway has 18 overlapping genes out of total 47 (p-value 2.66e-04). Kinetochore assembly pathway has 22 overlapping genes out of total 48 (p-value 5.10e-11). Metaphase/anaphase phase transition pathway has 13 overexpressed overlapping genes out of total 16 (p-value 2.07e-04). TGFB-/BMP-related pathways as well as chemokine related were also found to be activated in cultured bald DP cells in the dataset 1 (**S. Table 2**).

DNA repair is also activated process in bald DP cells. It is governed mostly by ATM/H2AFX double-strand repair mechanism. ATR/ATM is known as proteins that "recognize" DNA damage. In G1/S DNA damage checkpoint, these kinases phosphorylate TP53. TP53 stimulates the induction of CDKN1A, which results in CDKs inhibition and cell cycle arrest, preventing the replication of damaged DNA [123]. It is a probability that cell cycle arrest cannot be achieved in bald DP cells because CDKN1A strong underexpressed there, compared to nonbald ones as we found in datasets 1 and 2 (−4.94 log fold changed, p value 1.42e-88).

Though, underexpression of CDKN1A was not confirmed in analysis of differential expression in datasets 3–6. Androgen receptor could directly bind to the CDKN1A promoter [124]. AR was also involved in CDKN1A expression inhibition through LATS2 [85]. TGFB2 or BMP signaling pathways could effect on CDKN1A expression through SMAD and RUNX2 transcriptional factors [125]. ID1 and ID2 were shown to also down-regulate CDKN1A and promote cell cycle in prostate epithelial cells [126].

Also, in pathway analysis of datasets 1–2, there were canonical pathways of apoptosis and general signaling like TNF, TGFb, and NF-kb. Other groups of pathways were adiposal, bone, neuronal, or hematopoietic-specific pathways.

Pathway analysis with datasets 3–6 generally checked with the results of gene group's ontology analysis (**S. Table 2**). Cell-cycle-related pathway G0/G1 cell cycle phase transition (46% overlap, p-value 3.57093E-55) and single-strand nucleotide excision DNA repair (25% overlap, p-value 9.45E-10) were one of top pathways associated with bald DP cell samples. Apoptosis-associated TNF-alpha/TNFRSF1B signaling (64% overlap 1.80E-27) and TGF-beta signaling (32% overlap, p-value 3.04097E-27) also were on the top of the list. Estrogens/ESR1 nongenomic signaling (45% overlap, p-value 6.96E-06) and androgen receptor nongenomic signaling (14% overlap, 3.08E-05) also were found (**Figure 5**). A lot of pathways in the list were associated with canonical signaling pathways, such as ERK/MAPK canonical signaling or NF-κB canonical signaling (**Figure 6**). Pathways associated with chemokines signaling, adipose tissue, bone tissue, neuronal tissue, and hematopoietic cells were present.

3.4. Cross-talk between pathways affected in AGA DP cells

All noticed differences in molecular signaling pathways between DP cells from frontal and occipital scalp should help to define the general model of AR-related frontal scalp area hair follicle cycle switch in AGA. The results of microarray analysis suggest that androgen synthesis and metabolism are not affected in DP cells from AGA patients. Differential expression of such ferments from the androgen metabolism pathways as STS, HSD3B2, HSD17B1, and SRD5A2 is not changed in any time point in datasets 3–6. Though, expression of several proteins involved in the metabolism synthesis of cholesterol and estradiol had elevated. CYP1B1 differential expression was slightly elevated in bald DP cells with compare to nonbald DP cells at 1-, 3-, and 6-h time points.

BMP signaling is seemed to be activated both in bald and nonbald DP cell samples in the first 6 h after DHT treatment (while in bald DP cell samples, the activation was stronger). During the length of DHT treatment, the markers of BMB signaling DE genes ID1 and ID2 became underexpressed in bald DP cell samples (datasets 3–4) while not in nonbald DP cell samples. BMP2 was the only BMP ligand which differential expression had slightly changed (increase) in bald DP cells samples with compare to nonbald in the analysis of datasets 3–6. In mice, *Bmp4* has strong expression in catagen and early telogen and weak expression only before new anagen [9]. It is considered that in hair follicle, lowered activity of BMP signaling correlates with generally upregulated WNT signaling activity in the end of telogen due to existed reciprocal inhibition between WNT and BMP signaling [64, 70] (**Figure 6**). In mice hair follicle, low activity of BMP signaling in DP cells led to loosing signature characteristics of DP cells and failure in generating

http://dx.doi.org/10.5772/67845

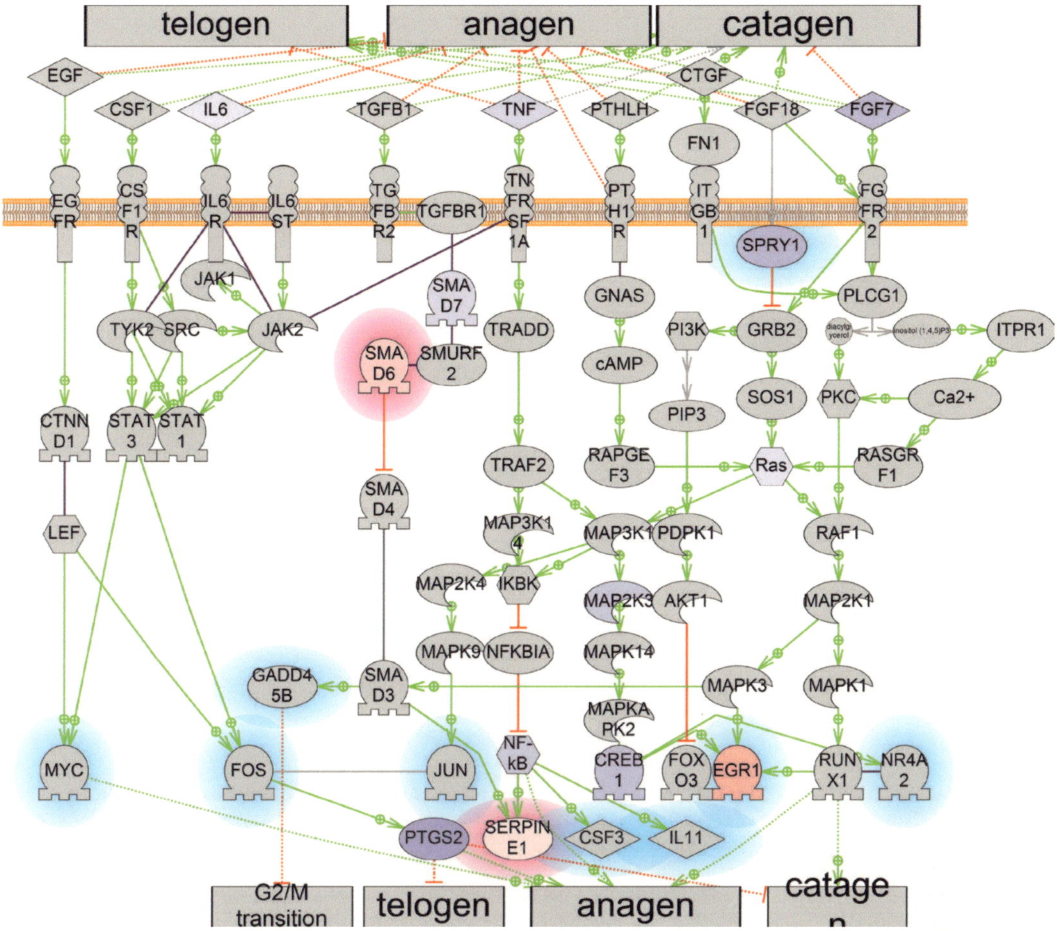

Figure 5. Signaling pathways of the regulation of transcription by growth factors and cytokines in AGA scalp. Pathways that include genes with changed expression in bald and nonbald DP cell samples after 12 hours of DHT treatment are shown. TNFa, CSF1, TGFb, EGF, FGF, PTHLH, CTGF, and IL6 ligand/receptor signaling pathways were the major affected pathways found in the pathway analysis. Only key proteins and relations of each ligand/receptor signaling are shown on the figure. Major transcription factors from dataset 3-4 (NF-kB, JUN-FOS, MYC, CREB1, and RUNX1) are shown on the bottom of the figure. Highlighted proteins correspond to underexpressed genes (SPRY1, NRHA2, EGR1, IL11, CSF3, JUN, FOS, GADD45B, and MYC) or overexpressed genes (SMAD6 and SERPINE1) in bald DP cells 12 hours after DHT treatment (datasets 3-4). IL6, TNF, FGF7, SPRY1, SMAD7, PTGS2, and CREB1 – underexpressed genes in datasets 5-6 (nonbald DP cells 12 hours after DHT treatment). SMAD6, EGR1, and SERPINE1 – overexpressed genes in datasets 5-6. The color saturation reflects the intensity of the differential expression within −0.5; 0.5 log-change interval, and 0.05 p-value cutoff.

new hair follicle cells [127]. Thereby, we may assume that the activity of WNT signaling should be lower in bald DP cell samples in first 6 h of DHT treatment. In nonbald "normal" DP cell samples, we found that WNT signaling was lowered but still activated in bald DP samples. DKK1 was suggested as one of the key player of triggering catagen in AGA [45]. We could not detect significant DE of DKK1 in dataset 1. We detected slight DKK1 underexpression in nonbald DP samples (dataset 5–6) at 1/3 h′ time point, whereas is not in bald DP cells. DKK4 is, vice versa, overexpressed in nonbald DP cells in the first 1 h.

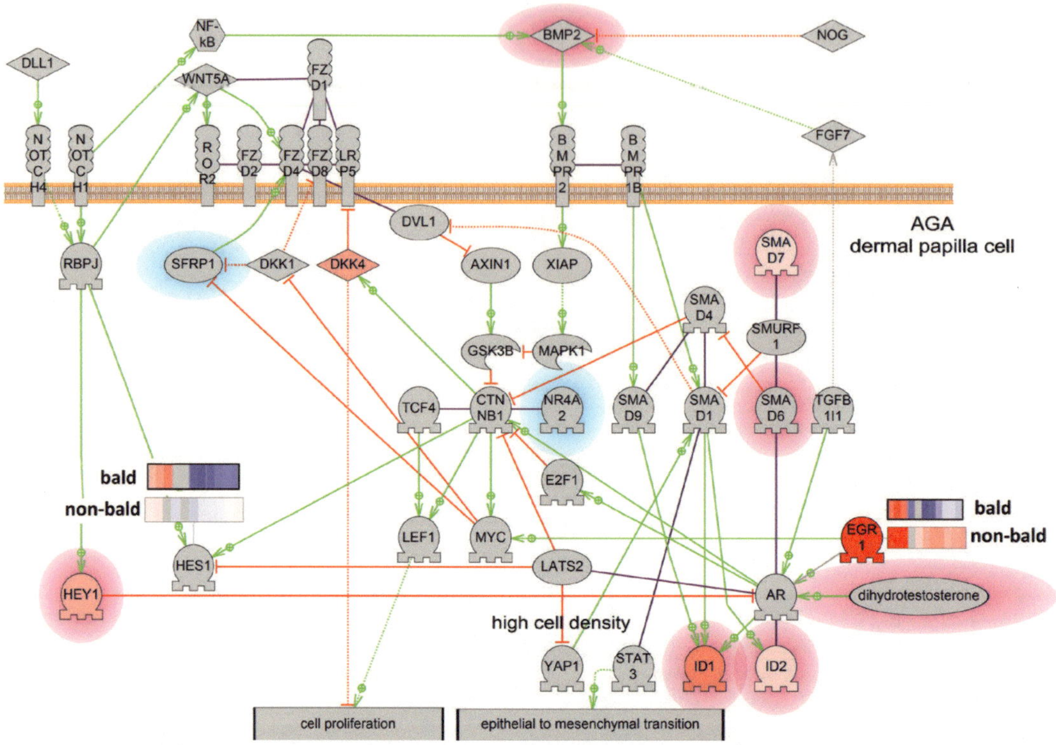

Figure 6. Model of BMP, WNT, NOTCH, and AR-related pathway cross-talk in AGA dermal papilla cell.DKK4, EGR1, HEY1 and ID1-2 are underexpressed genes in nonbald DP cells 1–3 h after DHT treatment (datasets 5–6). The higher color saturation reflects the higher degree of differential expression ([0.5; 0.5] log-change interval, 0.05 p-value cutoff). SFRP1 and NR4A2 are underexpressed genes in bald DP cells 1 and 3 h after DHT treatment (datasets 3–4). BMP2, SMAD6-7, HEY1, and ID1-2 are overexpressed genes. DKK1 and DKK4 inhibit WNT due to feedback loop in WNT signaling. AR regulates WNT pathway through LATS2, EGR1, and CTNNB1. BMP signaling inhibits activity of WNT pathway. BMP signaling in general inhibits WNT signaling. NOTCH pathway has negative effect on AR expression via HEY1. EGR1 and HES1 have significant changes in expression at all time points assessed after DHT treatment, so their expression is shown with heat maps.

Perhaps, larger amount of DHT is needed to stimulate AR-related DKK1 expression. High level of DKK1 was observed within 3–6 h after 50–100 nM DHT treatment previously [45]. In mice, DKK1 expression, similarly to BMP2/4 expression, is time-dependent in hair cycle and is changing according to hair follicle cycle phase [70]. We could not find severe relevant difference in the pattern of WNT signaling activity, which is not surprising, since fluctuations in these networks are closely associated with current hair cycle phase, which is, firstly, poorly studied in human, and secondly, impossible to verify in a culture of separated dermal papilla.

SFRP1 is one of the significant overexpressed in dataset 1 genes that could stimulate WNT pathway. Other speculations we developed on the basis of pathway analysis of current microarray data are shown (**Figure 6**).

As shown in **Figure 7**, numerous feedback loops regulate BMP/WNT crass-talk themselves, as well as intersections with AR and other signaling pathways, such as SHH, NOTCH, or Hippo/YAP1 [73].

http://dx.doi.org/10.5772/67845

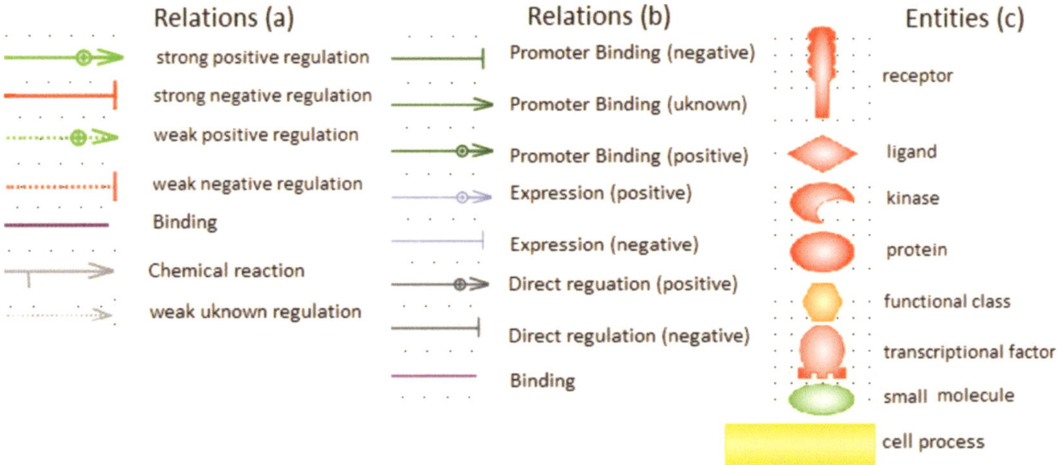

Figure 7. Legend for entities and relations displayed on pathways . Relations from ResNet® used in **Figures 1, 5**, and **6 (a)** and in **Figures 2** and **4 (b)** are shown. Shapes of entities from ResNet® used in **Figures 1–6** are shown **(c)**.

LATS2 is a DHT-responsible underexpressed gene in bald DP cell samples in current analysis. LATS2 phosphorylates and cause the degradation of the transcriptional co-activators Hippo/YAP1 and TAZ, which are in turn interact with RUNX1, SMAD7, and play role in TGF-beta/BMP/SMADs signaling inhibition [128]. SMAD7 and SMAD6 were detected slightly underexpressed in bald DP cell samples before 6-/12-h time point.

Overexpression of PTGDS in hair follicles during catagen was shown previously [55]. We detect overexpression of other type of synthase (PTGS2) of prostaglandins in current analysis (**Figure 5**). PTGS2 is DHT/AR-inducible expression target in skin [129]. Prostaglandin has different role, such as enhancing of the vascularization and chemotaxis.

In mice, FGF7 is one of the DP signature genes that elevated during telogen. FGF7 participates in instructing DP cells to proliferate and initiate the new hair cycle [64]. In current microarray, we did not detected significant overexpression of FGF7 in bald DP cells in datasets 3–6. FGF18 and its expression target RUNX1 were among SNEA regulators of underexpressed DE genes in dataset 3–4 at 12-h time point. SPRY1 may contribute to FGF signaling regulation in dermal cells. SPRY1 expression was shown to induce upon activation of the FGF receptor signaling pathway in cells of mesenchymal and epithelial origin [130]. In response to growth factors, SPRY1 binds GRB2 and inhibits downstream intracellular signaling. SPRY1 gene had negatively DE trend in bald samples after 1 h of DHT treatment (**Figure 5**).

4. Conclusion

Hair follicle miniaturization in androgenic alopecia is complex process induced by AR influence on dermal papilla cell function. Signaling pathways are useful models of complicated protein interactions in dermal papilla cell during hair follicle cycle. Cross-talks between AR and TGFB, BMP, and WNT signaling are believed to promote shortage on amount and functional activity of dermal papilla cells in bald scalp in AGA. WNT signaling is considered to be the main trigger of telogen anagen transition that drives repopulation of dermal papilla progenitor cells from bulge niche. Its impairment could potentially lead to AGA phenotype. Detailed understanding of molecular causes of hair loss in AGA is still has not been reached. New standardized studies of hair follicle cell cycle in human scalp are required to find human-specific information about dermal papilla and stem cells maintenance during their lifetime renewals.

Pathway analysis of cDNA microarray data from cultured immortalized human DP cells from balding (frontal) AGA scalps reveals activation of chromatin remodeling and metaphase-anaphase transition pathways. Observed slight up-regulation of cell cycle inhibitor protein CDKN2A confirms other studies and indicates up-regulation of DNA repairing pathways. Expression of AR-related genes NOS3, EGR1, SMAD6, BTG2, and LATS2 was significantly down-regulated exclusively after DHT treatment in frontal DP cells compared to occipital bald cells from AGA scalp. Differential expression of TGFB1I1, TGFB2, THBS1, PTHLH, and ANGPT2 was not changed dramatically, but they appeared among top 25 regulators of underexpressed genes in bald DP cells samples. TGFB1I1 is a reported AR cofactor. Ligands TGFB2, THBS1, PTHLH, and ANGPT2 launch receptors signaling related to catagen progression (and ligand CTGF to telogen). MIR106A was found among the top of significant miRNA regulators of DE genes in bald DP cells.

After 1 h of DHT treatment, EGR1 and EGR2 genes reduced their expression by more than 70% in balding versus nonbalding scalp. SPRY1 and CEPBD and NR4A2 genes had also negatively differential expression trend in bald samples. CYB1P1 and CTGF had positively increased in bald samples versus nonbald after 1 h of DHT treatment. DKK1 as WNT inhibitor was underexpressed in nonbald DP samples 1 h after DHT treatment. DKK4 was, vice versa, overexpressed in nonbald DP cells in the first 1 h. NR4A2, EGR1, HES1, and NR4A2 had remarkable difference in expression between bald and nonbald DP cell samples. Unfortunately, role of these proteins was acquired in cancer-related studies that make them hardly applicable to the hair follicle research. Further investigation is required.

The obtained results suggest that AGA dermal papilla in frontal scalp area differs from occipital ones unlikely due to downregulation of proliferation and increased expression of catagen triggers, but rather due to reduced expression of anagen triggers.

5. Methods

5.1. Pathway analysis

We chose several public studies about hair loss in men with AGA using microarray technology from GEO database (http://www.ncbi.nlm.nih.gov/geo/). Data from GSE66664 dataset were log2 transformed, quantile normalized, and then imported into Pathway Studio® software. We used Pathway Studio® version 9 with ResNet® database version 12.

Differentially expressed genes were identified with two-class unpaired T-test implemented in Pathway Studio®. Multiple probes were averaged by best p-value or maximum magnitude. Selection of differentially expressed genes was made using samples BAB (GSM1623702-72) and BAN (GSM1627372-441) after 0 min and after 15 min, 30 min, 3 **h**, 24 **h**, and 48 h after DHT treatment.

Cell processes and pathways enriched in over (under) DE genes were set up with GSEA algorithm or Fisher exact test. From DE list, significantly expressed genes were chosen with 0.05 p-value and 2-fold change of the expression (log change interval $[-1; 1]$) cutoffs. In GSEA, Mann-Whitney U-test with 0.05 p-value cutoff was applied, followed by expanding of the content of proteins groups. GO biological process groups and pathway collection from Pathway Studio were used as gene set. The pathway collection included Cell Process, Receptor Signaling, Expression targets, Canonical Signal Transduction Signaling, Immunology, Toxicity, and Disease sub-collections (2160 pathways in total). Moreover, 10 pathways were constructed specifically for analysis of hair follicle-specific genes expression. These are Dermal Papilla Cells Proliferation in Anagen; Dermal papilla Cell Regression in Catagen; Keratinocytes Apoptosis; Melanocytes Differentiation; Hair Stem Cells Maintenance; Androgen Synthesis in Sebocytes; Sebocytes Proliferation; Hair follicle in Telogen; Immune System Activation in AGA; Androgen Receptor Genomic, and Non-genomic Signaling (files with pathways available in Pathways Studio® or in XML format upon request). Total numbers of entities and relations in hair follicle-related pathways are 150 and 76, respectively.

To find statistically significant regulators of DE genes, SNEA algorithm was applied. SNEA is a sub-network analysis of DE genes or proteins based on GSEA method and 2 million biological relations in ResNet® database [71]. The choice of neighbors for sub-network generating was entities upstream of DE genes (proteins/genes, complexes, functional classes) connected by relations of "Expression" or "Promoter Binding" types. We used 0.05 p-value cutoff and limit of 100 generated sub-networks ranked by best p-value. We performed SNEA to find 100 significant miRNA regulators.

Pathways statistically enriched with discovered list of regulators were found with Fisher exact test. All images have been exported from Pathway Studio with special color specification (all overexpressed genes in experiment are red, all underexpressed genes are blue, entities not measured or filtered with p-value or log change cutoff are grey).

5.2. Signaling pathway reconstruction

Pathway Studio® software and ResNet® database from Elsevier were used for building hair follicle cells specific interactive model pathways. Model signaling pathways reconstruction was based on current scientific knowledge: settled facts and hypotheses (e.g., data acquired in animal models). Pathway creation relies on published papers and searching ResNet® database for neighbors, functions, and expression of chosen proteins and molecules.

Model of cell specific molecular interactions in this article consists in an interactive signaling pathway that is represented by the graphical scheme and the annotations. In the graphical representation, the members of interactions are shown linked together with functional relations. The annotations section includes the information about properties of pathway members and relations pulled out from ResNet® database. ResNet® database storages dictionary and ontology of biological-related entities (proteins, small molecules, diseases, cell processes, cells, treatments, etc.) linked together by relations (such as protein 1-protein 2 "binding") (**Figure 7**). Relations depict facts supporting by sentences (references) with scientific evidences which are extracted from more than 3 million articles and manually curated when adding to pathways. The relations indicate the effect of relation (negative or positive), the direction of the relation, mechanism of the relation (such as phosphorylation), etc. [71]. The method of the pathway reconstruction required looking for common relationships to entities in the database (common downstream cell process or disease, upstream regulators, downstream expression targets, etc.) and reviewing manually the results.

Supplemental Information:

Supplemental Table 1 and Supplemental Table 2 could be downloaded via link:

https://data.mendeley.com/datasets/yfnrkc7r9x/1

Author details

Anastasia Nesterova* and Anton Yuryev

*Address all correspondence to: a.nesterova@elsevier.com

Elsevier Life Sciences Solutions, Rockville, Maryland, USA

References

[1] Oh JW, Kloepper J, Langan EA, Kim Y, Yeo J, Kim MJ, et al. A guide to studying human hair follicle cycling in vivo. J Invest Dermatol. 2016;136:34–44. doi:10.1038/JID.2015.354

[2] Hamilton JB. Patterned loss of hair in man; types and incidence. Ann N Y Acad Sci. 1951;53:708–28

[3] Ludwig E. Classification of the types of androgenetic alopecia (common baldness) occurring in the female sex. Br J Dermatol. 1977;97:247–54. doi:10.1111/j.1365-2133.1977.tb15179.x

[4] Randall VA, Jenner TJ, Hibberts NA, De Oliveira IO, Vafaee T. Stem cell factor/c-Kit signalling in normal and androgenetic alopecia hair follicles. J Endocrinol. 2008;197:11–23. doi:10.1677/JOE-07-0522

[5] Sawaya ME, Price VH. Different levels of 5alpha-reductase type I and II, aromatase, and androgen receptor in hair follicles of women and men with androgenetic alopecia. J Invest Dermatol. 1997;109:296–300. doi:10.1111/1523-1747.ep12335779

[6] Brinkmann AO. Molecular mechanisms of androgen action—a historical perspective. Methods Mol Biol Clifton NJ. 2011;776:3–24. doi:10.1007/978-1-61779-243-4_1

[7] Ellis JA, Sinclair R, Harrap SB. Androgenetic alopecia: pathogenesis and potential for therapy. Expert Rev Mol Med. 2002;4:1–11. doi:10.1017/S1462399402005112

[8] Hibberts NA, Messenger AG, Randall VA. Dermal papilla cells derived from beard hair follicles secrete more stem cell factor (SCF) in culture than scalp cells or dermal fibroblasts. Biochem Biophys Res Commun. 1996;222:401–405. doi:10.1006/bbrc.1996.0756

[9] Plikus MV, Widelitz RB, Maxson R, Chuong C-M. Analyses of regenerative wave patterns in adult hair follicle populations reveal macro-environmental regulation of stem cell activity. Int J Dev Biol. 2009;53:857–68. doi:10.1387/ijdb.072564mp

[10] Rathnayake D, Sinclair R. Male androgenetic alopecia. Expert Opin Pharmacother. 2010;11:1295–304. doi:10.1517/14656561003752730

[11] Yuryev A, Kotelnikova E, Daraselia N. Ariadne's ChemEffect and Pathway Studio knowledge base. Expert Opin Drug Discov. 2009;4:1307–18. doi:10.1517/17460440903413488

[12] García-Campos MA, Espinal-Enríquez J, Hernández-Lemus E. Pathway analysis: state of the art. Front Physiol. 2015;6:383. doi:10.3389/fphys.2015.00383

[13] Henderson-Maclennan NK, Papp JC, Talbot CC, McCabe ERB, Presson AP. Pathway analysis software: annotation errors and solutions. Mol Genet Metab. 2010;101:134–40. doi:10.1016/j.ymgme.2010.06.005

[14] Müller-Röver S, Handjiski B, van der Veen C, Eichmüller S, Foitzik K, McKay IA, et al. A comprehensive guide for the accurate classification of murine hair follicles in distinct hair cycle stages. J Invest Dermatol. 2001;117:3–15. doi:10.1046/j.0022-202x.2001.01377.x

[15] Shimomura Y, Christiano AM. Biology and genetics of hair. Annu Rev Genomics Hum Genet. 2010;11:109–32. doi:10.1146/annurev-genom-021610-131501

[16] Alonso L, Fuchs E. The hair cycle. J Cell Sci. 2006;119:391–3. doi:10.1242/jcs.02793

[17] Paus R, Cotsarelis G. The biology of hair follicles. N Engl J Med. 1999;341:491–7. doi:10.1056/NEJM199908123410706

[18] Jackson EA. Hair disorders. Prim Care Clin Off Pract. 2000;27:319–32. doi:10.1016/S0095-4543(05)70198-6

[19] Plikus MV. New activators and inhibitors in the hair cycle clock: targeting stem cells' state of competence. J Invest Dermatol. 2012;132:1321–4. doi:10.1038/jid.2012.38

[20] Kligman AM. The comparative histopathology of male-pattern baldness and senescent baldness. Clin Dermatol. 1988;6:108–18. doi:10.1016/0738-081X(88)90074-0

[21] Jahoda C a. B. Cellular and developmental aspects of androgenetic alopecia. Exp Dermatol. 1998;7:235–48. doi:10.1111/j.1600-0625.2007.00666.x

[22] Jaworsky C, Kligman A m., Murphy G f. Characterization of inflammatory infiltrates in male pattern alopecia: implications for pathogenesis. Br J Dermatol. 1992;127:239–46. doi:10.1111/j.1365-2133.1992.tb00121.x

[23] Lattanand A, Johnson WC. Male pattern alopecia a histopathologic and histochemical study. J Cutan Pathol. 1975;2:58–70. doi:10.1111/j.1600-0560.1975.tb00209.x

[24] Kaufman KD. Androgen metabolism as it affects hair growth in androgenetic alopecia. Dermatol Clin. 1996;14:697–711

[25] Kaufman KD, Olsen EA, Whiting D, Savin R, DeVillez R, Bergfeld W, et al. Finasteride in the treatment of men with androgenetic alopecia. Finasteride Male Pattern Hair Loss Study Group. J Am Acad Dermatol. 1998;39:578–89.

[26] Ellis JA, Scurrah KJ, Cobb JE, Zaloumis SG, Duncan AE, Harrap SB. Baldness and the androgen receptor: the AR polyglycine repeat polymorphism does not confer susceptibility to androgenetic alopecia. Hum Genet. 2007;121:451–7. doi:10.1007/s00439-006-0317-8

[27] Schweikert HU, Wilson JD. Regulation of human hair growth by steroid hormones. II. Androstenedione metabolism in isolated hairs. J Clin Endocrinol Metab. 1974;39:1012–9. doi:10.1210/jcem-39-6-1012

[28] Chen W, Tsai S-J, Liao C-Y, Tsai R-Y, Chen Y-J, Pan B-J, et al. Higher levels of steroidogenic acute regulatory protein and type I 3beta-hydroxysteroid dehydrogenase in the scalp of men with androgenetic alopecia. J Invest Dermatol. 2006;126:2332–2335. doi:10.1038/sj.jid.5700442

[29] Inui S, Itami S. Molecular basis of androgenetic alopecia: From androgen to paracrine mediators through dermal papilla. J Dermatol Sci. 2011;61:1–6. doi:10.1016/j.jdermsci.2010.10.015

[30] Rutberg SE, Kolpak ML, Gourley JA, Tan G, Henry JP, Shander D. Differences in expression of specific biomarkers distinguish human beard from scalp dermal papilla cells. J Invest Dermatol. 2006;126:2583–2595. doi:10.1038/sj.jid.5700454

[31] Chew EGY, Tan JHJ, Bahta AW, Ho BS-Y, Liu X, Lim TC, et al. Differential expression between human dermal papilla cells from balding and non-balding scalps reveals new candidate genes for androgenetic alopecia. J Invest Dermatol. 2016;136:1559–67. doi:10.1016/j.jid.2016.03.032

[32] Goodarzi HR, Abbasi A, Saffari M, Fazelzadeh Haghighi M, Tabei MB, Noori Daloii MR. Differential expression analysis of balding and nonbalding dermal papilla microRNAs in male pattern baldness with a microRNA amplification profiling method. Br J Dermatol. 2012;166:1010–6. doi:10.1111/j.1365-2133.2011.10675.x

[33] Kim SJ, Dix DJ, Thompson KE, Murrell RN, Schmid JE, Gallagher JE, et al. Gene expression in head hair follicles plucked from men and women. Ann Clin Lab Sci. 2006;36:115–26.

[34] Midorikawa T, Chikazawa T, Yoshino T, Takada K, Arase S. Different gene expression profile observed in dermal papilla cells related to androgenic alopecia by DNA macroarray analysis. J Dermatol Sci. 2004;36:25–32. doi:10.1016/j.jdermsci.2004.05.001

[35] Hibberts NA, Howell AE, Randall VA. Balding hair follicle dermal papilla cells contain higher levels of androgen receptors than those from non-balding scalp. J Endocrinol. 1998;156:59–65.

[36] Hamada K, Randall VA. Inhibitory autocrine factors produced by the mesenchyme-derived hair follicle dermal papilla may be a key to male pattern baldness. Br J Dermatol. 2006;154:609–618. doi:10.1111/j.1365-2133.2006.07144.x

[37] Hunt DPJ, Morris PN, Sterling J, Anderson JA, Joannides A, Jahoda C, et al. A highly enriched niche of precursor cells with neuronal and glial potential within the hair follicle dermal papilla of adult skin. Stem Cells Dayt Ohio. 2008;26:163–72. doi:10.1634/stemcells.2007-0281

[38] Legué E, Nicolas J-F. Hair follicle renewal: organization of stem cells in the matrix and the role of stereotyped lineages and behaviors. Development. 2005;132:4143–54. doi:10.1242/dev.01975

[39] Zhang P, Kling RE, Ravuri SK, Kokai LE, Rubin JP, Chai J, et al. A review of adipocyte lineage cells and dermal papilla cells in hair follicle regeneration. J Tissue Eng. 2014;5:2041731414556850. doi:10.1177/2041731414556850

[40] Ohyama M, Kobayashi T, Sasaki T, Shimizu A, Amagai M. Restoration of the intrinsic properties of human dermal papilla in vitro. J Cell Sci. 2012;125:4114–25. doi:10.1242/jcs.105700

[41] Hoffmann R, Rot A, Niiyama S, Billich A. Steroid sulfatase in the human hair follicle concentrates in the dermal papilla. J Invest Dermatol. 2001;117:1342–8. doi:10.1046/j.0022-202x.2001.01547.x

[42] Zhuo FL, Xu W, Wang L, Wu Y, Xu ZL, Zhao JY. Androgen receptor gene polymorphisms and risk for androgenetic alopecia: a meta-analysis. Clin Exp Dermatol. 2012;37:104–11. doi:10.1111/j.1365-2230.2011.04186.x

[43] Lai J-J, Chang P, Lai K-P, Chen L, Chang C. The role of androgen and androgen receptor in skin-related disorders. Arch Dermatol Res. 2012;304:499–510. doi:10.1007/s00403-012-1265-x

[44] Kaliyadan F, Nambiar A, Vijayaraghavan S. Androgenetic alopecia: an update. Indian J Dermatol Venereol Leprol. 2013;79:613–625. doi:10.4103/0378-6323.116730

[45] Kwack MH, Kim MK, Kim JC, Sung YK. Dickkopf 1 promotes regression of hair follicles. J Invest Dermatol. 2012;132:1554–1560. doi:10.1038/jid.2012.24

[46] Yu M, Kissling S, Freyschmidt-Paul P, Hoffmann R, Shapiro J, McElwee KJ. Interleukin-6 cytokine family member oncostatin M is a hair-follicle-expressed factor with hair growth inhibitory properties. Exp Dermatol. 2008;17:12–19. doi:10.1111/j.1600-0625.2007.00643.x

[47] Kitagawa T, Matsuda K-I, Inui S, Takenaka H, Katoh N, Itami S, et al. Keratinocyte growth inhibition through the modification of Wnt signaling by androgen in balding dermal papilla cells. J Clin Endocrinol Metab. 2009;94:1288–1294. doi:10.1210/jc.2008-1053

[48] Kwack MH, Sung YK, Chung EJ, Im SU, Ahn JS, Kim MK, et al. Dihydrotestosterone-inducible dickkopf 1 from balding dermal papilla cells causes apoptosis in follicular keratinocytes. J Invest Dermatol. 2008;128:262–9. doi:10.1038/sj.jid.5700999

[49] Andl T, Reddy ST, Gaddapara T, Millar SE. WNT signals are required for the initiation of hair follicle development. Dev Cell. 2002;2:643–53.

[50] Inui S, Fukuzato Y, Nakajima T, Kurata S, Itami S. Androgen receptor co-activator Hic-5/ARA55 as a molecular regulator of androgen sensitivity in dermal papilla cells of human hair follicles. J Invest Dermatol. 2007;127:2302–6. doi:10.1038/sj.jid.5700883

[51] Kwack MH, Ahn JS, Kim MK, Kim JC, Sung YK. Dihydrotestosterone-inducible IL-6 inhibits elongation of human hair shafts by suppressing matrix cell proliferation and promotes regression of hair follicles in mice. J Invest Dermatol. 2012;132:43–49. doi:10.1038/jid.2011.274

[52] Gilliver SC, Ashworth JJ, Mills SJ, Hardman MJ, Ashcroft GS. Androgens modulate the inflammatory response during acute wound healing. J Cell Sci. 2006;119:722–32. doi:10.1242/jcs.02786

[53] Lee P, Zhu C-C, Sadick NS, Diwan AH, Zhang PS, Liu JS, et al. Expression of androgen receptor coactivator ARA70/ELE1 in androgenic alopecia. J Cutan Pathol. 2005;32:567–71. doi:10.1111/j.0303-6987.2005.00397.x

[54] Kollara A, Brown TJ. Expression and function of nuclear receptor co-activator 4: evidence of a potential role independent of co-activator activity. Cell Mol Life Sci CMLS. 2012. doi:10.1007/s00018-012-1000-y

[55] Garza LA, Liu Y, Yang Z, Alagesan B, Lawson JA, Norberg SM, et al. Prostaglandin D2 inhibits hair growth and is elevated in bald scalp of men with androgenetic alopecia. Sci Transl Med. 2012;4:126ra34–126ra34. doi:10.1126/scitranslmed.3003122

[56] Bahta AW, Farjo N, Farjo B, Philpott MP. Premature senescence of balding dermal papilla cells in vitro is associated with p16(INK4a) expression. J Invest Dermatol. 2008;128:1088–94. doi:10.1038/sj.jid.5701147

[57] Yang Y-C, Fu H-C, Wu C-Y, Wei K-T, Huang K-E, Kang H-Y. Androgen receptor accelerates premature senescence of human dermal papilla cells in association with DNA damage. PLoS One. 2013;8:e79434. doi:10.1371/journal.pone.0079434

[58] Ito M, Kizawa K, Hamada K, Cotsarelis G. Hair follicle stem cells in the lower bulge form the secondary germ, a biochemically distinct but functionally equivalent progenitor cell population, at the termination of catagen. Differentiation. 2004;72:548–557. doi:10.1111/j.1432-0436.2004.07209008.x

[59] Rahmani W, Abbasi S, Hagner A, Raharjo E, Kumar R, Hotta A, et al. Hair follicle dermal stem cells regenerate the dermal sheath, repopulate the dermal papilla, and modulate hair type. Dev Cell. 2014;31:543–58. doi:10.1016/j.devcel.2014.10.022

[60] Ohyama M, Terunuma A, Tock CL, Radonovich MF, Pise-Masison CA, Hopping SB, et al. Characterization and isolation of stem cell-enriched human hair follicle bulge cells. J Clin Invest. 2006;116:249–60. doi:10.1172/JCI26043

[61] Najafzadeh N, Esmaeilzade B, Dastan Imcheh M. Hair follicle stem cells: In vitro and in vivo neural differentiation. World J Stem Cells. 2015;7:866–72. doi:10.4252/wjsc.v7.i5.866

[62] Inoue K, Aoi N, Sato T, Yamauchi Y, Suga H, Eto H, et al. Differential expression of stem-cell-associated markers in human hair follicle epithelial cells. Lab Invest. 2009;89:844–56. doi:10.1038/labinvest.2009.48

[63] Poblet E, Jiménez F, Godínez J m., Pascual-Martín A, Izeta A. The immunohistochemical expression of CD34 in human hair follicles: a comparative study with the bulge marker CK15. Clin Exp Dermatol. 2006;31:807–12. doi:10.1111/j.1365-2230.2006.02255.x

[64] Greco V, Chen T, Rendl M, Schober M, Pasolli HA, Stokes N, et al. A two-step mechanism for stem cell activation during hair regeneration. Cell Stem Cell. 2009;4:155–69. doi:10.1016/j.stem.2008.12.009

[65] Garza LA, Yang C-C, Zhao T, Blatt HB, Lee M, He H, et al. Bald scalp in men with androgenetic alopecia retains hair follicle stem cells but lacks CD200-rich and CD34-positive hair follicle progenitor cells. J Clin Invest. 2011;121:613–622. doi:10.1172/JCI44478

[66] Myung P, Ito M. Dissecting the bulge in hair regeneration. J Clin Invest. 2012;122:448–454. doi:10.1172/JCI57414

[67] Goldstein J, Horsley V. Home sweet home: skin stem cell niches. Cell Mol Life Sci. 2012;69:2573–82. doi:10.1007/s00018-012-0943-3

[68] DasGupta R, Fuchs E. Multiple roles for activated LEF/TCF transcription complexes during hair follicle development and differentiation. Dev Camb Engl. 1999;126:4557–68.

[69] Blanpain C, Fuchs E. Epidermal stem cells of the skin. Annu Rev Cell Dev Biol. 2006;22:339–73. doi:10.1146/annurev.cellbio.22.010305.104357

[70] Plikus MV, Baker RE, Chen C-C, Fare C, de la Cruz D, Andl T, et al. Self-organizing and stochastic behaviors during the regeneration of hair stem cells. Science. 2011;332:586–9. doi:10.1126/science.1201647

[71] Genander M, Cook PJ, Ramsköld D, Keyes BE, Mertz AF, Sandberg R, et al. BMP signaling and its pSMAD1/5 target genes differentially regulate hair follicle stem cell lineages. Cell Stem Cell. 2014;15:619–33. doi:10.1016/j.stem.2014.09.009

[72] Kandyba E, Hazen VM, Kobielak A, Butler SJ, Kobielak K. Smad1 and 5 but not Smad8 establish stem cell quiescence which is critical to transform the premature hair follicle during morphogenesis toward the postnatal state. Stem Cells Dayt Ohio. 2014;32:534–47. doi:10.1002/stem.1548

[73] Chen D, Zhao M, Mundy GR. Bone morphogenetic proteins. Growth Fact. 2004;22:233–241. doi:10.1080/08977190412331279890

[74] Schneider MR, Schmidt-Ullrich R, Paus R. The hair follicle as a dynamic miniorgan. Curr Biol. 2009;19:R132–42. doi:10.1016/j.cub.2008.12.005

[75] Sakaki-Yumoto M, Katsuno Y, Derynck R. TGF-β family signaling in stem cells. Biochim Biophys Acta. 2013;1830:2280–96. doi:10.1016/j.bbagen.2012.08.008

[76] Walsh C, Hu P, Batt J, Santos C. Microarray meta-analysis and cross-platform normalization: integrative genomics for robust biomarker discovery. Microarrays. 2015;4:389–406. doi:10.3390/microarrays4030389

[77] Sivachenko AY, Yuryev A, Daraselia N, Mazo I. Molecular networks in microarray analysis. J Bioinform Comput Biol. 2007;5:429–56. doi:10.1142/S0219720007002795

[78] Subramanian A, Tamayo P, Mootha VK, Mukherjee S, Ebert BL, Gillette MA, et al. Gene set enrichment analysis: a knowledge-based approach for interpreting genome-wide expression profiles. Proc Natl Acad Sci U S A. 2005;102:15545–50. doi:10.1073/pnas.0506580102

[79] Barrett T, Wilhite SE, Ledoux P, Evangelista C, Kim IF, Tomashevsky M, et al. NCBI GEO: archive for functional genomics data sets—update. Nucleic Acids Res. 2013;41:D991–5. doi:10.1093/nar/gks1193

[80] Chen W, Yang C-C, Tsai R-Y, Liao C-Y, Yen Y-T, Hung C-L, et al. Expression of sex-determining genes in the scalp of men with androgenetic alopecia. Dermatology. 2007;214:199–204. doi:10.1159/000099583

[81] Yamaguchi Y, Itami S, Watabe H, Yasumoto K-I, Abdel-Malek ZA, Kubo T, et al. Mesenchymal-epithelial interactions in the skin: increased expression of dickkopf1 by palmoplantar fibroblasts inhibits melanocyte growth and differentiation. J Cell Biol. 2004;165:275–85. doi:10.1083/jcb.200311122

[82] Klokk TI, Kurys P, Elbi C, Nagaich AK, Hendarwanto A, Slagsvold T, et al. Ligand-specific dynamics of the androgen receptor at its response element in living cells. Mol Cell Biol. 2007;27:1823–43. doi:10.1128/MCB.01297-06

[83] Mao B, Zhang Z, Wang G. BTG2: a rising star of tumor suppressors (review). Int J Oncol. 2015;46:459–64. doi:10.3892/ijo.2014.2765

[84] Banno T, Gazel A, Blumenberg M. Effects of tumor necrosis factor-alpha (TNF alpha) in epidermal keratinocytes revealed using global transcriptional profiling. J Biol Chem. 2004;279:32633–42. doi:10.1074/jbc.M400642200

[85] Suzuki H, Yabuta N, Okada N, Torigata K, Aylon Y, Oren M, et al. Lats2 phosphorylates p21/CDKN1A after UV irradiation and regulates apoptosis. J Cell Sci. 2013;126:4358–68. doi:10.1242/jcs.125815

[86] Visser S, Yang X. LATS tumor suppressor: a new governor of cellular homeostasis. Cell Cycle Georget Tex. 2010;9:3892–903. doi:10.4161/cc.9.19.13386

[87] Kang J-I, Kim S-C, Kim M-K, Boo H-J, Kim E-J, Im G-J, et al. Effects of dihydrotestosterone on rat dermal papilla cells in vitro. Eur J Pharmacol. 2015;757:74–83. doi:10.1016/j.ejphar.2015.03.055

[88] Yang S-Z, Abdulkadir SA. Early growth response gene 1 modulates androgen receptor signaling in prostate carcinoma cells. J Biol Chem. 2003;278:39906–11. doi:10.1074/jbc.M307250200

[89] Xie B, Wang C, Zheng Z, Song B, Ma C, Thiel G, et al. Egr-1 transactivates Bim gene expression to promote neuronal apoptosis. J Neurosci Off J Soc Neurosci. 2011;31:5032–44. doi:10.1523/JNEUROSCI.5504-10.2011

[90] Lee JH, Gaddameedhi S, Ozturk N, Ye R, Sancar A. DNA damage-specific control of cell death by cryptochrome in p53-mutant ras-transformed cells. Cancer Res. 2013;73:785–91. doi:10.1158/0008-5472.CAN-12-1994

[91] Gobinet J, Carascossa S, Cavaillès V, Vignon F, Nicolas J-C, Jalaguier S. SHP represses transcriptional activity via recruitment of histone deacetylases. Biochemistry (Mosc). 2005;44:6312–20. doi:10.1021/bi047308d

[92] Ayadi A, Suelves M, Dollé P, Wasylyk B. Net, an Ets ternary complex transcription factor, is expressed in sites of vasculogenesis, angiogenesis, and chondrogenesis during mouse development. Mech Dev. 2001;102:205–8. doi:10.1016/S0925-4773(01)00289-1

[93] Fukuda T, Kanomata K, Nojima J, Urakawa I, Suzawa T, Imada M, et al. FGF23 induces expression of two isoforms of NAB2, which are corepressors of Egr-1. Biochem Biophys Res Commun. 2007;353:147–51. doi:10.1016/j.bbrc.2006.12.011

[94] Yu J, Akishita M, Eto M, Koizumi H, Hashimoto R, Ogawa S, et al. Src kinase-mediates androgen receptor-dependent non-genomic activation of signaling cascade leading to endothelial nitric oxide synthase. Biochem Biophys Res Commun. 2012;424:538–43. doi:10.1016/j.bbrc.2012.06.151

[95] Cui Y, Qin L, Wu J, Qu X, Hou C, Sun W, et al. SIRT3 enhances glycolysis and proliferation in SIRT3-expressing gastric cancer cells. PLoS One. 2015;10:e0129834. doi:10.1371/journal.pone.0129834

[96] Yang F, Li X, Sharma M, Sasaki CY, Longo DL, Lim B, et al. Linking beta-catenin to androgen-signaling pathway. J Biol Chem. 2002;277:11336–44. doi:10.1074/jbc.M111962200

[97] Bazzi H, Fantauzzo KA, Richardson GD, Jahoda CAB, Christiano AM. The Wnt inhibitor, Dickkopf 4, is induced by canonical Wnt signaling during ectodermal appendage morphogenesis. Dev Biol. 2007;305:498–507. doi:10.1016/j.ydbio.2007.02.035

[98] Piscopo DM, Johansen EB, Derynck R. Identification of the GATA factor TRPS1 as a repressor of the osteocalcin promoter. J Biol Chem. 2009;284:31690–703. doi:10.1074/jbc.M109.052316

[99] Fantauzzo KA, Christiano AM. Trps1 activates a network of secreted Wnt inhibitors and transcription factors crucial to vibrissa follicle morphogenesis. Dev Camb Engl. 2012;139:203–14. doi:10.1242/dev.069971

[100] Schlake T. Krox20, a novel candidate for the regulatory hierarchy that controls hair shaft bending. Mech Dev. 2006;123:641–8. doi:10.1016/j.mod.2006.06.001

[101] Fang F, Shangguan AJ, Kelly K, Wei J, Gruner K, Ye B, et al. Early growth response 3 (Egr-3) is induced by transforming growth factor-β and regulates fibrogenic responses. Am J Pathol. 2013;183:1197–208. doi:10.1016/j.ajpath.2013.06.016

[102] Collins S, Waickman A, Basson A, Kupfer A, Licht JD, Horton MR, et al. Regulation of CD4+ and CD8+ effector responses by Sprouty-1. PLoS One. 2012;7:e49801. doi:10.1371/journal.pone.0049801

[103] Thisse B, Thisse C. Functions and regulations of fibroblast growth factor signaling during embryonic development. Dev Biol. 2005;287:390–402. doi:10.1016/j.ydbio.2005.09.011

[104] Munkley J, Lafferty NP, Kalna G, Robson CN, Leung HY, Rajan P, et al. Androgen-regulation of the protein tyrosine phosphatase PTPRR activates ERK1/2 signalling in prostate cancer cells. BMC Cancer. 2015;15:9. doi:10.1186/s12885-015-1012-8

[105] Yueh M-F, Li T, Evans RM, Hammock B, Tukey RH. Triclocarban mediates induction of xenobiotic metabolism through activation of the constitutive androstane receptor and the estrogen receptor alpha. PLoS One. 2012;7:e37705. doi:10.1371/journal.pone.0037705

[106] DuSell CD, Nelson ER, Wittmann BM, Fretz JA, Kazmin D, Thomas RS, et al. Regulation of aryl hydrocarbon receptor function by selective estrogen receptor modulators. Mol Endocrinol Baltim Md. 2010;24:33–46. doi:10.1210/me.2009-0339

[107] Jung S, Li C, Duan J, Lee S, Kim K, Park Y, et al. TRIP-Br1 oncoprotein inhibits autophagy, apoptosis, and necroptosis under nutrient/serum-deprived condition. Oncotarget. 2015;6:29060–75. doi:10.18632/oncotarget.5072

[108] Ao J, Meng J, Zhu L, Nie H, Yang C, Li J, et al. Activation of androgen receptor induces ID1 and promotes hepatocellular carcinoma cell migration and invasion. Mol Oncol. 2012;6:507–15. doi:10.1016/j.molonc.2012.06.005

[109] Liao G, Chen L-Y, Zhang A, Godavarthy A, Xia F, Ghosh JC, et al. Regulation of androgen receptor activity by the nuclear receptor corepressor SMRT. J Biol Chem. 2003;278:5052–61. doi:10.1074/jbc.M206374200

[110] O'Kane M, Markham T, McEvoy AN, Fearon U, Veale DJ, FitzGerald O, et al. Increased expression of the orphan nuclear receptor NURR1 in psoriasis and modulation following TNF-alpha inhibition. J Invest Dermatol. 2008;128:300–10. doi:10.1038/sj.jid.5701023

[111] Auld KL, Berasi SP, Liu Y, Cain M, Zhang Y, Huard C, et al. Estrogen-related receptor α regulates osteoblast differentiation via Wnt/β-catenin signaling. J Mol Endocrinol. 2012;48:177–91. doi:10.1530/JME-11-0140

[112] Pérez-Sieira S, López M, Nogueiras R, Tovar S. Regulation of NR4A by nutritional status, gender, postnatal development and hormonal deficiency. Sci Rep. 2014;4:4264. doi:10.1038/srep04264

[113] Pulido-Salgado M, Vidal-Taboada JM, Saura J. C/EBPβ and C/EBPδ transcription factors: Basic biology and roles in the CNS. Prog Neurobiol. 2015;132:1–33. doi:10.1016/j.pneurobio.2015.06.003

[114] Lindqvist A, Rodriguez-Bravo V, Medema RH. The decision to enter mitosis: feedback and redundancy in the mitotic entry network. J Cell Biol. 2009;185:193–202. doi:10.1083/jcb.200812045

[115] Yu DW, Yang T, Sonoda T, Gong Y, Cao Q, Gaffney K, et al. Osteopontin gene is expressed in the dermal papilla of pelage follicles in a hair-cycle-dependent manner. J Invest Dermatol. 2001;117:1554–8. doi:10.1046/j.0022-202x.2001.01568.x

[116] Li H, Li T, Wang S, Wei J, Fan J, Li J, et al. miR-17-5p and miR-106a are involved in the balance between osteogenic and adipogenic differentiation of adipose-derived mesenchymal stem cells. Stem Cell Res. 2013;10:313–24. doi:10.1016/j.scr.2012.11.007

[117] Li D, Yu W, Liu M. Regulation of KiSS1 gene expression. Peptides. 2009;30:130–8. doi:10.1016/j.peptides.2008.09.025

[118] Raveh E, Cohen S, Levanon D, Negreanu V, Groner Y, Gat U. Dynamic expression of Runx1 in skin affects hair structure. Mech Dev 2006;123:842–50. doi:10.1016/j.mod.2006.08.002

[119] Kong X, Ma S, Guo J, Ma Y, Hu Y, Wang J, et al. Ubiquitously expressed transcript is a novel interacting protein of protein inhibitor of activated signal transducer and activator of transcription 2. Mol Med Rep. 2015;11:2443–8. doi:10.3892/mmr.2014.3023

[120] Kerosuo L, Bronner ME. Biphasic influence of Miz1 on neural crest development by regulating cell survival and apical adhesion complex formation in the developing neural tube. Mol Biol Cell. 2014;25:347–55. doi:10.1091/mbc.E13-06-0327

[121] Li Y, Yang J, Luo J-H, Dedhar S, Liu Y. Tubular epithelial cell dedifferentiation is driven by the helix-loop-helix transcriptional inhibitor Id1. J Am Soc Nephrol JASN. 2007;18:449–60. doi:10.1681/ASN.2006030236

[122] Mita P, Savas JN, Djouder N, Yates JR, Ha S, Ruoff R, et al. Regulation of androgen receptor-mediated transcription by RPB5 binding protein URI/RMP. Mol Cell Biol. 2011;31:3639–52. doi:10.1128/MCB.05429-11

[123] Sancar A, Lindsey-Boltz LA, Unsal-Kaçmaz K, Linn S. Molecular mechanisms of mammalian DNA repair and the DNA damage checkpoints. Annu Rev Biochem. 2004;73:39–85. doi:10.1146/annurev.biochem.73.011303.073723

[124] Lu S, Jenster G, Epner DE. Androgen induction of cyclin-dependent kinase inhibitor p21 gene: role of androgen receptor and transcription factor Sp1 complex. Mol Endocrinol Baltim Md. 2000;14:753–60. doi:10.1210/mend.14.5.0461

[125] Vitolo MI, Anglin IE, Mahoney WM, Renoud KJ, Gartenhaus RB, Bachman KE, et al. The RUNX2 transcription factor cooperates with the YES-associated protein, YAP65, to promote cell transformation. Cancer Biol Ther. 2007;6:856–63. doi:10.4161/cbt.6.6.4241

[126] Schmidt M, Asirvatham AJ, Chaudhary J. Inhibitor of differentiation 1 (ID1) promotes cell survival and proliferation of prostate epithelial cells. Cell Mol Biol Lett. 2010;15:272–95. doi:10.2478/s11658-010-0007-3

[127] Rendl M, Lewis L, Fuchs E. Molecular dissection of mesenchymal-epithelial interactions in the hair follicle. PLoS Biol. 2005;3:e331. doi:10.1371/journal.pbio.0030331

[128] Ferrigno O, Lallemand F, Verrecchia F, L'Hoste S, Camonis J, Atfi A, et al. Yes-associated protein (YAP65) interacts with Smad7 and potentiates its inhibitory activity against TGF-beta/Smad signaling. Oncogene. 2002;21:4879–84. doi:10.1038/sj.onc.1205623

[129] Simanainen U, Ryan T, Li D, Suarez FG, Gao YR, Watson G, et al. Androgen receptor actions modify skin structure and chemical carcinogen-induced skin cancer susceptibility in mice. Horm Cancer. 2015;6:45–53. doi:10.1007/s12672-014-0210-1

[130] Nadeau RJ, Toher JL, Yang X, Kovalenko D, Friesel R. Regulation of Sprouty2 stability by mammalian Seven-in-Absentia homolog 2. J Cell Biochem. 2007;100:151–60. doi:10.1002/jcb.21040

Section 5

Cicatricial Alopecia

Chapter 10

Cicatricial Alopecias

Ibrahim Halil Yavuz, Goknur Ozaydin Yavuz and
Serap Gunes Bilgili

Additional information is available at the end of the chapter

http://dx.doi.org/10.5772/67277

Abstract

Primary cicatricial alopecias (PCA) are a rare group of disorders in which the hair follicle is the main target of destructive inflammation resulting in irreversible hair loss with scarring of affected lesions. Inflammation may predominantly involve lymphocytes or neutrophils. Cicatricial alopecias that mainly involve lymphocytic inflammation include lichen planopilaris, discoid lupus erythematosus, pseudopelade (Brocq), central centrifugal alopecia, alopecia mucinosa, and keratosis follicularis spinulosa decalvans. Cicatricial alopecias that are due to predominantly neutrophilic inflammation include folliculitis decalvans and dissecting cellulitis of the scalp. Acne keloidalis, acne necrotica, and erosive pustular dermatosis are cicatricial alopecias with a mixed inflammatory infiltrate.

Keywords: cicatricial alopecia, lichen planopilaris, discoid lupus erythematosus

1. Introduction

Cicatricial alopecias are the result of various diseases of the scalp. It is usually circumscribed but may be widespread [1]. It presents as areas of hair loss in which the underlying scalp is scarred, sclerosed, or atrophic [1, 2]. In early stages, the underlying disease is usually diagnosable clinically and histologically, but in later stages, only scarring may be evident [3–5]. The scarring is the result of the destruction and fibrosis of hair follicles [1, 6, 7]. The primary cicatricial alopecias, which are the focus of this chapter, can be particularly challenging clinically. Several classification schemes for primary cicatricial alopecia exist in the literature. Workshop sponsored by the North American Hair Research Society, a working classification of primary cicatricial alopecias based on the predominant inflammatory cellular infiltrate was developed (**Table 1**) [8].

1—Lymphocytic
Lichen planopilaris
Classic lichen planopilaris
Frontal fibrosing alopecia
Graham-Little syndrome
Chronic cutaneous lupus erythematosus
Classic pseudopelade
Central centrifugal cicatricial alopecia
Alopecia mucinosa
Keratosis follicularis spinulosa decalvans
2—Neutrophilic
Folliculitis decalvans
Dissecting cellulitis
3—Mixed
Acne keloidalis
Acne necrotica
Erosive pustular dermatosis
4—Nonspecific

Table 1. Classification of primary cicatricial alopecias.

2. Lymphocytic cicatricial alopecias

2.1. Lichen planopilaris

Lichen planopilaris is a rare disease characterized by autoreactive lymphocytic destruction of the hair follicle and is the cause of progressive cicatricial alopecia. Perifollicular erythema, squams, and keratotic follicular papules are commonly encountered clinical findings of LPP (**Figure 1**) [4, 9]. Although diagnosis can be made clinically and histopathologically in the early stages, it becomes more difficult to diagnose in the late stages due to the absence of specific findings [1, 5]. Lichen planopilaris can be subdivided into three groups including classic lichen planopilaris, frontal fibrosing alopecia, and Graham-Little syndrome [4, 6]. Classic lichen planopilaris presents as scalp hair involvement and is sometimes accompanied by extracranial lichen forms. Frontal fibrosing alopecia is characterized by band-like scarring alopecia of the frontal hairline that usually affects middle-aged women. Graham-Little syndrome, also known as Graham-Little-Piccardi-Lasseur syndrome, is a disease having a triad of cicatricial alopecia, lichen planus spinulosus, and nonscarring hair loss of axillary and pubic area [1].

http://dx.doi.org/10.5772/67277

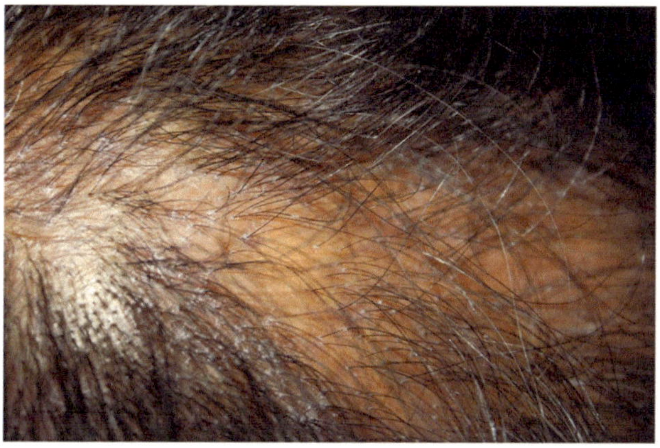

Figure 1. Lichen planopilaris.

2.1.1. Classic lichen planopilaris

It was initially described by Pringle. It is more common in women than in men. Light-skinned individuals are more frequently affected than dark-skinned individuals. Most patients visit a doctor in the first year [1, 4, 10]. Although the etiology of lichen planopilaris is poorly understood, the most widely accepted theory states that it is an autoimmune disorder in which Langerhans cells-activated T lymphocytes destroy keratinocytes. In LPP, most T lymphocytes are located around the bulge area. It is seen that cells in the bulge area are multipotent and are important in generating anagen hair follicle. Destruction of follicular stem cells localized in the bulge area is found to be significant in lichen planopilaris [4, 11]. Contact sensitizers such as metals can enhance a T cell inflammatory reaction. Commonly encountered metals are gold, mercury, and cobalt. The role of infection is determined in the development of LPP. These infections include hepatitis C, HIV, HSV type 2, Helicobacter pylori, and HPV. It was observed that antimalarial agents, beta-blockers, thiazides, ACE inhibitors aggravate lichen planopilaris, and classic lichen planus [1, 3, 4, 12]. Although the pathogenesis of lichen planopilaris shows extensive similarities to the lichen planus, some reports point out differences in immunoreactant deposition. Lichenoid dermatitis is histopathologically detected at the dermoepidermal junction around follicular infundibulum and isthmus. Occasionally similar lichenoid changes may be observed at the papillary dermis between surface epithelium and hair follicles. Mild to severe dyskeratosis and lymphocytic infiltration are encountered. However, epidermal and dermal mucin accumulation seen in DLE are not found [3, 4]. Immunofluorescence evaluation may demonstrate the deposition of fibrinogen, IgM or rarely C3, and IgA at the follicular basement membrane zone of the follicle in a linear pattern. Histopathological findings vary according to disease progression and sometimes it may be difficult to diagnose. It is especially difficult to diagnose in the late stages due to follicular scar. The biopsy site selection is an important process to establish an exact diagnosis. It is recommended to perform biopsy in areas particularly having active lesions. Active inflammatory areas are squamous, erythematous, and also symptomatic [3,

13, 14]. First signs of LPP include alopecia and pruritus. Rarely pain, burning, and seborrheic dermatitis are observed. The most frequent clinical forms are perifollicular erythema and affinitative, violescent brown, hyperkeratotic follicular papules and flat, atrophic, polygonal-sided alopecic plaques are subsequently appeared following the aggregation of papules. Scalp lesions may be single or multiple, focal, or wide. They are most frequently involved in the vertex and parietal area. Tiny alopecic patches slowly proceed and bind with other patches causing reticular pattern. Pull test is positive in the active periods [1, 4, 15]. Distinctive diagnosis of classic lichen planopilaris is carried out with DLE, pseudopelade of Brocq, folliculitis decalvans, keratosis pilaris spondiloza, alopecia mucinosa, and seborrheic dermatitis. The lack of pustules supports the distinction from folliculitis decalvans. In the clinical manifestation, histopathologic and immunohistochemical properties of LPP facilitate the differentiation from other diseases.

LPP is difficult to treat. Local and systemic therapies are used. Local therapies are initially selected in most cases since they are relatively safe. The aim of therapy is to reduce subjective symptoms and to prevent inflammation and progression [4, 15]. Topical and intralesional corticosteroids are often chosen as the first-line therapy. However, best regimen of treatment for topical corticosteroids in LPP is not known. High potent corticosteroids are mainly selected. If there is no response to corticosteroid therapy, other alternative drugs should be considered. Intralesional corticosteroid injections reduce inflammation significantly. However, atrophy can occur. In progressive patients, prednisone, an oral corticosteroid, can be given at 1 mg/kg/day over 2–4 months. Relapse may occur following the withdrawal of systemic corticosteroid therapy. Hydroxychloroquine has an immunomodulatory property and is well tolerated. Effects of treatment are initiated within 2–3 months and maximal clinical efficacy may take up to 6–12 months. 400 mg/day of oral hydroxychloroquine therapy is recommended after liver function test, complete blood count, and ophthalmologic examination. Adverse reactions are rare, but include abdominal pain, anorexia, nausea, myalgia, skin hyperpigmentation, and ophthalmologic damage. Smoking may decrease efficacy. Cyclosporine is effective in lichen planus. There are reports with mycophenolate mofetil especially in patients unresponsive to corticosteroids and hydroxychloroquine therapy demonstrating its efficacy and lower side effect profile [3, 16]. Other treatment options include retinoids, tetracycline, griseofulvin, thalidomide, dapsone, topical tacrolimus, and minoxidil. However, there effectiveness is still controversial [4, 9].

2.1.2. Frontal fibrosing alopecia

Frontal fibrosing alopecia (FFA), first described by Kossard in 1994, is a form of lichen planopilaris characterized by cicatricial alopecia at the frontoparietal hairline and it occurs primarily in postmenopausal women. Although the disease occurred typically in postmenopausal women, it is rarely seen in men too. A total of 80 cases have been reported so far [17, 18]. Etiopathogenesis of FFA is not fully understood. As most of the cases are postmenopausal, hormone-related triggering mechanisms are thought to play role in the etiopathogenesis. In some cases, successful usage of 5-alpha reductase inhibitors supports the latter. Some reports state that the occurrence of familial cases of FFA points to a possible genetic contribution. The most characteristic clinical feature of frontal fibrosing alopecia is the progressive recession of

http://dx.doi.org/10.5772/67277

the frontal and parietal hairline. All FFA patients exhibit this finding which is required to diagnose [17, 19, 20]. Hairline recession usually occurs symmetrically and bilaterally, giving rise to a band of alopecia between 0.5 and 8 cm from its original site. The progression is relatively slow, and erythema and hyperkeratosis papules indistinguishable from that seen in LPP are common findings. Eyebrow loss or thinning was reported in 62.82% of patients. Despite 50% of lichen planus lesions are observed in lichen planopilaris, the prevalence is only 5% in FFA [3, 17, 21]. Histopathological and immunofluorescence evaluations are similar to classic lichen planopilaris. However, it is harder to diagnose in the late stages. Causes of cicatricial alopecia should be considered in the differential diagnosis of FFA. Clinical features of FFA differ from other alopecias by its histopathological features [1, 4, 22]. Precise, effective treatment options are limited. There are no randomized clinical studies. Corticosteroids are proper approach in the early stages. Systemic corticosteroids can be administered in the dose of 0.5–3 mg/kg per day for a period of 3–18 months. Some studies demonstrated that topical corticosteroids were not effective. Intralesional corticosteroid treatment used in the advanced stages may even worsen the disease rather than improvement. Topical minoxidil revealed controversial results. Mono- or combination therapy of finasteride produced successful results. Other treatment options including griseofulvin, isotretinoin, tacrolimus, pimecrolimus, cyclosporin, hydroxychloroquine do not show promising results [3, 19, 23].

2.1.3. *Graham-Little syndrome (Piccardi-Lasseur syndrome)*

It was first described by Piccardi in 1914 and the components of the disease were described by Graham-Little in 1915. It has a triad of cicatricial alopecia of the scalp, noncicatricial alopecia of axillae and pubic region and keratotic follicular papules over body and extremities [24]. Patients are generally females aged 30–70 years. The rate of incidence is four times higher in women. Its exact etiology is not known, but it is thought to be a variant of lichen planopilaris [24, 25]. Cellular immunity seems to play a role in the clinical manifestation. However, in a number of cases, hepatitis B vaccination and genetic patterns were thought to be the causes [26, 27]. In the early stages, alopecic patches-like lesions, perifollicular erythema occur in the periphery of scalp [1, 22]. Atrophy is not observed even there is no loss in the hair follicles in the axillae and pubic region. Follicular keratosis occurring mostly over body and extremities is rarely observed on the eyebrows. Histopathological findings include follicular orthokeratotic hyperkeratosis in the early lesions, perifollicular infiltrate of lymphocytes, and loss in pilosebaceous unit. Similar to other cicatricial alopecias, fibrosis is observed in the advanced stages [24, 25]. Treatment options may include topical and systemic corticosteroids, and cyclosporine [24, 28].

2.2. Discoid lupus erythematosus

Cutaneous lupus erythematosus is a widespread disease group. It may be categorized into three main entities: acute, subacute, and chronic. Discoid lupus erythematosus (DLE), is often related to the cicatricial alopecia. Discoid lupus erythematosus most often affects women in 4th and 5th decade of life. Its etiology is not fully understood [4, 29]. It seems that disease occurs following the exposure to UV light of sensitive individuals accompanied by the increase in keratinocyte apoptosis and the induction of reactive T cell or immunocomplex-mediated response [30, 31]. Compared to other lupus erythematosus forms, the course is benign and transformation to systemic lupus erythematosus is less than 10%. Generalized forms of discoid lupus tend to transform into systemic forms [1, 30, 31].

Approximately 20% of men with DLE and 50% of women exhibit cicatricial alopecia. Lesions are clinically transformed from definite macules and papules into adhesive squams followed by discoid plaques (coin-like shape). Plaques may be painful and itchy. In the course of time, these lesions transform into atrophic plaques having peripheral hyperpigmentation, depigmentation in the middle. Exposure to sun light and trauma may induce the disease [1, 30, 32]. Lesions evolved to squamous cell carcinoma over years. Scalp hair involvement occurred during the first year of disease. Patients generally consult a physician with complaints in hair loss increase and itching. Rarely stinging, burning or scalp sensitivity may occur. Lesions are generally at the vertex localization. Coupled with the centrifugal progression of lesions, plaques containing follicular plugs are formed. Telangiectasia and atrophy are observed on plaques. Approximately 35% of DLE patients manifest a positive antinuclear antibody. Lupus band test is positive in 90% of DLE lesions [4, 31, 32]. Histopathology of DLE reflects its clinical presentation. Epidermis is generally atrophic. Vacuolar degeneration in basal keratinocytes and thickening in the basal membrane are confirmed. Lymphocytic infiltrate is observed around veins and adnexal structures in the dermis. Mucin accumulation is the most significant indicator of cutaneous lupus erythematosus. Collagen and elastic fibrils may get damaged. Lymphocytic infiltrate may diffuse to the subcutaneous fatty tissue. In more than 90% of biopsies IgG and C3 depositions are demonstrated immunopathologically. It is hard to presume the prognosis and course of DLE. Newly diagnosed patients should be evaluated in terms of SLE. Complete physical examination, routine blood tests, urine analysis and anti-dsDNA antibodies are examined. If it is negative, it is regarded as skin-limited form [3, 29, 31, 33].

Differential diagnosis should consider lupus vulgaris, actinic keratosis, sarcoidosis, rosacea, psoriasis, lichen planus granuloma annulare, tinea faciei, and seborrheic dermatitis. Clinically, histopathological and immunological tests are favorable in differentiating from other diseases [1, 4].

First step of the therapy is to recommend sun protection. First-line therapy options include corticosteroids and antimalarial agents. Corticosteroids are administered in forms of potent topical corticosteroids or intralesional triamcinolone acetonide (4–10 mg/mL, monthly injections). Most frequently used antimalarial drug, hydroxychloroquine should be initially started in doses of 200–400 mg daily. Pediatric posology is 4–6 mg/kg. Basal ophthalmological examination and complete blood count should be performed. Side effects are rare and include abdominal pain, anorexia, nausea, myalgia, skin hyperpigmentation, hematologic changes, and ophthalmological damage. Oral corticosteroids can be used until efficacy has been proven (1 mg/kg, tapering in 8 weeks). Oral retinoids can be tried in unresponsive cases. For this purpose, acitretin (50 mg per day) or isotretinoin (40 mg per day) are used. Moreover, topical immunomodulatory agents (e.g., tacrolimus), thalidomide, dapsone, and oral vitamin C may be considered. If none of these treatments are found to be effective, oral immunosuppressant therapies (mycophenolate mofetil, methotrexate, and azathioprine) are initiated [31, 34–36].

http://dx.doi.org/10.5772/67277

2.3. Classic pseudopelade of Brocq

It was first described by Brocq in 1888. It is frequently characterized as slowly progressing disease with cicatricial alopecic patches without chronic inflammation [37–39]. The cause is not known. There are many debates on accounting the disease. While some researchers believe that Pseudopelade of Brocq is clinicopathologically different disease, some reported that it the last phase of primary cicatricial alopecias. Consequently, successful determination of the disease is not available until this date. The epidemiology is not known. Although Pseudopelade of Brocq may occur in both genders, it is more frequent in women over 40 years of age. It is very rare in pediatric population. Although its etiopathogenesis is not fully understood, the possible causes include genetics, autoimmunity, and infections [1, 38]. Pseudopelade of Brocq is a chronic, and insidious form of primary cicatricial alopecia. There are usually no symptoms. Mild itching may be present. Three clinical forms were identified by Brocq including scattered small plaques, large plaques, and a combination of both. Vertex involvement is frequently observed in all three forms. Patients rarely have squams. Small plaques showed confetti-like scattering. Classic Pseudopelade of Brocq involves scalp, however, beard involvement occurs too. The course of disease is slow and progressive but some cases rarely exhibit fast progression [3, 38]. Biopsy is significant to diagnose histopathologically. Two deep punch biopsies along clinically active alopecic areas should be taken. To differentiate from other cicatricial alopecias patients should undergo both routine and direct immunofluorescence examination. Pseudopelade of Brocq does not have pathognomonic histopathological properties. In the early lesions, there is mild perivascular and perifollicular lymphocyte infiltrate. However, interphase changes are not present. Sebaceous glands are diminished or absent. Follicular epithelial atrophy is present two deep punch biopsies along clinically active alopecic areas should be taken two deep punch biopsies along clinically active alopecic areas should be taken [40, 41]. As alopecia develops, atrophy becomes evident in the infundibular epithelium. Direct immunofluorescence findings are usually negative. In the advanced stages, atrophic epidermis is seen on the dermis containing follicular fibrotic bands extending to the subcutaneous tissue [42, 43]. Differential diagnosis should include alopecia areata, lichen planopilaris, discoid lupus erythematosus, and central centrifugal alopecia.

Treatment objective is to prevent clinical remission and progression of the disease. Unfortunately, the progression still continues even after treatment [38, 44, 45]. Choice of therapy depends mainly on activity, extent, and tolerance of the disease. In patients having less than 10% scalp involvement, topical or intralesional corticosteroid therapy is the first choice. There are reports stating the efficacy of topical tacrolimus and topical minoxidil therapies. In addition, there are also reports indicating that systemic prednisolone, hydroxychloroquine, isotretinoin therapies are effective [36, 43, 44].

2.4. Central centrifugal cicatricial alopecia

It was first described by LoPresti et al. and also referred to as hot comb alopecia and follicular degeneration syndrome [46]. It is the most common form of cicatricial alopecia in African American females. Although its etiopathogenesis is not fully understood, the causes include usage of hot comb, styling practices, chemical agents, infections, autoimmune diseases, and genetics [47, 48]. Clinically disease initiated at the vertex and middle of the scalp, as it progresses, it can cause centrifugal baldness. Symptoms such as itching or pain are often absent or mild. Most of patients are adult black women [48, 49]. Histopathologic features include perifollicular lymphocytic infiltrate, and fibrosis in the early stages. Terminal follicle count is diminished. In the advanced stages, sebaceous gland and follicle loss are observed. Dyskeratosis and epidermal mucin accumulation are absent. Perifollicular erythema and follicular keratosis is usually absent. Pigment incontinence is minimal. Histopathology in the last stage is similar to other cicatricial alopecias [48, 50]. Moreover, chronic transitional alopecia, androgenic alopecia, alopecia areata, trichotillomania, folliculitis decalvans should be excluded [1, 49, 51].

Treatment objective is to stop progression rather than hair growth. Regrowth is not possible due to the formation of scar tissue. This is related to styling methods and even though this relation is not confirmed, natural hair care techniques not causing trauma are recommended. Hair care method involving chemicals and techniques causing traction should be eliminated [3, 49–53]. Until the disease is stabilized, daily topical corticosteroids usage followed by three times a week posology is recommended. 10 mg/ml doses of intralesional corticosteroids are applied once a month for at least 6 months. The therapy is then continued depending upon the symptoms. Especially in severe cases, oral anti-inflammatory drugs such as tetracycline are applied for at least 6 months. In order to reduce itching and desquamation, seborrhoeic dermatitis-like therapy (shampoos containing zinc pyrithione and/or ketoconazole) is recommended. Antimalarial agents, minoxidil, thalidomide, cyclosporine, mycophenolate mofetil, vitamins, and several herbal treatments are found to be effective. The treatment should be continued at least 6 months and following enhancement, it should be lasted for a year until the remission. Besides, hair transplantation may be performed. Wigs can also be used [1, 36, 43, 49].

2.5. Alopecia mucinosa

It is also known as follicular mucinosis and characterized by the follicular papillary erythema and squam formation in the perifollicular zone [4, 54]. All age groups can be affected and its initiation can go to the infiltrate period. Its etiopathogenesis is not fully understood. Antigenic stimulus T cell-related follicular response formed in hair follicles is thought to increase the folliculotropic response.

Occurrence of lymphoproliferative diseases in 30% of adult patients is an important step in the etiopathogenesis. Its course includes sharp-edged erythematous squamous plaques. The most significant involvement occurs in the head and neck. Alopecia is seen when lesion affects hair follicles. Dysesthesia and anesthesia can be observed in lesions [1, 55, 56]. Clinically, acne-formed, hypopigmented, eczematous plaques and endured nodule forms are reported. Clinically there are 3 types. Primary or benign type occurs in young patients and it is the only lesion tending to improve in several years. Secondary or malignant type occurs in the elderly and it is characterized by many lesions. Third type is chronic benign form having properties of both [4, 55, 57]. The most malignity associated with alopecia mucinosa is mycosis fungoides. Other malignities include leukemia, Hodgkin lymphoma, renal carcinoma, lymphosarcoma. Its

http://dx.doi.org/10.5772/67277

pathology reveals several mucin accumulation in follicular epithelium and sebaceous tissues, perivascular, and perifollicular lymphocyte infiltrates. Dyskeratosis and lameller fibrosis are absent [55, 57].

Differential diagnosis is performed by alopecia areata, telogen effluvium, lichen planopilaris, morphea, tinea capitis, subcutaneous panniculitis-like T cell lymphoma, and dissecting folliculitis.

The most effective therapy in benign type alopecia mucinosa is intralesional steroid treatment. There are a wide range of therapy options. These are topical oral antibiotics, topical retinoids, steroids, dapsone, methotrexate, immunosuppressive agents, nitrogen mustard, and PUVA. In the malignity-associated alopecia mucinosa direct malignity treatment should be performed. Long term follow-ups are needed in chronic alopecia mucinosa [3, 36, 57, 58].

2.6. Keratosis follicularis spinulosa decalvans

Keratosis follicularis spinulosa decalvans (KFSD) is also known as keratosis pilaris decalvans. It was first described by Siemens in 1926. It is characterized by scalp follicular hyperkeratosis and photophobia. The end point is atrophy and cicatricial alopecia. Transition depending on X and sporadic cases also occur. It is thought to be a part of keratosis pilaris atrophicans [59–61]. Its etiology is not known. It is usually initiated around facial with follicular hyperkeratosis in the early life. Later on, it spreads on scalp, hair, and eyelashes. Patch-like alopecia on scalp, hair, and eyelashes occurs and it is followed by cicatrices is observed on alopecic areas. Reddish-brown telangiectasia on lesions can be seen. Moderate itching is present. *Staphylocuccus aureus*-related pustule infections can worsen the disease. The disease is generally more severe in men [4, 62, 63]. Histopathologic examination revealed intrafollicular and perifollicular edema and neutrophil infiltrate. As the disease progresses, mucin accumulation around the top of follicles and perivascular and perifollicular lymphocyte infiltration are detected [3, 61, 62].

Differential diagnosis should include KID syndrome, lichen planopilaris, and folliculitis decalvans.

Treatment should be done especially in childhood where the disease is active. Unfortunately, there is no specific treatment. Topical and intralesional corticosteroids, oral retinoids, and dapsone can be used [63, 64].

3. Neutrophilic cicatricial alopecias

3.1. Folicullitis decalvans

Foliculitis decalvans is a disease occurred in pustules on scalp. The cause is not known. Some researchers blame isolation of *S. aureus* in the pustular lesions as its etiology. Immune interaction between microorganisms and the host is thought to be the most significant factor in folliculitis development. Its epidemiology is not fully known. It is one of most important causes of cicatricial alopecia. The prevalence is same in both genders [65–67]. Clinically initial lesion is erythema follicular pustule and papule. These can be painful and itchy. Later, new pustules are observed and accumulated to form pustular milier abscess (**Figure 2**). Consequently, cicatricial alopecia plaques have been formed [67]. Tufted folliculitis is characterized by having more than one hair on dilated orificial follicles. It is often seen in folliculitis decalvans [67, 68]. Concurrently DLE, LPP, acne keloid, and tinea capitis can occur during the course. In order to diagnose folliculitis decalvans, biopsy must be taken from pustules. Although pathognomonic findings are absent in the histopathological evaluation, follicular neutrophilic pustules in the early stages, plasma cells in chronic period are seen. As a response to follicular damage, foreign matter granules can be formed and consequently common fibrosis occurs. Careful histological and clinical evaluation should be carried out even after the diagnosis since the disease can overlap with other alopecias. Diagnosis should take into consideration of dissecting folliculitis, acne keloid, erosive pustular dermatosis, acne necrotica, DLE, CCCPA, LPP, and pseudopelade [67, 68].

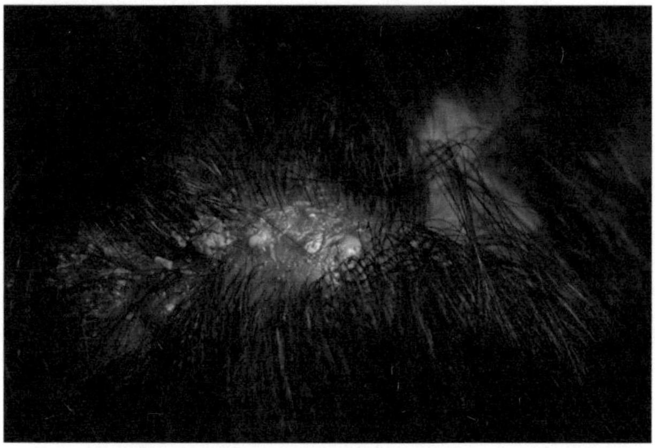

Figure 2. Folliculitis decalvans; pustules on the scalp are noticed.

Bacterial cultures should be taken from each patient and antibiotic resistance should be determined prior treatment. Long-term antibiotics targeting *S. Auerus* must be used. Tetracycline, coloxylin, erythromycin is used as first-line therapy. Antibiotic treatment is initiated as in acne and reduced according to the response. The disadvantage of antibiotic therapy is recurrence. Clindamycin and rifampicin is used in combination in unresponsive patients. Other effective choice of therapy is isotretinoin. It can be administered intralesionally in fast progressive cases. Other treatments include dapsone, hydroxychloroquine, adalimumab, infliximab. Wigs can be recommended as cosmetic camouflage in patients with cicatricial alopecia [36, 69, 70].

3.2. Dissecting cellulitis

Described by Hoffman in 1908, it is also known as perifolliculitis capitis abscedens et suffodiens. It forms follicular occlusion triad along with acne conglobate and hidradenitis suppurativa. If pilonidal cysts are added to the picture, they all referred as tetrad. Dissecting cellulitis most commonly affects young black men with an average age of 18–40 years. Although its etiopathogenesis remains shrouded in mystery, *S. aureus*-induced neutrophilic response is the cause. It seems genetically transferred disease since familial cases have been reported [71, 72]. Initial lesion is generally follicular pustules at the vertex. Later, these are transformed into painful nodules. Accumulated nodules form tubular bridges. Seropurulent discharge can occur on nodules. Skin can be covered by crut and squams. Hypertrophic and keloid scar atrophy and cicatricial alopecia may occur in patients treated insufficiently. Although spontaneous remission occurs, relapse is frequent. Cervical and occipital lymphadenopathy may be observed [1, 3, 72].

In its histopathology, perifolliculitis formed by lymphocyte around follicles, histiocyte and polymorphous nuclear cells is present. Superficial fat tissue and abscess formation may be observed in dermis. Intensive fibrosis occurs in the late stages [71, 72].

Medical treatment of dissecting folliculitis involves high doses of isotretinoin. Antibiotics such as minocycline, tetracycline, erythromycin, clindamycin along with zinc sulfate, dapsone, colchicine, corticosteroids can be recommended as other treatment options. In persistent cases, surgical interventions such as excision and grafting may be considered [73–76].

4. Mixed cicatricial alopecias

4.1. Acne keloidalis

Acne keloidalis was first described in 1869 by Kohn. This disease is also known as folliculitis keloidalis nuchae or folliculitis keloidalis. The term acne keloidalis is somewhat of a misnomer since the condition is neither a kind of acne nor keloidal in nature. Acne keloidalis is most often seen in African Americans. The prevalence in American football players is 15%. Mechanical trauma, infections, autoimmunity, and drugs are the causes in its etiopathogenesis [76–78]. It is clinically developed in the early stages on the occipital scalp and on the nape of the neck as reddish-brown colored papules with smooth surface. Occasionally, these papules transformed into nodules and plaques. Pustules and abscesses are rarely occurred. Intrafollicular and perifollicular lymphocytes and plasma cell infiltrates are histopathologically involved in the early lesions. In the advanced stages, follicular destruction develops. Sebaceous glands disappear. Differential diagnosis should include folliculitis decalvans, acne necrotica, and dissecting folliculitis [1, 76].

First-line therapy of acne keloidalis is prevention. Preventing trauma and infections is important. In mild cases, combination of potent topical corticosteroids with topical antibiotics is advantageous. Oral tetracycline may be added to the monthly injections of intralesional corticosteroids. Partial response can be obtained by cryotherapy and laser therapy. Effective lasers include carbon dioxide, 1064 nm Nd:YAG or 810 nm diode. Surgical excision may be needed for common keloidal plaques. Surgical approaches include excision with primary closure or secondary intention healing. Deep surgical excision is more efficient. Surgical excision is an effective option [36, 79, 80].

4.2. Acne necrotica

Acne necrotica is also known as folliculitis necrotica. It is a mysterious disease not understood by many dermatologists. Infections are routinely mentioned in its etiology but evidence cannot be demonstrated. Drugs and food allergies are also thought to be the cause. Mechanical factors such as itching only spread the disease. Most of patients are women. Lesions are generally observed on the scalp along face and hairline. They are rarely occurred on nose and cheeks [4, 81, 82]. Initial lesions are umbilicated follicular papules. Not long after, they transformed into pustules. Consequently, varioliform scars may develop. Initially perivascular and perifollicular lymphocytic infiltrate, subepidermal edema is apparent. In the advanced stages, necrosis is observed in the follicular epithelium and epidermis [3, 81]. Neutrophiles can be seen in superficial dermis. Differential diagnosis should also include folliculitis decalvans, dissecting folliculitis, colitis, eczema herpeticum, and molluscum contagiosum [81, 82].

Treatment with oral tetracycline, antistaphylococcal antibiotics may be effective. They should be used in long term. In patients not having complete response, topical or intralesional corticosteroid can be added. Isotretinoin treatment may prolong the remission period [4, 43].

4.3. Erosive pustular dermatosis

The disease was first described in 1979 by Pye et al. and about 100 cases have been reported so far [83]. The disease most commonly occurs in elderly and females. Sun damage, local trauma (surgery, cryotherapy, herpes zoster), and autoimmunity are blamed in its etiology. Lesions with crusts and pustules on atrophic skin are clinically observed. The number of pustules can vary remarkably, and in some cases they are absent. Pain and pruritus in the lesions are not observed. However, cicatricial alopecia may develop in the advanced stages. Histopathology is uncharacteristic and not very helpful in confirming the diagnosis [84, 85]. Histopathological examination is crucial to exclude other diseases. Histopathology shows subcorneal pustules, epidermal atrophy, and erosions. In addition, these findings can be accompanied by a polymorphous dermal inflammatory infiltrate and in some cases leukocytoclastic vasculitis might be present. The differential diagnosis should consider tinea capitis, Gram-negative folliculitis, pyoderma gangrenosum, DLE, pemphigus vulgaris, and SCC. High-potency topical steroids reduce the inflammation significantly [1, 85].

Steroids must be used more than 6 months for better responses. Other treatment options include tacrolimus, dapsone, calcipotriol, and acitretin. Sun protection is reported to be effective since disease etiology includes actinic damage [86, 87].

5. Conclusion

Cicatricial alopecia forms an important group of disorders that end up with scarring and persistent hair loss. An elaborate physical examination, skin biopsies and blood tests can be helpful in order to establish the accurate diagnosis and to suggest the most appropriate treatment for the hair loss. Many patients do not respond to the first treatment they receive and the condition frequently relapses when treatment is stopped. Some clinics offer surgical treatment, such as scalp reduction surgery and hair transplantation, but it may not be suitable for all patients. Patients often have significant psychosocial impact and management of these patients should address not only their physical but also psychological aspects.

Author details

Ibrahim Halil Yavuz*, Goknur Ozaydin Yavuz and Serap Gunes Bilgili

*Address all correspondence to: ihalilyavuz@gmail.com

Department of Dermatology, Faculty of Medicine, Yuzuncu Yil University, Van, Turkey

References

[1] Ross EK, Tan E, Shapiro J. Update on primary cicatricial alopecias. J Am Acad Dermatol. 2005;**53**(1):1–37. DOI: http://dx.doi.org/10.1016/j.jaad.2004.06.015

[2] Mirmirani P, Willey A, Headington JT, Stenn K, McCalmont TH, Price VH. Primary cicatricial alopecia: histopathologic findings do not distinguish clinical variants. J Am Acad Dermatol. 2005;**52**(4):637–43. DOI: http://dx.doi.org/10.1016/j.jaad.2004.07.069

[3] Sperling LC. Alopecias. In: Bolognia JL, Jorizzo JL, Rapini RP, editors. Dermatology. 2nd ed. New York: Elsevier, 2008; pp. 987–1005.

[4] Sinclair RD. Acquired cicatricial alopecias. In: Burns DA, Breathnach SM, Cox NH, et al. editors. Rook's Textbook of Dermatology. 7th ed. Oxford: Blackwell Publishing, 2004; pp. 63.1–63.120.

[5] Ohyama M. Primary cicatricial alopecia: recent advances in understanding and management. J Dermatol. 2012;**39**:18–26. DOI: 10.1111/j.1346-8138.2011.01416.x.

[6] Rigopoulos D, Stamatios G, Ioannides D. Primary scarring alopecias. Curr Probl Dermatol. 2015;**47**:76–86. DOI: 10.1159/000369407.

[7] Dogra S, Sarangal R. What's new in cicatricial alopecia? Indian J Dermatol Venereol Leprol. 2013;**79(5)**:576–90. DOI: 10.4103/0378-6323.116726.

[8] Olsen EA, Bergfeld WF, Cotsarelis G, Price VH, Shapiro J, Sinclair R, Solomon A, Sperling L, Stenn K, Whiting DA, Bernardo O, Bettencourt M, Bolduc C, Callendar V, Elston D, Hickman J, Ioffreda M, King L, Linzon C, McMichael A, Miller J, Mulinari F, Trancik R. Workshop on Cicatricial Alopecia. Summary of North American Hair Research Society (NAHRS)-sponsored Workshop on Cicatricial Alopecia, Duke University Medical Center, February 10 and 11, 2001. J Am Acad Dermatol. 2003;**48(1)**:103–10. DOI: 10.1067/mjd.2003.68

[9] Kang H, Alzolibani AA, Otberg N, Shapiro J. Lichen planopilaris. Dermatol Ther. 2008;**21 (4):**249–56. DOI: 10.1111/j.1529-8019.2008.00206.x.

[10] Nayar M, Schomberg K, Dawber RP, Millard PR. A clinicopathological study of scarring alopecia. Br J Dermatol. 1993;**128(5**):533–36. DOI: 10.1111/j.1365-2133.1993.tb00230.x.

[11] Mobini N, Tam S, Kamino H. Possible role of the bulge region in the pathogenesis of inflammatory scarring alopecia: lichen planopilaris as the prototype. J Cutan Pathol. 2005;**32**:675–79. DOI: 10.1111/j.0303-6987.2005.00399.x

[12] Meinhard J, Stroux A, Lünnemann L, Vogt A, Blume-Peytavi U. Lichen planopilaris: Epidemiology and prevalence of subtypes—a retrospective analysis in 104 patients. J Dtsch Dermatol Ges. 2014;**12(3**):229–35. DOI: 10.1111/ddg.12264.

[13] Grace PM. Living with lichen planopilaris. Dermatol Nurs. 2007;**19**: 184–85. PMID: 17526308

[14] Rosina P, Chieregato C, Magnanini M, Barba A. Lichen planopilaris and autoimmune thyroiditis. J Eur Acad Dermatol Venereol. 2002; **16(6)**: 648–49. DOI: 10.1046/j.1468-3083.2002.00653_10.x

[15] Chieregato C, Zini A, Barba A, Magnanini M, Rosina P. Lichen planopilaris: report of 30 cases and review of the literature. Int J Dermatol. 2003;**42(5**):342–45. DOI: 10.1046/j.1365-4362.2003.01695.x

[16] Tursen U, Api H, Kaya T, Ikizoglu G. Treatment of lichen planopilaris with mycophenolate mofetil. Dermatol Online J. 2004: **10**:24. PMID: 15347506

[17] Kossard S. Postmenopausal frontal fibrosing alopecia. Scarring alopecia in a pattern distribution. Arch Dermatol. 1994;**130(6**):770–74. DOI:10.1001/archderm.1994.01690060100013

[18] Kossard S, Lee MS, Wilkinson B. Postmenopausal frontal fibrosing alopecia: a frontal variant of lichen planopilaris. J Am Acad Dermatol. 1997;**36(1)**:59–66. DOI: http://dx.doi.org/10.1016/S0190-9622(97)70326-8

[19] Tan KT, Messenger AG. Frontal fibrosing alopecia: clinical presentations and prognosis. Br J Dermatol. 2009;**160(1**):75–79. DOI: 10.1111/j.1365-2133.2008.08861.x.

[20] MacDonald A, Clark C, Holmes S. Frontal fibrosing alopecia: a review of 60 cases. J Am Acad Dermatol. 2012; **67(5**):955–61. DOI: 10.1016/j.jaad.2011.12.038.

[21] Tziotzios C, Fenton DA, Stefanato CM, McGrath JA. Familial frontal fibrosing alopecia. J Am Acad Dermatol. 2015;**73(1**):e37. DOI: 10.1016/j.jaad.2015.01.057.

[22] Miteva M, Whiting D, Harries M, Bernardes A, Tosti A. Frontal fibrosing alopecia in black patients. Br J Dermatol. 2012;**167(1):**208–10. DOI: 10.1111/j.1365-2133.2012.10809.x.

[23] Rallis E, Gregoriou S, Christofidou E, Rigopoulos D. Frontal fibrosing alopecia: to treat or not to treat? J Cutan Med Surg. 2010;**14(4):**161–66. DOI: 10.2310/7750.2010.09041

[24] Ghafoor R, Khoso BK, Anwar MI, Hashmi SF. Graham-Little-Piccardi-Lassueur syndrome: a rare case report and review of literature. J Pak Assoc Dermatol. 2015;**25 (4):**327–330.

[25] Zegarska B, Kallas D, Schwartz RA, Czajkowski R, Uchanska G, Placek W. Graham-Little syndrome. Acta Dermatovenerol Alp Pannonica Adriat. 2010;**19(3)**:39–42. PMID: 20976421

[26] Vega-Gutierrez J, Miranda-Romero A, Perez-Milan F, Martinez-Garcia G. Graham Little-Piccardi-Lassueur syndrome associated with androgen insensitivity syndrome (testicular feminization). J Eur Acad Dermatol Venereol. 2004;**18(4):**463–66. DOI: 10.1111/j.1468-3083.2004.00945.x

[27] Bardazzi F, Landi C, Orlandi C, Neri I, Varotti C. Graham Little-Piccardi-Lasseur syndrome following HBV vaccination. Acta Derm Venereol 1999; **79(1)**:93. PMID: 10086877

[28] Bianchi L, Paro Vidolin A, Piemonte P, Carboni I, Chimenti S. Graham Little-Piccardi-Lassueur syndrome: effective treatment with cyclosporin-A. Clin Exp Dermatol. 2001;**26 (6):**518–20. DOI: 10.1046/j.1365-2230.2001.00881.x

[29] Okon LG, Werth VP. Cutaneous lupus erythematosus: diagnosis and treatment. Best Pract Res Clin Rheumatol. 2013;**27(3)**:391–404. DOİ: 10.1016/j.berh.2013.07.008.

[30] Walling HW, Sontheimer RD. Cutaneous lupus erythematosus: issues in diagnosis and treatment. Am J Clin Dermatol. 2009;**10(6):**365–81. DOI: 10.2165/11310780-000000000-00000.

[31] Gordon KA, Tosti A. Alopecia: evaluation and treatment. Clin Cosmet Investig Dermatol. 2011;**4:**101–6. DOI: 10.2147/CCID.S10182.

[32] Parodi A, Massone C, Cacciapuoti M, Aragone MG, Bondavalli P, Cattarini G, Rebora A. Measuring the activity of the disease in patients with cutaneous lupus erythematosus. Br J Dermatol. 2000;**142(3):**457–60. DOI: 10.1046/j.1365-2133.2000.03356.x

[33] Crowson AN, Magro C. The cutaneous pathology of lupus erythematosus: a review. J Cutan Pathol. 2001;**28(1)**:1–23. DOI: 10.1034/j.1600-0560.2001.280101.x

[34] Kuhn A, Gensch K, Haust M, Meuth AM, Boyer F, Dupuy P, Lehmann P, Metze D, Ruzicka T. Photoprotective effects of a broad-spectrum sunscreen in ultraviolet-induced cutaneous lupus erythematosus: a randomized, vehicle-controlled, double-blind study. J Am Acad Dermatol. 2011;**64(1):**37–48. DOI: 10.1016/j.jaad.2009.12.053.

[35] Chang AY, Werth VP. Treatment of cutaneous lupus. Curr Rheumatol Rep. 2011;**13 (4):**300–7. DOI: 10.1007/s11926-011-0180-z.

[36] Otberg N, Wu WY, McElwee KJ, Shapiro J. Diagnosis and management of primary cicatricial alopecia: part I. Skinmed. 2008;**7(1):**19–26. PMID: 18174797

[37] Dawber R. What is pseudopelade? Clin Exp Dermatol. 1992;**17(5):**305–6. DOI: 10.1111/j.1365-2230.1992.tb00216.x

[38] Alzolibani AA, Kang H, Otberg N, Shapiro J. Pseudopelade of Brocq. Dermatol Ther. 2008;**21(4):**257–63. DOI: 10.1111/j.1529-8019.2008.00207.x.

[39] Olsen E, Stenn K, Bergfeld W, Cotsarelis G, Price V, Shapiro J, Sinclair R, Solomon A, Sperling L, Whiting D. Update on cicatricial alopecia. J Invest Dermatol Symp Proc. 2003;**8(1)**:18–19. DOI: http://dx.doi.org/10.1046/j.1523-1747.2003.12166.x

[40] Amato L, Mei S, Massi D, Gallerani I, Fabbri P. Cicatricial alopecia; a dermatopathologic and immunopathologic study of 33 patients (pseudopelade of Brocq is not a specific clinico-pathologic entity). Int J Dermatol. 2002;**41(1):**8–15. DOI: 10.1046/j.1365-4362.2002.01331.x

[41] Sperling LC. Brocq's alopecia (pseudopelade of Brocq) and „burnt out" scarring alopecia. In: Sperling LC, editor. An Atlas of Hair Pathology with Clinical Correlations. New York: Parthenon Publishing, 2003; pp. 115–118.

[42] Moretti S, Amato L, Massi D, Bianchi B, Gallerani I, Fabbri P. Evaluation of inflammatory infiltrate and fibrogenic cytokines in pseudopelade of Brocq suggests the involvement of T-helper 2 and 3 cytokines. Br J Dermatol. 2004;**151(1):**84–90. DOI: 10.1111/j.1365-2133.2004.05976.x

[43] Pincelli C, Girolomoni G, Benassi L. Pseudopelade of Brocq: an immunologically mediated disease? Dermatologica. 1987;**174(1):**49–50. PMID: 3803675

[44] Bergfeld WF, Elston DM. Cicatricial alopecia. In: Olsen E, editor. Disorders of Hair Growth: Diagnosis and Treatment, 2nd ed. New York: McGraw-Hill, 2003; pp. 363–398.

[45] Madani S, Trotter MJ, Shapiro J. Pseudopelade of Brocq in beard area. J Am Acad Dermatol. 2000;**42**:895–6. DOI: http://dx.doi.org/10.1016/S0190-9622(00)90266-4

[46] LoPresti P, Papa CM, Kligman AM. Hot comb alopecia. Arch Dermatol. 1968;**98(3**):234–8. DOI:10.1001/archderm.1968.01610150020003

[47] McMichael AJ. Ethnic hair update: past and present. J Am Acad Dermatol. 2003;**48(6 Suppl)**:S127–33. DOI: 10.1067/mjd.2003.278

[48] Herskovitz I, Miteva M. Central centrifugal cicatricial alopecia: challenges and solutions. Clin Cosmet Investig Dermatol. 2016;**9:**175–81. DOI: 10.2147/CCID.S100816.

[49] Whiting DA, Olsen EA. Central centrifugal cicatricial alopecia. Dermatol Ther. 2008;**21 (4)**:268–78. DOI: 10.1111/j.1529-8019.2008.00209.x.

[50] Sperling LC. Central centrifugal scarring alopecia. In: Sperling LC, editor. An Atlas of Hair Pathology with Clinical Correlations. New York: Parthenon Publishing, 2003; pp. 91–100.

[51] Davis EC, Reid SD, Callender VD, Sperling LC. Differentiating central centrifugal cicatricial alopecia and androgenetic alopecia in African American men: report of three cases. J Clin Aesthet Dermatol. 2012;**5(6):**37–40. PMID: 22768355

[52] Gathers RC, Lim HW. Central centrifugal cicatricial alopecia: past, present, and future. J Am Acad Dermatol. 2009;**60(4):**660–8. DOI: 10.1016/j.jaad.2008.09.066.

[53] Bin Saif GA, McMichael A, Kwatra SG, Chan YH, Yosipovitch G. Central centrifugal cicatricial alopecia severity is associated with cowhage-induced itch. Br J Dermatol. 2013;**168(2):**253–6. DOI: 10.1111/bjd.12043.

[54] Hempstead RW, Ackerman AB. Follicular mucinosis. A reaction pattern in follicular epithelium. Am J Dermatopathol. 1985;**7(3):**245–57. PMID: 2932031

[55] Cerroni L, Fink-Puches R, Bäck B, Kerl H. Follicular mucinosis: a criticalreappraisal of clinicopathologic features and association with mycosis fungoides and Sézary syndrome. Arch Dermatol. 2002;**138(2)**:182–9. DOI: 10.1001/archderm.138.2.182

[56] Rupnik H, Podrumac B, Zgavec B, Lunder T. Follicular mucinosis in a teenage girl. Acta Dermatovenerol Alp Pannonica Adriat. 2005;**14(3)**:111–4. PMID: 16200337

[57] Brown HA, Gibson LE, Pujol RM, Lust JA, Pittelkow MR. Primary follicular 5-mucinosis: long-term follow-up of patients younger than 40 years with and without clonal T-cell receptor gene rearrangement. J Am Acad Dermatol. 2002;**47(6)**: 856–62. DOI: 10.1067/mjd.2002.124604

[58] Parker SR, Murad E. Follicular mucinosis: clinical, histologic, and molecular remission with minocycline. J Am Acad Dermatol. 2010;**62(1)**:139–41. DOI: 10.1016/j.jaad.2009.01.031

[59] Eramo LR, Esterly NB, Zieserl EJ, Stock EL, Herrmann J. Ichthyosis follicularis with alopecia and photophobia. Arch Dermatol. 1985;**121(9)**:1167–74. DOI: 10.1001/archderm.1985.01660090081019

[60] Romine KA, Rothschild JG, Hansen RC. Cicatricial alopecia and keratosis pilaris. Keratosis follicularis spinulosa decalvans. Arch Dermatol. 1997;**133(3)**:381–4. DOI: 10.1001/archderm.1997.03890390121018

[61] Baden HP, Byers HR. Clinical findings, cutaneous pathology, and response to therapy in 21 patients with keratosis pilaris atrophicans. Arch Dermatol. 1994;**130(4)**:469–75. DOI: 10.1001/archderm.1994.01690040073011

[62] Castori M, Covaciu C, Paradisi M, Zambruno G. Clinical and genetic heterogeneity in keratosis follicularis spinulosa decalvans. Eur J Med Genet. 2009;**52(1)**:53–8. DOI: 10.1016/j.ejmg.2008.09.005.

[63] Kunte C, Loeser C, Wolff H. Folliculitis spinulosa decalvans: successful therapy with dapsone. J Am Acad Dermatol. 1998;**39(5 Pt 2**):891–3. DOI: http://dx.doi.org/10.1016/S0190-9622(98)70374-3

[64] Hallai N, Thompson I, Williams P, Anstey AV. Folliculitis spinulosa decalvans: failure to respond to oral isotretinoin. J Eur Acad Dermatol Venereol. 2006;**20(2)**:223–4. DOI: 10.1111/j.1468-3083.2005.01367.x

[65] Brooke RC, Griffiths CE. Folliculitis decalvans. Clin Exp Dermatol. 2001;**26(1)**:120–2. DOI: 10.1046/j.1365-2230.2001.00746.x

[66] Otberg N, Kang H, Alzolibani AA, Shapiro J. Folliculitis decalvans. Dermatol Ther. 2008;**21(4)**:238–44. DOI: 10.1111/j.1529-8019.2008.00204.x.

[67] Karakuzu A, Erdem T, Aktas A, Atasoy M, Gulec AI. A case of folliculitis decalvans involving the beard, face and nape. J Dermatol. 2001;**28**: 329–31. DOI: 10.1111/j.1346-8138.2001.tb00143.x

[68] Powell JJ, Dawber RP, Gatter K. Folliculitis decalvans including tufted folliculitis: clinical, histological and therapeutic findings. Br J Dermatol. 1999;**140:** 328–33. DOI: 10.1046/j.1365-2133.1999.02675.x

[69] Mihaljević N, von den Driesch P. Successful use of infliximab in a patient with recalcitrant folliculitis decalvans. J Dtsch Dermatol Ges. 2012;**10(8):**589–90. DOI: 10.1111/j.1610-0387.2012.07972.x

[70] Bastida J, Valerón-Almazán P, Santana-Molina N, Medina-Gil C, Carretero-Hernández G. Treatment of folliculitis decalvans with tacrolimus ointment. Int J Dermatol. 2012;**51 (2):**216–20. DOI: 10.1111/j.1365-4632.2011.05212.x

[71] Stites PC, Boyd AS. Dissecting cellulitis in a white male: a case report and review of the literature. Cutis. 2001;**67(1):**37–40. DOI: PMID: 11204602

[72] Wu WY, Otberg N, McElwee KJ, Shapiro J. Diagnosis and management of primary cicatricial alopecia: part II. Skinmed. 2008;**7(2):**78–83. PMID: 18326998

[73] Scheinfeld N. Dissecting cellulitis (Perifolliculitis Capitis Abscedens etSuffodiens): a comprehensive review focusing on new treatments and findings of the last decade with commentary comparing the therapies and causes of dissecting cellulitis to hidradenitis suppurativa. Dermatol Online J. 2014;**20(5):**22692. PMID: 24852785

[74] Bolz S, Jappe U, Hartschuh W. Successful treatment of perifolliculitis capitis abscedens et suffodiens with combined isotretinoin and dapsone. J Dtsch Dermatol Ges. 2008;**6(1):**44–7. DOI: 10.1111/j.1610-0387.2007.06399.x

[75] Khaled A, Zeglaoui F, Zoghlami A, Fazaa B, Kamoun MR. Dissecting cellulitis of the scalp: response to isotretinoin. J Eur Acad Dermatol Venereol. 2007;**21(10):**1430–1. DOI: 10.1111/j.1468-3083.2007.02239.x

[76] Brandt HR, Malheiros AP, Teixeira MG, Machado MC. Perifolliculitis capitis abscedens et suffodiens successfully controlled with infliximab. Br J Dermatol. 2008;**159(2):**506–7. DOI: 10.1111/j.1365-2133.2008.08674.x.

[77] Ogunbiyi A, George A. Acne keloidalis in females: case report and review of literature. J Natl Med Assoc. 2005;**97(5):**736–8. PMID: 15926654

[78] Knable AL Jr, Hanke CW, Gonin R. Prevalence of acne keloidalis nuchae in football players. J Am Acad Dermatol. 1997;**37(4):**570–4. DOI: http://dx.doi.org/10.1016/S0190-9622(97)70173-7

[79] Adegbidi H, Ogunbiyi A. Keloid acne of the neck: epidemiological studies over 10 years. Int J Dermatol. 2005;**44 (Suppl. 1):**49–50. DOI: 10.1111/j.1365-4632.2005.02815.x

[80] Quarles FN, Brody H, Badreshia S, Vause SE, Brauner G, Breadon JY, SwinehartJ, Epps RE. Acne keloidalis nuchae. Dermatol Ther. 2007;**20(3):**128–32. DOI: 10.1111/j.1529-8019.2007.00123.x

[81] Fisher DA. Acne necroticans (varioliformis) and Staphylococcus aureus. J Am Acad Dermatol. 1988;**18(5 Pt 1):**1136–8. PMID: 2968375

[82] Kossard S, Collins A, McCrossin I. Necrotizing lymphocytic folliculitis: the early lesion of acne necrotica (varioliformis). J Am Acad Dermatol. 1987;**16(Pt 1):**1007–14. PMID: 2953765

[83] Pye RJ, Peachey RD, Burton JL. Erosive pustular dermatosis of the scalp. Br J Dermatol. 1979;**100(5)**:559–66. DOI: 10.1111/j.1365-2133.1979.tb05581.x

[84] Grattan CE, Peachey RD, Boon A. Evidence for a role of local trauma in the pathogenesis of erosive pustular dermatosis of the scalp. Clin Exp Dermatol. 1988;**13(1)**:7–10. DOI: 10.1111/j.1365-2230.1988.tb00639.x

[85] Vaccaro M, Guarneri C, Barbuzza O, Guarneri B. Erosive pustular dermatosis of the scalp: an uncommon condition typical of elderly patients. J Am Geriatr Soc. 2008;**56 (4)**:761–2. DOI: http://dx.doi.org/10.1016/S0190-9622(97)70173-7

[86] Zahdi MR, Seidel GB, Soares VC, Freitas CF, Mulinari-Brenner FA. Erosive pustular dermatosis of the scalp successfully treated with oral prednisone and topical tacrolimus. An Bras Dermatol. 2013;**88(5)**:796–8. DOI: 10.1590/abd1806-4841.20132109

[87] Ena P, Lissia M, Doneddu GM, Campus GV. Erosive pustular dermatosis of the scalp in skin grafts: report of three cases. Dermatology. 1997;**194(1)**:80–4. PMID: 9031801

Section 6

Scalp Disorders

Chapter 11

Infections, Infestations and Neoplasms of the Scalp

Filiz Canpolat

Additional information is available at the end of the chapter

http://dx.doi.org/10.5772/67278

Abstract

This chapter reviews common cutaneous infections, infestations, and neoplasms of the scalp. Infections of the scalp are subdivided into three major groups. The most seen are: (1) Bacterial: Folliculitis, folliculitis decalvans, tufted hair folliculitis and acne keloidalis nuchae. (2) Fungal: Tinea capitis, favus and kerion celsi. (3) Protozoal: Syphilitic alopecia. Pediculosis capitis is the most common worldwide infestation of the scalp. The neoplasms of the scalp are large group of different diseases due to arising different origin. In the following section, trichilemmal cyst, proliferating trichilemmal cyst, nevus sebaceous and cylindroma are discussed in detail.

Keywords: infection, infestation, neoplasm, scalp

1. Introduction

Scalp diseases are one of the most seen reasons for admission to dermatology clinics. There is a wide spectrum of different aetiologies for scalp lesions. This chapter will review cutaneous infections, infestations and neoplasms of the scalp. Examples of bacterial infections include folliculitis, folliculitis decalvans, tufted hair folliculitis and acne keloidalis nuchae. There will be some detailed information about fungal infections, such as tinea capitis, favus and kerion celsi. The neoplasms of the scalp represent a varied group of dermatoses. This review focuses on trichilemmal cyst, proliferating trichilemmal cyst, nevus sebaceous and cylindroma.

2. Bacterial infections of scalp

There are several types of infections of the scalp including chronic scalp folliculitis [SF], folliculitis decalvans [FD], tufted folliculitis [TF], acne nuchae keloidalis [ANK] and dissecting cellulitis [DCS]. These infections have similar features like chronic scarring folliculocentric pustules localised to the scalp. Many of these conditions show the presence of *Staphylococcus aureus* [SA] and response to antibiotic therapy [1].

2.1. Scalp folliculitis

Folliculitis is a pyoderma that begins within the hair follicle. It is classified according to the microbial aetiology, including bacteria, viruses and fungi, as well as many other non-infectious ones. The most seen folliculitis of scalp are *Staphylococcus aureus* [*S. aureus*] folliculitis, Herpes simplex virus folliculitis and dermatophytic folliculitis [Tinea capitis]. Some of the predisposing factors are hyperhidrosis, maceration, friction, overweight, medications such as corticosteroids and halogenated compounds, as well as occlusive hair care products and topical hydrocarbons, such as oils and tars. In addition, immunodeficiencies such as HIV/AIDS and diabetes mellitus are also predisposed to folliculitis [2].

S. aureus is the most common cause of folliculitis. The major cause is either contagion or autoinoculation from a carrier focus, usually nasal or perianal region. The typical lesion of folliculitis is a small inflamed, dome-shaped papule or pustule which can be drained spontaneously. Both pruritus and pain can be seen. Systemic symptoms, such as fever or lymphadenopathy, may occur when the involvement is widespread. Biopsy is rarely needed to distinguish between fungal or viral folliculitis. Biopsy shows neutrophils in the dermis and follicular wall damage. Many of the patients may carry *S. aureus*, so nasal and perineal cultures should be taken. Other forms of folliculitis can be identical in appearance, so this possibility should always be taken into consideration. Treatment options include topical antibiotic or disinfectant solutions such as mupirocin cream, triclosan [2%] or chlorhexidine [1%] and antistaphylococcal systemic antibiotics [1, 2].

2.2. Folliculitis decalvans

Folliculitis decalvans [FD] is a rare type of cicatricial alopecia and was first described by Quinquaud in 1881 [3]. It is an inflammatory disease characterised by follicular pustules and haemorrhagic crusting, leading to scarring hair loss. Although in most patient FD started in the vertex, other sites such as the occipital or midscalp area may also be affected. At the periphery of lesion, follicular pustules continue to form. Tufting of hairs may be seen [4]. Clinically, the majority of the patients were generally healthy, without any systemic symptoms or any signs of immunosuppression. Although the exact cause remains unknown, *S. aureus* is usually cultured from these pustules [5]. The disease shows a chronic and relapsing course. Histologically, early lesions show dense perifollicular inflammatory infiltrates consisting mostly of neutrophils. In later stages, follicular rupture, lymphocytes, histiocytes and plasma cells are seen, as well as perifollicular and interstitial dermal fibrosis [6, 7]. Differential diagnosis of FD consists of follicular degeneration syndrome or central centrifugal scarring alopecia.

As FD is usually associated with infection of *S. aureus* [5, 6], systemic antibiotics are the mainstay of disease [e.g., cephalexin, minocycline, tetracycline, clindamycin, rifampicin, ciprofloxacin].

http://dx.doi.org/10.5772/67278

Because of its high lipid solubility, and it is said to be the best antistaphylococcal antibiotic, rifampicin has been successfully used in combination with various other antibiotics [5, 7]. Rifampicin is not recommended for lone use. Rifampicin 300 mg b.i.d and clindamycin 300 mg b.i.d is the preferred regimen. Shampooing with antibacterial wash products and topical corticosteroids may also be useful. Varying results have been reported after treatment with prednisolone, isotretinoin, human immunoglobulin and more recently biologics [e.g., infliximab and adalimumab] [8, 9], neodymium: yttrium aluminium-garnet [Nd:YAG] laser [10] and photodynamic therapy [PDT] [11]. There is very limited evidence that FD can be treated with dapsone, minoxidil or radiation therapy [12].

2.3. Tufted hair folliculitis

Tufted hair folliculitis [THF] was first described by Smith and Sanderson in 1978 [7]. It is characterised by scarring bacterial folliculitis of the scalp associated with multiple bundles of hair emerging from a single dilated follicular orifice in a 'doll's hair' pattern. Infection with *S. aureus* is thought to be initial causative factor [13]. Tufting of hair is caused by clustering of adjacent follicular unit due to a fibrosing process and to retention of telogen hairs within a dilated follicular orifice [14]. The patients were 20–60 years old, the peak incidence occurring in 30 years [4]. It affects male more frequently than female.

Clinically, it presents erythematous, infiltrated plaque of cicatricial alopecia and enlarged follicular openings with tufts containing 20–30 apparently normal hair shafts (**Figure 1**). The lesions are usually found in the occipital and parietal areas [8]. Frequently reported subjective symptoms are pruritus, pain and scales adherent to the scalp and hair. Regional lymph node enlargement [occipital, pre- or retroauricular] may also be noticed [9]. *S. aureus* is most often cultured from the lesions [10]. Underlying differences in follicular anatomy or host response may be responsible for the lesion [15]. Histopathological studies reveal scarring with perifollicular inflammation of plasma cells, lymphocytes and neutrophils around the upper portions of the follicles sparing at the hair root level. Multiple hairs are seen emerging from a single follicular opening (**Figure 2**) [13].

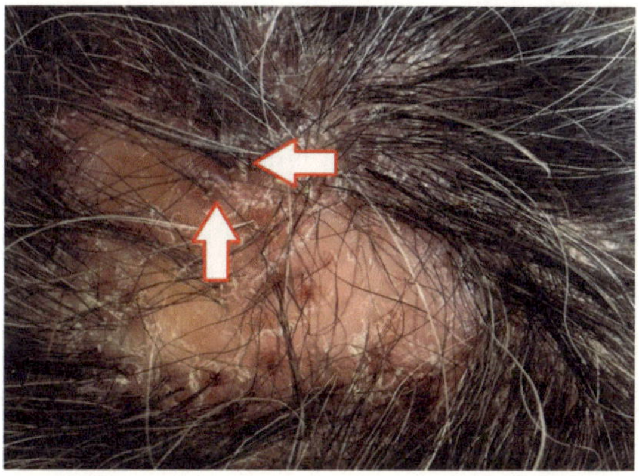

Figure 1. Cicatricial alopecia with tufted folliculitis.

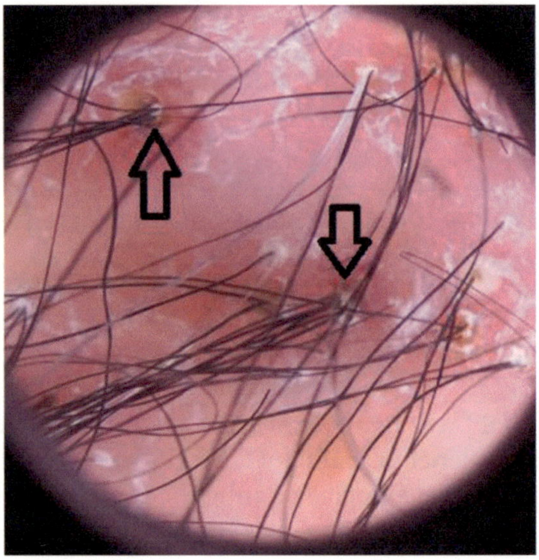

Figure 2. Dermoscopic image of the scalp with tufted folliculitis characterised by multiple hairs emerging from one single dilated follicular orifice.

THF may be seen with dissecting cellulitis of the scalp, folliculitis decalvans, acne keloidalis, Melkersson-Rosenthal syndrome and hidradenitis suppurativa [16]. In some case reports it has been described that tufted folliculitis in association with medication use, specifically with cyclosporine and lapatinib [17, 18]. Differential diagnosis consists of folliculitis decalvans, folliculitis keloidalis nuchae, kerion celsi, dissecting cellulitis of scalp, trichostasis spinulosa, follicular lichen planus and relapsing staphylococcal folliculitis [19].

The course of THF is chronic and the patient may experience intermittent flares and remissions. Treatment of this relapsing condition is notoriously difficult. As *S. aureus* is the initial causative agent, systemic antibiotics including ciprofloxacin, erythromycin, flucloxacillin and amoxicillin/clavulanic acid are regarded the standard therapy. Rifampicin and nadifloxacin have been proven as more effective than other therapeutic modality to control the pustular phase of the disease, of the best antibiotics active against *S. aureus*, as well as to prevent possible recurrences [4, 20]. Rifampicin can be used with a dose of 450 mg twice per day for 4 weeks or 600 mg daily for 10 weeks [20, 21]. Recently, a case of tufted hair folliculitis being treated with trastuzumab, a selective HER2 inhibitor, has been reported [22]. Good results with excision of the areas of scarring have also been described [13, 15].

2.4. Acne keloidalis nuchae

Acne keloidalis nuchae [AKN] is a chronic scarring folliculitis characterised by fibrotic, keloid-like papules and plaques on the occipital scalp and posterior neck. The term acne keloidalis was given to this condition in 1872 by Bazin [23].

Early AKN lesions are seen as mildly pruritic papules and pustules arranged in irregularly linear groups just below the hairline. With continued inflammation or infection the

http://dx.doi.org/10.5772/67278

papules tend to coalesce and form hypertrophic scars or keloids that may be painful and disfiguring (**Figures 3** and **4**). In advanced cases, abscesses and sinus tracts with purulent discharge may develop [24, 25]. Actually AKN is not a form of acne vulgaris and unlike true acne vulgaris, comedones are not a feature of AKN. It is very common in individuals of African descent. Its prevalence ranges from 1 to 16% and the male to female ratio is at least 20:1. The probable onset age of AKN is 15–25 years and reduces after 55 years of age [26].

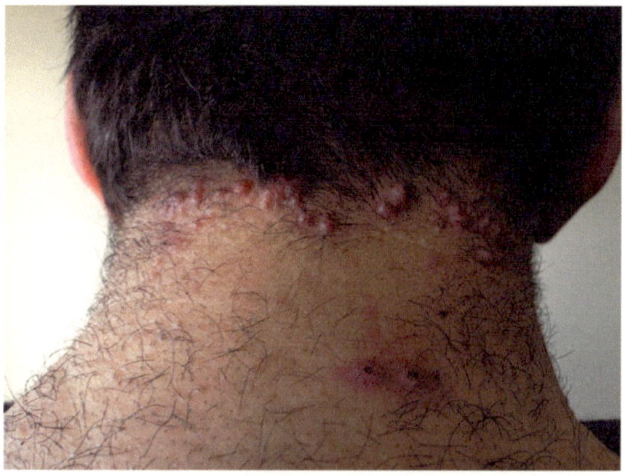

Figure 3. Acne keloidalis nuchae. Papules are seen below the hairline.

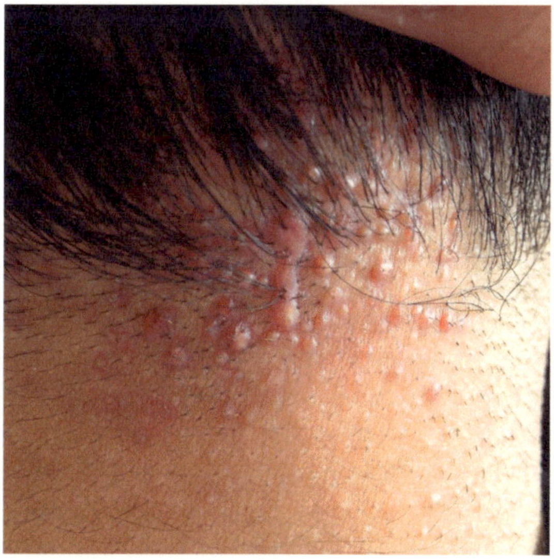

Figure 4. Acne keloidalis nuchae. Papules and hypertrophic scars are noticed on the occipital region.

The exact aetiology of AKN is unclear but it is associated with several factors including androgen excess, chronic mechanical trauma such as close haircuts and chronic rubbing of the area by clothing stimulating an inflammatory reaction, secondary bacterial infection, mast cell density and medications such as antiepileptic drugs or cyclosporine [24, 26–28].

Histological studies show evidence of follicular and perifollicular infiltrate at the upper one-third of the hair follicle in early lesions, whereas more advanced lesions reveal disrupted hair follicles, a foreign-body reaction with granulomatous inflammation and fibrotic dermis [25, 29]. Differential diagnosis of AKN consists of the other chronic scarring folliculocentric pustules localised to the scalp.

First step in treatment is patient education. It should be advised that the patient should avoid from mechanical irritation from clothing for prevention. Prognosis becomes good if the treatment begins at early stage. However, once major scarring develops, therapy is more difficult and morbidity is increased. If pathogenic microorganism with culture are identified, appropriate antibiotics should be prescribed. Conventional treatment modalities usually involve use of topical, intralesional or systemic steroids in combination with retinoids and/or oral antibiotics such as doxycycline or minocycline to decrease inflammation. Oral isotretinoin of 20 mg daily may be used alone or in combination with topical fusidic acid and oral cefadroxil [500 mg twice daily for 2 weeks] to treat the patient [30]. Other treatment options are cryotherapy and targeted ultraviolet B [290–320 nm] phototherapy. Combination of cryotherapy and intralesional steroid may help to reduce the size and firmness of papules and nodules [31]. Radiation therapy and intralesional 5-fluorouracil are alternative treatment strategies for refractory cases [32]. Recently, laser treatment such as CO_2 laser, 1064-nm Nd:YAG laser, 59-nm pulse dye laser [PDL] and 810-nm diode laser have been used which allow for 82–95% improvement in one to five sessions [33]. Patients who present with big fibrotic nodules would benefit most from surgical excision. Excision with primary closure may be used for excellent cosmetic results for the management of extensive cases of AKN [23, 28, 34].

3. Fungal infections of scalp

3.1. Tinea capitis

Tinea capitis (TC) is a disease caused by dermatophytes of the skin of the scalp with a propensity for attacking hair shafts and follicles. It occurs predominantly in pre-pubertal children aged between 3 and 7 years. It is reported more in boys than in girls within pre-pubertal age. Tinea capitis is the most seen pediatric dermatophyte infection worldwide [35]. All species of *Trichophyton* and *Microsporum* can cause TC. *Microsporum canis* is the cause of the most seen dermatophyte worldwide, whereas in the United States *Tricophyton tonsurans* is the most common organism. Transmission occurs by direct head-to-head contact through fomites, from animals to humans, and, least commonly, acquired from soil. Asymptomatic carriers of *Tricophyton tonsurans* are common, making it difficult to treat [36].

From the site of inoculation, the fungal hyphae grow centrifugally in the stratum corneum. According to the patterns of contamination, tinea of the scalp is classified into two types: ectothrix and endothrix. In an ectothrix infection, the fungi continue downward

http://dx.doi.org/10.5772/67278

growth into the follicle and they invade the keratin part of the hairs. Ectothrix invasion is usually associated with *Trichophyton verrucosum, Trichophyton mentagrophytes* and all *Microsporum* species. The endothrix hair invasion caused by *Trichophyton tonsurans* and *Trichophyton violaceum* is characterised by the development of the fungi within the hair shaft only. While the ectothrix-infected hairs can be of fluoresce bright green or yellow green caused by the destruction of the cuticle of the hair, the endothrix infection do not fluoresce, because the cuticle of the hair remains intact in endothrix infection. The hair is very fragile and breaks the surface of the scalp. Therefore, leaves the infected dark stubs visible in the follicular orifices. Thus, endothrix infection is often described as a 'black dot' appearance [37].

Among predisposing factors for dermatophyte infections are humid environment, atopic diathesis, such as cell-mediated immune deficiency, systemic immunocompromised states, prolonged immunosuppression with the use of topical glucocorticoids and broad-spectrum antibiotic use [38].

Typical clinical features are small areas of fine scale with minimal hair loss. 'Moth-eaten' alopecia is seen. When *Tricophyton tonsurans* is responsible, black dots are seen. Erythema is also a clue for *Microsporum canis*. Shedding of fungal spores may continue several months despite active treatment; therefore, children with tinea capitis may attend school. Also, short haircuts and wearing a cap during treatment are not necessary. Clinical manifestations of TC may resemble pityriasis amiantacea, seborrheic dermatitis, bacterial folliculitis, pediculosis capitis, trichotillomania, alopecia areata or pustular psoriasis, which are often treated incorrectly [39].

Definitive diagnosis of TC is made through 10–20% potassium hydroxide [KOH] examination and culture from lesions. The turn-around time for culture may take several weeks. Wood light examination is also helpful to demonstrate fungal fluoresce. Infected hair produces bright green or yellow green fluorescence. It should be kept in mind that endothrix organisms do not fluoresce. Trichoscopy is an additional tool for the diagnosis of tinea capitis. Comma shaped hairs, corkscrew hairs and zigzag shaped hairs are the diagnostic trichoscopic features of tinea capitis [40, 41]. Skin biopsy can be done for differential diagnosis. Fungal hyphae in the stratum corneum can be demonstrated histopathologically.

As the dermatophyte penetrate the hair follicle, oral antifungals is required for the treatment of TC. Basically, three different groups of systemic antifungals are used to eliminate TC: Griseofulvin, azoles [itraconazole, fluconazole, ketoconazole] and allylamines [terbinafine]. Of these agents, itraconazole and terbinafine are most commonly used. Griseofulvin [10–25 mg/kg/day for 6–8 weeks] is the most frequently used antifungal agent, but recently it has also been reported that newer agents such as terbinafine [10–20 kg: 62.5 mg/day; 20–40 kg: 125 mg/day; >40 kg: 250 mg/day for 2–4 weeks], itraconazole [5 mg/kg/day for 2–6 weeks] and fluconazole [first dose 6–12 mg/kg, then 3–6 mg/kg/day for 2–4 weeks] to be effective. Selenium sulphide, zinc pyrithione, povidone iodine or ketoconazole shampoos have been shown to help to decrease the shedding of fungal spores. Common recommendations are to use these shampoos two to four times weekly for 2–4 weeks [42, 43].

3.2. Favus

Favus or tinea favosa is the most severe form of tinea capitis. It is caused by *Tricophyton schoenleinii*. The disease frequently occurs in children and is seen rarely in adults. If untreated, the disease persists forever. Favus is seen almost exclusively in Africa, the Mediterranean and the Middle East and, rarely, in North America and South America [44].

The most common clinical manifestations on the scalp are yellowish cup-shaped crusts termed scutula, which surround the infected hair follicles. The scutula have an unpleasant mousy odour. Besides the scalp, it may involve glabrous skin, hairy regions and nails. If not treated properly, the lesion advances peripherally and it can leave scarring alopecia [45, 46].

The diagnosis is confirmed by direct mycological examination and culture. A greyish-green fluorescence may be observed with Wood's lamp examination. Optical microscopy with KOH preparation shows invasion by the fungus, hyphae parallely arranged to the axis, air spaces and a few spores.

In presence of scaly patches without alopecia, favus is misdiagnosed as seborrheic dermatitis, psoriasis, tinea amiantacea or lichen planus [47, 48].

The treatment of tinea favosa lies on the combination of an oral and topical antifungal agents. The local treatment consists in cutting of hair around the alopecia patches and applying once or twice a day of antifungal imidazol [shampoo, foam gel, lotion and spray]. Griseofulvin terbinafine and itraconazole could be used in systemic therapy [44, 45].

3.3. Kerion

Kerion celsi [KC] [so-called deep tinea capitis] is an uncommon inflammatory presentation of tinea capitis [TC], which appears as a boggy, large inflammatory painful mass studded with broken hairs, pustules and, often, purulent drainage from its surface (**Figure 5**). Hair loss is frequently seen in KC. It is usually solitary but multiple lesions may be found. Reactive lymphadenopathy, especially cervical or suboccipital, is a very common associated feature. KC often occurs in children but it has been described in elderly patients [49–51]. The higher

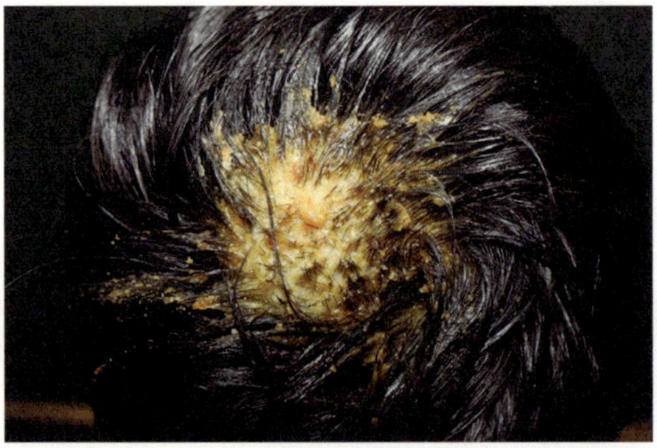

Figure 5. Boggy, large inflammatory painful plaque lesion is seen.

prevalence in females may be related to fact that they generally have longer hair [52]. KC is a markedly inflammatory type of TC secondary to a vigorous host immune response. It is generally caused by zoophilic dermatophytes [*Microsporum canis and Trichophyton mentagrophytes*], but also by anthropophilic [*Trichophyton rubrum*] and rarely by geophilic [*Microsporum gypseum*] species. KC is thought to be the result of a hypersensitivity reaction to dermatophytes [49].

The main source of the fungi responsible for KC is from humans or animals, though dermatophytes may spread via fomites [combs, hairbrushes, hats and contaminated wearing materials]. Although the gold standard diagnostic method is fungal culture, conventional sampling of a kerion can be difficult. Negative results are not uncommon in these cases. The diagnosis of kerion is usually made clinically. A moistened standard bacteriological swab taken from the pustular areas and inoculated onto the culture plate may yield a positive result [53].

Id reactions [so-called dermatophytid] are noted in patients with KC. This is an often pruritic dermatitis based on sensitisation to fungal antigens, reported in 4–5% of fungal infection. Although it may mimic an allergic reaction, it should not lead to discontinuation of antifungal treatment [54]. Acute vesicular dermatitis of the hands and feet is the most common type of id reaction. Other less common types of id reactions include annular erythema and erythema nodosum. These patients have a strong delayed-type hypersensitivity [DTH] reaction to intradermal trichophytin. EN is thought to be due either the deposition of immune complexes in capillaries and venules of the dermal and adipose plexus, or to a DTH reaction to an antigen [55, 56].

The principal differential diagnoses consist of impetigo and bacterial or sterile folliculitis or abscesses. KC is usually misdiagnosed as bacterial abscesses. However, bacterial infections do not cause alopecia, and hairs plucked from a kerion are painless. Diagnostic errors causes patients to undergo unnecessary surgery or antibiotic treatment. However, there is little evidence to support the use of antibiotics for severe KC [49]. Kerion celsi requires treatment with systemic antifungals to penetrate the affected hair shafts. Early short course of glucocorticosteroids with a dose of 1 mg/kg/day were often used in severe KC to reduce inflammation. Oral steroid is tapered to withdraw in 10 days. Manual pressure to remove pus from sinuses was an adjuvant therapy to systemic oral antifungal agents for severe KC.

4. Protozoal infection of scalp

4.1. Syphilitic alopecia

Syphilis is a sexually transmitted disease caused by *Treponema pallidum*. Syphilitic alopecia [SA] is an uncommon feature of secondary syphilis with an incidence of 2.9–11.2% [57]. The physical examination findings include numerous non-scarring, non-inflammatory, irregular in size without defined borders, 'moth-eaten' patches of alopecia of the scalp [58]. The eyebrows and beard may also be involved. SA can be seen with other mucocutaneous symptoms of secondary syphilis. Hair loss usually occurs late in the secondary syphilis, about 8–12 weeks after the first signs of secondary syphilis [59].

According to the patterns of McCarthy made in 1940, secondary SA is classified into two types: symptomatic SA and essential SA. The other cutaneous manifestations of syphilis is not seen in essential SA. Essential SA, characterised by alopecia without any other visible syphilitic lesions on the scalp, may appear as one of three different clinical patterns: 'moth-eaten' alopecia, diffuse alopecia and mixed pattern of alopecia [58, 60]. The 'moth-eaten' pattern alopecia [alopecia syphilitica] is considered the most common and characteristic form of secondary syphilis [61, 62].

The diagnosis of SA is confirmed by both patient's sexual history and positive serological tests for RPR and TPPA. The histopathology findings of SA usually include a normal epidermis with areas of follicular hyperkeratosis. While the number of anagen follicles are reduced markedly, the number of catagen and telogen follicles increase. A perivascular and perifollicular [especially in the peribulbar region] lymphocytic dermal infiltration with scattered plasma cells is observed in some cases [63].

The differential diagnosis of 'moth-eaten' alopecia includes alopecia areata, trichotillomania and tinea capitis except from syphilis [64]. Under trichoscopy black dots, focal atrichia, hypopigmentation of hair shaft and yellow dots are observed in the hair loss region. Alopecia areata, tinea capitis and trichotillomania differ from SA with absence of exclamation hair, coma hair, flame hairs or v-sign, respectively [57].

The antisyphilitic treatment with a weekly dose of 2.4 million units of benzathine penicillin for 3 weeks or procaine penicillin 600,000 units i.m. daily for 10 days leads to complete resolution of alopecia. Hair growth is observed about 6–12 weeks after the start of the treatment [57, 65, 66].

5. Infestations of scalp

5.1. Pediculosis capitis

Pediculosis capitis [PC] [head lice] is a major worldwide infestation caused by *Pediculus humanus capitis* seen in school-aged children of 3–12 years of age. The prevalence of PC is usually higher in girls and women and varies greatly from country to country. It is 0.7–59% in Turkey, 0.48–22.4% in Europe, 37.4% in England, 13% in Australia, up to 58.9% in Africa and 3.6–61.4% in the Americas [67]. There are estimates that 6–12 million children in the United States are infected with PC annually [68]. The prevalence in 5318 elementary school children, aged 8–16 years in Mersin, Turkey, was 6.8% [69]. In another study of 1569 school children, aged 7–14 years, the prevalence of head lice was 16.6% [70]. It tends to be more prevalent in children because they have a high incidence of head-to-head contact with other children. Girls were at a greater risk for head lice because of their tendency to have longer hair than boys and social behaviour [close contact].

The lice are spread by direct head-to-head contact as well as by the sharing of clothing, headgear, hats, combs, hairbrushes, hair barrettes and pillows. PC affects all socioeconomic classes. Although direct contact with an infested individual can cause PC, personal and environmental hygiene are not risk factors for PC [71].

The head louse [plural-lice] is an ectoparasite whose only host is humans for survival. There are three stages that comprise the life cycle of the louse: egg, nymp and adult. Adult female louse lays their eggs [nits] on hair shafts. The nits are usually laid close to scalp for warmth, because they must stay warm in order to hatch. These nits cannot be moved along the hair shaft in contrast to pseudonits. Only in warmer climates, nits can be found 15 cm or more from the scalp, especially favour the nape of the neck. They are of size 0.8 mm × 0.3 mm, oval and usually yellow to white and are located 6 mm from scalp. Nits take about 1 week to hatch [range 6–9 days]. The nit hatches and release a single nymph. Nymph becomes an adult after three molts, about 7–10 days after hatching. Each instar molts every 3–4 days, and after the third molt, it becomes adult louse (**Figure 6**). The first and second instar or nymph forms are relatively immobile. Mobile forms are the third instar forms and adults form. The mature adult louse is approximately the size of a sesame seed [2–3 mm] and is tan to greyish-white [68, 72, 73]. Female lice are larger than males and must take blood before copulation. After copulation she lays between 5 and 10 eggs a day. The adult males usually do not survive after copulation. The adult louse lives only up to 36 hours away from its host. Head lice can travel up to 23 cm/min by crawling. The head lice do not attach firmly to smooth surfaces [e.g., glass, metal, plastic, synthetic leathers] [72, 74].

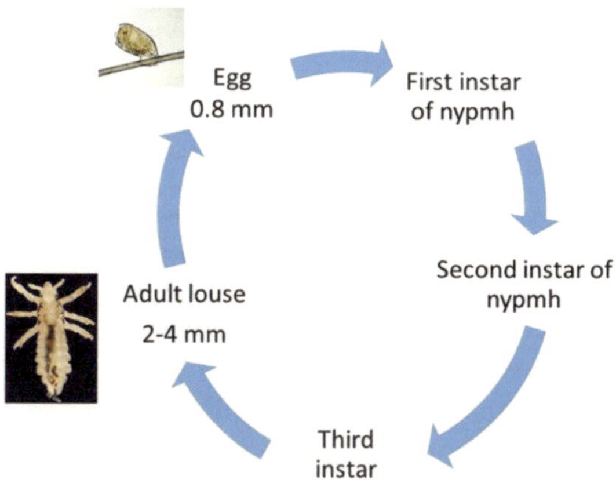

Figure 6. Schematic representation of life cycle of head louse.

The head louse takes a blood meal [hematophagia] usually 4–5 times per day. Chronic and heavy lice infestation can rarely lead to anaemia, especially in females. Pruritus is the most common complaint and is believed to be the result of a hypersensitivity reaction to the saliva of lice. On examination, nits are seen that firmly attached to hair shaft within 6 mm from the scalp skin especially in the occipital pit [louse pit] and retro-auricular areas. Scratches on the skin may lead to secondary bacterial infection and impetiginisation. Serous purulent discharge may result in the formation of a plica [plica polonica or plica neuropathica]. There are innumerable nits and live lice in patients with plica polonica. Cervical lymphadenopathy and conjunctivitis may also be seen. Lice infestation can cause allergic reactions within the nasal cavity manifested by nasal obstruction and rhinorrhea [72, 74, 75].

The diagnosis of head lice infestation is made through finding viable eggs [nits], nymphs and live adult lice. For the diagnosis, the use of a louse comb is more efficient than direct visual examination of the scalp [76]. Examining suggestive particles under the microscope may be helpful to confirm the diagnosis. Non-contact dermoscopy is also a useful instrument for differentiate nymph-containing eggs from empty cases or pseudonits [72]. Histology is rarely required for diagnosis. Examination of a louse bite reveals intradermal haemorrhage and a deep, wedge-shaped infiltrate with many eosinophils and lymphocytes.

Differential diagnosis of head lice includes seborrheic scales, hair casts [inner root sheath remnants], pityriasis amiantacea, white piedra, black piedra, impetigo, pili torti and monilethrix. It should kept in mind that, in contrast to nits, hair casts are freely movable along hair shaft [72].

Basically, therapeutic wet combing, topical application of a pediculicide and oral treatment [Trimethoprim-sulfamethoxazole and ivermectin] are used to eliminate head lice. Wet combing is a mechanical removal of the lice. The patients must comb their wet hair with a fine-toothed comb every 3–4 days for a total of 2 weeks. If all young lice are combed out a few days after hatching, the infestation can be eradicated completely. Pediculicides are the most effective treatment for head lice. They can be divided into three types. Pediculisides with neurotoxic mode of action are permetrin [Nix®], pyrethrin [Rid®], malathion [Ovide®], carbaryl, lindan [Kwell®] and spinosad [Natroba®]. Dimeticones [Nyda®, Hedrin®], isopropyl myristate [Resultz®] and 1,2-octanediol are the pediculicides with physical mode of action. The other group of pediculicides is plant-based pediculicides. All topical preparations are used for two or three applications, 1 week apart [68, 71].

Because permetrin and pyretrin are non-ovicidal, they should be reapplied on days 7 and 13–15. Permethrin 1% is a synthetic pyrethroid and is approved for use in children aged 2 months or older. It shows neurotoxic effect by inhibiting the sodium ion flux through nerve cell membrane channels [68]. It should be applied on damp unconditioned hair for 10 min and then rinsed off. Pruritus, erythema and edema are its usual side effects [77]. Pyretrin is used for children aged 2 years and older. Malathion is a cholinesterase inhibitor. It is approved for use in individuals aged 6 years or older. Both malathion and lindan are ovicidal. Spinosad is ovicidal, killing both eggs and lice and also kills permethrin-resistant populations of lice. It is approved in patients aged 4 years and older [78]. Oral ivermectin is administered a single dose of 200 μg/kg and repeated in 10 days. It is restricted to children older than 5 years and weighing at least 15 kg [71].

Resistance of lice to the pediculocides is an important problem. Spinosad, benzyl alcohol 5% or malathion 0.5% may also be used, in case of resistance, for those older than 6 and 24 months, respectively. Another treatment option is manual removal of nits [especially the ones within 1 cm of the scalp]. It is recommended after treatment with any product. Besides these treatments, occlusive agents such as petroleum jelly, vinegar, isopropyl alcohol, olive oil, mayonnaise and melted butter can been used once per week for 3 weeks to suffocate the lice [68, 78].

Patients with head lice should have laundered potential fomites [e.g., towels, pillowcases, sheets, hats, toys] with hot water [at least 130°F/55°C] and then dried in a dryer using the

http://dx.doi.org/10.5772/67278

hottest cycle. For items that are not machine washable, dry-cleaning may be an effective alternative or storing for 2 weeks in a plastic bag. Children should also be educated not to share combs, brushes, hair accessories and towels and to avoid head-to-head contact [72, 73, 78].

6. Neoplasms of scalp

The neoplasms of the scalp consist of large group of different diseases due to arising different origin. They can be divided into two groups: benign and malignant. They can be categorised as shown in **Table 1**. The common benign swellings of the scalp are the epidermoid cysts, trichilemmal cysts, lipomas, dermoid cyst, pilomatrixoma, steatocystoma multiplex and cylindroma. In this section, neoplasms especially which is most seen and is arising from scalp are discussed in detail.

Benign neoplasms	Malignant neoplasms
Epidermoid cysts	Basal cell carcinoma
Trichilemmal cyst	Squamous cell carcinoma
Proliferating trichilemmal cyst	Melanoma
Seborrheic keratosis	Proliferating trichilemmal cyst
Lipoma	Angiosarcoma
Dermoid cyst	Cutaneous lymphoma
Pilomatricoma	Cutaneous metastases
Steatocystoma multiplex	
Actinic keratosis	
Nevus sebaceous	
Melanocytic nevus	
Cylindroma	
Angiolymphoid hyperplasia with eosinophilia	
Neurothekeoma	
Infantile myofibromatosis	
Hemangioma	

Table 1. The neoplasms of the scalp.

6.1. Trichilemmal cyst

Trichilemmal cyst [TC] also known as 'pilar cyst' is an adnexal tumour that arises from outer root sheath of the hair follicle. It is almost always benign but may be locally aggressive. Malignant transformation is very rare but may lead to distant metastases [77, 79].

It affects 5–10% of the population with a female preponderance [77, 80]. TC may be sporadic or they may be inherited as an autosomal dominant trait. It presents as an asymptomatic or mildly painful firm nodule but frequently they are multiple. The cysts are classically located in areas bearing hair follicle, mostly on the scalp and rarely the face, trunk and extremities may be involved. They are usually 1–2 cm in size but can be much larger.

Histopathologic evaluation can confirm the diagnosis. Histopathologically TCs are lined by stratified squamous epithelial cells and consist homogenous eosinophilic material that frequently show foci of calcification and abrupt keratinisation without an intervening granular layer.

TC may be misdiagnosed as epidermal cyst clinically but unlike epidermal cyst, no punctum is seen. Treatment is by complete excision. Trichilemmal cysts typically can be extracted more easily than epidermoid cysts [77, 79, 80].

6.2. Proliferating trichilemmal cyst

Proliferating trichilemmal cyst [PTC] also known as proliferating pilar tumour is a rare neoplasm arising from the isthmus region of the outer root sheath of the hair follicle. It can be inherited in an autosomal dominant pattern. It occurs most commonly on the scalp in women older than 50 years. Most tumours arise within a pre-existing trichilemmal cyst but some PTCs arise *de novo* [81]. They have different clinical and histologic features from trichilemmal cyst. PCTs may slowly or rapidly grow into a large, solitary, well-circumscribed painless mass overlying alopecia. The size may range from 1 to 10 cm, although there have been reports of lesions exceeding 25 cm in diameter. Inflammation, ulceration, bleeding and/or yellowish discharge may occur and may be clinically confused with squamous cell carcinoma. They usually behave in a benign nature but malignant transformation with local invasion and metastasis has also been described [82, 83].

Broad anastomosing bands and lobules of squamous epithelium in the cyst wall are the histologic features of PCT. PTC shows features of typical trichilemmal cyst, but additionally shows extensive epithelial proliferation, variable cytologic atypia and mitotic activity. Complete excision is recommended for the treatment of PCT owing to their potential for locally aggressive behaviour and malignant transformation [81, 83]. If malignant PTC with multi-nodal metastasis is identified, wide local excision with 1-cm margins should be performed, followed by adjuvant chemotherapy and radiation to prevent recurrence [84].

6.3. Nevus sebaceous

Nevus sebaceous [NS] is uncommon hamartomatous lesions that exhibits epidermal, follicular, sebaceous and apocrine malformation to varying degrees. It was first described by Jadassohn in 1895. It occurs most commonly on the head and neck while similar lesions elsewhere on the body are termed verrucous epidermal nevi. It often presents at birth with an incidence of 0.5–1% [85]. The characteristic clinical feature is a well-circumscribed, flesh-coloured, bald patch on the scalp at birth. At puberty, lesion grows proportionally with the patient and tends to be slightly yellow or orange, thick, velvety and verrucous surface. Familial cases have been reported [86].

Development of benign or malignant adnexal neoplasms may occur in NS, usually in adulthood. Syringocystadenoma papilliferum and trichoblastoma are the most common benign tumours arising in NS [87]. Other benign tumours include trichilemmoma, sebaceous adenoma, apocrin adenoma and poroma. Malignant transformation can develop in 10–15% of lesions in some series and basal cell carcinoma is the most seen malignant tumour. Actually, this rate is less than 1% of cases. Development of six different tumours has also been reported in one solitary lesion [88].

Histologically, early lesions show few abnormal features. A few misshapen hair follicles and small apocrine glands may be identifiable during childhood. At adolescence, as the lesions clinically thicken, NS looks like an epidermal nevus, with papillated epidermal hyperplasia, abortive hair follicles and enlarged apocrine glands.

The lesions must be distinguished from aplasia cutis congenita, congenital nevi, epidermal nevus syndrome and seborrheic keratosis. Although there is no consensus regarding the NS, increasing to the possibility of malignant tumour outgrowth from a NS with age, it is necessary to prophylactic excision especially in adulthood. Photodynamic therapy with topical aminolevulinic acid is another treatment option for non-surgical treatment [89].

6.4. Cylindroma

Cylindroma is a benign skin adnexal tumour differentiating towards either the eccrine or apocrine line. It has two different clinical presentations, solitary and multiple. Solitary cylindroma is a slow growing, benign tumour effecting the scalp especially the capillitium and neck region. Solitary cylindromas affect middle-aged and elderly persons and female-to-male ratios are 6:1 and 9:1 [90].

Multiple cylindromas are very rare and inherited in an autosomal dominant pattern by mutations in CYLD1, a tumour suppressor gene. They frequently occur on the scalp and rarely on the trunk. The term turban tumour is used to describe multiple cylindromas. Since the nodules enlarge and coalesce on the scalp, the patient looks as wearing a turban. Multiple cylindromas should suggest of Brook-Spiegler syndrome, which has been characterised by the development of multiple skin appendage tumours, such as cylindromas, trichoepitheliomas and spiradenomas [91, 92].

Histopathology is diagnostic with islands of basaloid cells in a jigsaw puzzle-like pattern separated by hyaline basement membrane material that is PAS positive. Eosinophilic PAS-positive hyaline material in globules is also seen within the lobules [93].

Differential diagnosis of cylindroma includes trichilemmal cysts, basal cell carcinoma, spiradenoma and dermatofibroma. Under dermatoscopy, cylindromas demonstrates arborising telangiectasia and scattered white globules on a background of white to salmon-pink. Vascular branches can be seen at the periphery which may extend into the centre of the lesion [94].

For solitary lesions, the treatment option is complete excision. Other treatments include electrodesiccation/curettage, cryotherapy and carbon dioxide laser. The patients with multiple cylindromas should follow up because of the tendency for new lesions to develop [95].

Author details

Filiz Canpolat

Address all correspondence to: filizcanpolat@hotmail.com

Sağlık Bilimleri Üniversitesi Yıldırım Beyazıt Dışkapı Eğitim Araştırma Hastanesi Dermatoloji Kliniği, Ankara, Turkey

References

[1] Lee AH, Cho SY, Yam TS, Harris K, Ardern-Jones MR. Staphylococcus aureus and chronic folliculocentric pustuloses of the scalp—cause or association? Br J Dermatol. 2016; **175**: 410–13. doi: 10.1111/bjd.14518

[2] Abeck D. Staphylococal and Streptococcal Diseases. In: Burgdorf WHC, Plewig G, Wolff HH, Landthaler M, editors. Braun-Falco's Dermatology. 3rd ed. Italy, Springer; 2009. p 126.

[3] Quinquaud E. Bull Mem Soc Hop Paris. 1888; **5**: 395–8.

[4] Powell JJ, Dawber RPR, Gatter K. Folliculitis decalvans including tufted folliculitis: clinical, histological and therapeutic findings. Br J Dermatol. 1999; **140**: 328–33.

[5] Bunagan MJK, Banka N, Shapiro JJ. Retrospective review of folliculitis decalvans in 23 patients with course and treatment analysis of long-standing cases. Cutan Med Surg. Vol. 2015; **19**: 45–49.

[6] Stefanato C. Histopathology of alopecia: a clinicopathologic approach to diagnosis. Histopathology. 2010; **56**: 24–38.

[7] Sperling LC, Cowper SE. The histopathology of primary cicatricial alopecia. Semin Cutan Med Surg. 2006; **25**: 41–50.

[8] Mihaljevic N, von den Driesch P. Successful use of infliximab in a patient with recalcitrant folliculitis decalvans. J Dtsch Dermatol Ges. 2012; **10**: 589–90.

[9] Kreutzer K, Effendy I. Therapy-resistant folliculitis decalvans and lichen planopilaris successfully treated with adalimumab. J Dtsch Dermatol Ges. 2014; **12**: 74–6.

[10] Meesters AA, van der Veen JP, Wolkerstorfer A. Long-term remission of folliculitis decalvans after treatment with long-pulsed Nd:YAG laser. J Dermatolog Treat. 2014; **25**: 167–8.

[11] Castano-Suarez E, Romero-Mate A, Arias-Palomo D, Borbujo J. Photodynamic therapy for the treatment of folliculitis decalvans. Photodermatol Photoimmunol Photomed. 2012; **28**: 102–4.

http://dx.doi.org/10.5772/67278

[12] Powell J, Dawber RPR. Successful treatment regime for folliculitis decalvans despite uncertainty of all etiologic factors. Br J Dermatol. 2001;**144**:428–9.

[13] Broshtilova V, Bardarov E, Kazandjieva J, Marina S. Tufted hair folliculitis: a case report and literature review. Acta Dermatovenerol Alp Pannonica Adriat. 2011; **20**: 27–9.

[14] Ekmekci TR, Koslu A. Tufted hair folliculitis causing skullcap-pattern cicatricial alopecia. J Eur Acad Dermatol Venereol. 2006; **20**: 227–9.

[15] Trüeb RM, Pericin M, Hafner J, Burg G. Tufted hair folliculitis. Hautarzt.1997; **48**: 266–9.

[16] Gungor S, Yuksel T, Topal I. Tufted hair folliculitis associated with Melkersson-Rosenthal syndrome and hidradenitis suppurativa. Indian J Dermatol Venereol Leprol. 2014; **80**: 484.

[17] Farhi D, Buffard V, Ortonne N, Revuz J. Tufted folliculitis of the scalp and treatment with cyclosporine. Arch Dermatol. 2006; **142**: 251–2.

[18] Ena P, Fadda GM, Ena L, Farris A, Santeufemia DA. Tufted hair folliculitis in a woman treated with lapatinib for breast cancer. Clin Exp Dermatol. 2008; **33**: 790–1.

[19] Petronić-Rosić V, Krunić A, Mijusković M, Vesić S. Tufted hair folliculitis: a pattern of scarring alopecia? J Am Acad Dermatol. 1999; **41**: 112–4.

[20] Pranteda G, Grimaldi M, Palese E, Di Napoli A, Bottoni U. Tufted hair folliculitis: complete enduring response after treatment with rifampicin. J Dermatol Treat. 2004; **15**: 396–8.

[21] Brozena SJ, Cohen LE, Fenske NA. Folliculitis decalvans—response to rifampicin. Cutis. 1988; **42**: 512–5.

[22] Rosman IS, Anadkat MJ. Tufted hair folliculitis in a woman treated with trastuzumab. Target Oncol. 2010; **5**: 295–6.

[23] Gloster HM Jr. The surgical management of extensive cases of acne keloidalis nuchae. Arch Dermatol. 2000; **136**: 1376–9.

[24] Ogunbiyi A, Adedokun B. Perceived aetiological factors of folliculitis keloidalis nuchae [acne keloidalis] and treatment options among Nigerian men. Br J Dermatol. 2015; **173** [Suppl. 2]: 22–25.

[25] Shah GK. Efficacy of diode laser for treating acne keloidalis nuchae. Indian J Dermatol Venereol Leprol. 2005; **71**: 31–4.

[26] Okoye GA, Rainer BM, Leung SG, et al. Improving acne keloidalis nuchae with targeted ultraviolet B treatment: a prospective, randomized, split-scalp comparison study. Br J Dermatol. 2014; **171**: 1156–63.

[27] George AO, Akanji AO, Nduka EU, Olasode JB, Odusan O. Clinical, biochemical and morphologic features of acne keloidalis in a black population. Int J Dermatol. 1993; **32**: 714–6.

[28] Ogunbiyi A, George A. Acne keloidalis in females: case report and review of literature. J Natl Med Assoc. 2005; **97**: 736–8.

[29] Luz Ramos M, Munoz-Perez MA, Pons A, Ortega M, Camacho F. Acne keloidalis nuchae and tufted hair folliculitis. Dermatology. 1997; **194**: 71–3.

[30] Janjua SA, Iftikhar N, Pastar Z, Hosler GA. Keratosis follicularis spinulosa decalvans associated with acne keloidalis nuchae and tufted hair folliculitis. Am J Clin Dermatol. 2008;**9**:137–40.

[31] Quarles FN, Brody H, Badreshia S, et al. Acne keloidalis nuchae. Dermatol Ther. 2007; **20**: 128–32.

[32] Millán-Cayetano JF, Repiso-Jiménez JB, Del Boz J, de Troya-Martín M. Refractory acne keloidalis nuchae treated with radiotherapy. Australas J Dermatol. 2015 Jul 29. doi: 10.1111/ajd.12380. [Epub ahead of print]

[33] Maranda EL, Simmons BJ, Nguyen AH, Lim VM, Keri JE. Treatment of acne keloidalis nuchae: a systematic review of the literature. Dermatol Ther [Heidelb]. 2016; **6**: 363–78.

[34] Bajaj V, Langtry JAA. Surgical excision of acne keloidalis nuchae with secondary intention healing. Clin Exp Dermatol. 2008; **33**: 53–5.

[35] Seebacher C, Bouchara JP, Mignon B. Updates on the epidemiology of dermatophyte infections. Mycopathologia. 2008; **166**: 335–52.

[36] Pomeranz AJ, Sabnis SS, McGrath GJ, Esterly NB. Asymptomatic dermatophyte carriers in the households of children with tinea capitis. Arch Pediatr Adolesc Med. 1999; **153**: 483–6.

[37] Fu M, Ge Y, Chen W, Feng S, She X, Li X, et al. Tinea faciei in a newborn due to Trichophyton tonsurans. J Biomed Res. 2013; **27**: 71–4.

[38] Zaraa I, Hawilo A, Trojjet S, El Euch D, Mokni M, Ben Osman A. Letter: Tinea capitis in infants in their first 2 years of life: a 12-year study and a review of the literature. Dermatol Online J. 2012; **18**: 16.

[39] Koussidou-Eremondi T, Devliotou-Panagiotidou D, Mourellou-Tsatsou O, Fotidou D, Minas A. Tinea capitis in children in northern Greece during the period 1981-1995. Mycoses. 1999; **42**: 319–22.

[40] El-Taweel AE, El-Esawy F, Abdel-Salam O. Different trichoscopic features of tinea capitis and alopecia areata in pediatric patients. Dermatol Res Pract. 2014; **2014**: 848763.

[41] Brasileiro A, Campos S, Cabete J, Galhardas C, Lencastre A, Serrão V. Trichoscopy as an additional tool for the differential diagnosis of tinea capitis: a prospective clinical study. Br J Dermatol. 2016; **175**: 208–9.

[42] González U, Seaton T, Bergus G, Jacobson J, Martínez-Monzón C. Systemic antifungal therapy for tinea capitis in children. Cochrane Database Syst Rev. 2007 Oct 17;[4]: CD004685. Review. Update in: Cochrane Database Syst Rev. 2016;[5]:CD004685.

[43] Gupta AK, Cooper EA. Update in antifungal therapy of dermatophytosis. Mycopathologia. 2008; **166**: 353–67.

[44] Ilkit M. Favus of the scalp: an overview update. Mycopathologia. 2010; **170**: 143–154.

[45] Vallarelli AFA. Goya and tinea favosa. An Bras Dermatol. 2014; **89**: 992–4.

[46] Niczyporuk W, Krajewska-Kulak E, Lukaszuk C. Tinea capitis favosa in Poland. Mycoses. 2004; **47**: 257–60.

[47] Anane S, Chtourou O. Tinea capitis favosa misdiagnosed as tinea amiantacea. Med Mycol Case Rep. 2012; **28**; 2:29–31.

[48] Poppe H, Kolb-Mäurer A, Wobser M, Trautmann A. Pitfall scarring alopecia: favus closely mimicking lichen planus. Mycoses. 2013; **56**: 382–4.

[49] Liu ZH, Zhang Y, Zhu J, Dai YQ, Shen H. Successful treatment of severe kerion celsi in an immunocompromised girl with evacuation of pus, terbinafine and short course glucocorticosteroids. J Mycol Med. 2016; **26**: 42–5.

[50] Feetham JE, Sargant N. Kerion celsi: a misdiagnosed scalp infection. Arch Dis Child. 2016; **101**: 503.

[51] Larralde M, Gomar B, Boggio P, Abad ME, Pagotto B. Neonatal kerion celsi: report of three cases. Pediatric Dermatol. 2010; **27**: 361–3.

[52] Tanuma H, Doi M, Abe M, Kume H, Nishiyama S, Katsuoka K. Case report. Kerion celsi effectively treated with terbinafine. Characteristics of kerion celsi in the elderly in Japan. Mycoses. 1999; **42**: 581–5.

[53] Friedlander SF, Pickering B, Cunningham BB, Gibbs NF, Eichenfield LF. Use of the cotton swab method in diagnosing Tinea capitis. Pediatrics. 1999; **104**: 276–9.

[54] Jaspers GJ, Werrij1 BG, Jagtman BA, Loza B. Severe kerion celsi due to Trichophyton mentagrophytes: a case report. Acta Paediatrica. 2011; **100**: e181–e183.

[55] Castriota M, Ricci F, Paradisi A, Fossati B, De Simone C, Capizzi R, Guerriero C. Erythema nodosum induced by kerion celsi of the scalp in a child: a case report and mini-review of literature. Mycoses. 2013; **56**: 200–3.

[56] Bassi N, Kersey P. Erythema nodosum complicating a case of kerion celsi of the scalp due to *Trichophyton mentagrophytes*. Clin Exper Dermatol. 2009; **34**: 621–38.

[57] Ye Y, Zhang X, Zhao Y, Gong Y, Yang J, Li H, Zhang X. The clinical and trichoscopic features of syphilitic alopecia. J Dermatol Case Rep. 2014; **8**: 78–80.

[58] Hernández-Bel P, Unamuno B, Sánchez-Carazo JL, Febrer I, Alegre V. Syphilitic alopecia: a report of 5 cases and a review of the literature. Actas Dermosifiliogr. 2013; **104**: 512–7.

[59] Pareek SS. Syphilitic alopecia and Jarisch-Herxheimer reaction. Br J Vener Dis. 1977; **53**: 389–90.

[60] Lee JY, Hsu ML. Alopecia syphilitica, a simulator of alopecia areata: histopathology and differential diagnosis. J Cutan Pathol. 1991; **18**: 87–92.

[61] Cuozzo DW, Benson PM, Sperling LC, Skelton HG 3rd. Essential syphilitic alopecia revisited. J Am Acad Dermatol. 1995; **32**: 840–3.

[62] Friedli A, Chavaz P, Harms M. Alopecia syphilitica: report of two cases in Geneva. Dermatology. 2001; **202**: 376–7.

[63] Lee JW, Jang WS, Yoo KH, et al. Diffuse pattern essential syphilitic alopecia: an unusual form of secondary syphilis. Int J Dermatol. 2012; **51**: 1006–7.

[64] Bi MY, Cohen PR, Robinson FW, Gray JM. Alopecia syphilitica: report of a patient with secondary syphilis presenting as motheaten alopecia and a review of its common mimickers. Dermatol Online J 2009; **15**: 6.

[65] Pareek SS. Unusual location of syphilitic alopecia: a case report. Sex Transm Dis. 1982; **9**: 43–4.

[66] Abdul Gaffoor PM. Syphilitic alopecia. Indian J Sex Transm Dis. 1990; **11**: 66–7.

[67] Falagas ME, Matthaiou DK, Rafailidis PI, Panos G, Pappas G. Worldwide prevalence of head lice. Emerg Infect Dis. 2008; **14**: 1493–4.

[68] Wadowski L, Balasuriya L, Price HN, O'Haver J. Lice update: new solutions to an old problem. Clin Dermatol. 2015; **33**: 347–54.

[69] Kokturk A, Baz K, Bugdayci R, Sasmaz T, Tursen U, Kaya TI, Ikizoglu G. The prevalence of pediculosis capitis in schoolchildren in Mersin, Turkey. Int J Dermatol. 2003; **42**: 694–8.

[70] Akisu C, Aksoy U, Delibas SB, Ozkoc S, Sahin S. The prevalence of head lice infestation in school children in Izmir, Turkey. Pediatr Dermatol. 2005; **22**: 372–3.

[71] Feldmeier H. Treatment of pediculosis capitis: a critical appraisal of the current literature. Am J Clin Dermatol. 2014; **15**: 401–12.

[72] Madke B, Khopkar U. Pediculosis capitis: an update. Indian J Dermatol Venereol Leprol 2012; **78**: 429–38.

[73] Head Lice. Centers for Disease Control and Prevention Web site. http://www.cdc.gov/parasites/lice/head. 2013 Sep 24; Accessed: August 2, 2014.

[74] Bartosik K, Buczek A, Zając Z, Kulisz J. Head pediculosis in schoolchildren in the eastern region of the European Union. Ann Agric Environ Med. 2015; **22**: 599–603.

[75] Pavithran K. Plica neuropathica causing traction alopecia. Indian J Dermatol Venereol Leprol. 1990; **56**: 141–2.

[76] Jahnke C, Bauer E, Hengge UR, Feldmeier H. Accuracy of diagnosis of pediculosis capitis: visual inspection vs wet combing. Arch Dermatol. 2009; **145**: 309–13.

[77] Jha AK, Sinha R, Prasad S, Kumar S. Multiple trichilemmal cysts of the scalp in a young male. Int J Trichol. 2015; **7**: 167–9.

[78] Verma P, Namdeo C. Treatment of pediculosis capitis. Indian J Dermatol. 2015; **60**: 238–47.

[79] Dewanda NK, Midya M. Baker's dozen on the scalp: an interesting case of multiple trichilemmal cyst. J Cutan Aesthet Surg. 2014; **7:** 67–8.

[80] Weiss J, Heine M, Grimmel M, Jung EG. Malignant proliferating trichilemmal cyst. J Am Acad Dermatol. 1995; **32**: 870–3.

[81] Poiares Baptista A, Garcia E, Silva L, Born MC. Proliferating trichilemmal cyst. J Cutan Pathol.1983;**10**: 178–87.

[82] Ye J, Nappi O, Swanson PE, Patterson JW, Wick MR. Proliferating pilar tumors: a clinicopathologic study of 76 cases with a proposal for definition of benign and malignant variants. Am J Clin Pathol. 2004; **122**: 566–74.

[83] Alam K, Gupta K, Maheshwari V, Varshney M, Jain A, Khan AH. A large proliferating trichilemmal cyst masquerading as squamous cell carcinoma. Indian J Dermatol. 2015; **60**: 104.

[84] Alici O, Keles MK, Kurt A. A rare cutaneous adnexal tumor: malignant proliferating trichilemmal tumor. Case Rep Med. 2015; **2015**: 742920.

[85] Kamyab-Hesari K, Seirafi H, Jahan S, Aghazadeh N, Hejazi P, Azizpour A,Goodarzi A. Nevus sebaceus: a clinicopathological study of 168 cases and review of the literature. Int J Dermatol. 2016; **55**:193–200.

[86] Happle R, Konig A. Familial naevus sebaceus may be explained by paradominant transmission. Br J Dermatol. 1999; **141**: 377.

[87] Jaqueti G, Requena L, Sanchez Yus E. Trichoblastoma is the most common neoplasm developed in nevus sebaceus of Jadassohn: a clinicopathologic study of a series of 155 cases. Am J Dermatopathol. 2000; **22**: 108–18.

[88] Gozel S, Donmez M, Akdur NC, Yikilkan H. Development of six tumors in a sebaceus nevus of jadassohn: report of a case. Korean J Pathol. 2013; **47**: 569–74.

[89] Gaitan-Gaona F, Said MC, Galvan-Linares A, Palafox-Vigil G, Valdes-Rodriguez R. Rapidly growing pigmented tumor on a scalp nevus sebaceous of a pediatric patient: observation or excision. Dermatol Online J. 2014; **15**; 20[7].

[90] Massoumi R, Podda M, Fässler R, Paus R. Cylindroma as tumor of hair follicle origin. J Invest Dermatol. 2006; **126**: 1182–4.

[91] Manicketh I, Singh R, Ghosh PK. Eccrine cylindroma of the face and scalp. Indian Dermatol Online J. 2016; **7**: 203–5.

[92] Akgul GG, Yenidogan E, Dinc S, Pak I, Colakoglu MK, Gulcelik MA. Malign cylindroma of the scalp with multiple cervical lymph node metastasis—a case report. Int J Surg Case Rep. 2013; **4**: 589–92.

[93] Weedon D. Tumors of cutaneous appendages. In: Weedon D, editor. Weedon's Skin Pathology. 3rd ed. China: Churchill Livingstone Elsevier; 2010. pp. 785–6.

[94] Cohen YK, Elpern DJ. Dermatoscopic pattern of a cylindroma. Dermatol Pract Concept. 2014; **4**: 67–8.

[95] Retamar RA, Stengel F, Saadi ME, et al. Brooke-Spiegler syndrome—report of four families: treatment with CO_2 laser. Int J Dermatol. 2007; **46**: 583–6.

Section 7

Psychocutaneous Disorders of Hair

Chapter 12

Trichotillomania and Traction Alopecia

Tugba Kevser Uzuncakmak, Melek Aslan Kayıran,
Burak Tekin and Filiz Cebeci

Additional information is available at the end of the chapter

http://dx.doi.org/10.5772/66746

Abstract

Trichotillomania and traction alopecia are chronic habitual disorders characterized by repetitive pulling of hair that results in alopecia. They are commonly observed in children and adolescents but may present in adults due to occupational or traditional behavioral patterns. Trichotillomania (hair-pulling disorder) has been described more than a century ago, but we still have very limited data about its etiology and treatment. It is classified under the obsessive-compulsive and related disorders along with hoarding disorder, skin-picking disorder (excoriation) and body dysmorphic disorder in the *Diagnostic and Statistical Manual of Mental Disorders*, Fifth Edition (DSM-5; American Psychiatric Association, May 2013). Traction alopecia is defined as loss of hair caused by repetitive or continuous and prolonged tension applied to the hair, usually on the scalp periphery and associated with mechanical traction of hair due to occupational behavioral patterns such as ballerinas or traditional behavioral patterns of hairstyles that cause tension. We aim to overview the clinical and diagnostic features of trichotillomania and traction alopecia and review the therapeutic options of these disorders in this chapter.

Keywords: alopecia, hair loss, psychosomatic disorders, traction alopecia, trichotillomania

1. Trichotillomania

1.1. Introduction

Trichotillomania is the disorder of repetitively pulling out one's hair from different areas of the body that results in noticeable hair loss [1]. The name trichotillomania was given to this behavior by a French dermatologist, Francois Henri Hallopeau, in 1889; however, the disorder also appears in the literature in the works of Hippocrates. It is even found in plays by William Shakespeare such as Romeo and Juliet and The Life and Death of King John. The name is derived from the combination of Greek *thrix* for hair; *tillein*, plucking; and *mania*, madness.

Trichotillomania is classified under the obsessive-compulsive and related disorders along with hoarding disorder, skin-picking disorder (excoriation) and body dysmorphic disorder in the *Diagnostic and Statistical Manual of Mental Disorders* Fifth Edition (DSM-5; American Psychiatric Association, May 2013) [2] (**Table 1**). It is also grouped under obsessive-compulsive disorders in the eleventh revision of the World Health Organization's International Classification of Diseases and Related Health Problems (ICD-11) [3].

• Recurrent pulling out of one's hair, resulting in hair loss
• Repeated attempts to decrease or stop the pulling out of hair
• The hair pulling causes clinically significant distress or impairment in social, occupational, or other important areas of functioning
• The hair pulling or hair loss is not attributable to another medical condition
• The hair pulling is not better explained by the symptoms of another mental disorder

Table 1. Diagnostic criteria (DSM-5) [2].

1.2. Epidemiology

Trichotillomania occurs more frequently in females. The lifetime prevalence is 3.4% for women and 1.5% for men [4]. The typical age of onset is between 5 and 12 years or early childhood to adolescence, but it may occur in any age.

1.3. Pathogenesis

The onset of trichotillomania often occurs after a stressful event such as the divorce of parents, loss of a loved one or unemployment [5]. Occasionally, trichotillomania is only seen while sleeping, a condition known as sleep-isolated trichotillomania [6].

1.4. Diagnosis

1.4.1. Clinical features

Patients may have other problems with self-mutilation such as nail-biting or dermatitis artefacta. Approximately one-third of the patients chew or swallow the hair they pull out, which is called trichophagia and some of them develop trichobezoars, which is the accumulation of the patients' own hair in the intestines. These trichobezoars may result in a "tail" that lies along the duodenum, a phenomenon which is called *Rapunzel Syndrome*. Around 1% of trichobezoar patients may need surgical intervention [4].

Symptom severity can be measured by using different validated instruments including Massachusetts General Hospital Hair Pulling Scale that has seven parameters, rating symptom

http://dx.doi.org/10.5772/66746

severity from 0 to 4 and assessing various aspects of plucking during the past seven days: actual pulling, urge to pull, associated distress and perceived control, The Yale-Brown Obsessive-Compulsive Scale, The Psychiatric Institute Trichotillomania Scale, The Trichotillomania Scale for Children, The Milwaukee Inventory for Styles of Trichotillomania-Child Version [7]. The MGHHS includes seven parameters, rating symptom severity from 0 to 4 and assesses several aspects of hair pulling during the previous 7 days: urge to pull, actual pulling, perceived control and associated distress. The MGHHS and its Dutch adaptation have been reported to provide good psychometric properties [7].

Three subtypes of hair pulling have been described (**Table 2**).

• Early onset: occurring in young children, mostly under the age of 8; usually does not need any treatment.
• Automatic: occurring when the individual is busy with other activities, such as reading. This type affects 75% of patients.
• Focused: occurs with the patient's attention and is associated with strong impulses to pull hair.

Table 2. Subtypes of trichotillomania.

Any part of the hair may be affected, but the targeted hair is mostly on the scalp (75%). The eyelashes (53%), eyebrows (42%), pubic region (17%) and beard (10%) may also be involved, but sometimes there is more than one location (17%) [8, 9]. The most affected scalp areas are the frontoparietal region and vertex, while the least affected region is the occiput. The lower eyelid is usually not involved; this is helpful to distinguish trichotillomania from alopecia areata [10].

Alopecic plaques are usually located on the contralateral side of the dominant hand. There may be more than one plaque. These plaques of hair loss most often have irregular shapes and contain many broken hairs of varying lengths. The margins have normal and long hair.

The plucked hairs have fiber fractures and feel rough on examination. There are usually no signs of inflammation in the plaques, but there may also be signs of excoriation, lichenification and post-inflammatory hyperpigmentation in some cases.

1.4.2. Dermoscopy

Trichoscopy may also be utilized for differential diagnosis. The trichotillomania plaque includes broken and irregular coiled hair and hair density is decreased. Black dots, follicular hemorrhages and V-sign may be seen [11]. Trichoscopy is very useful in the differential diagnosis of trichotillomania from alopecia areata where exclamation mark hairs, yellow dots and proximal tapering hairs could be seen, in contrast with trichotillomania where trichoptilosis, pointed hairs, flame hairs, V-sign, hook hairs, hair powder, follicular microhemorrhage and tulip hairs are more characteristic. Follicular microhemorrhage meaning a red dot that corresponds to a follicular ostium stuffed with blood clot, may support local trauma, a clue for trichotillomania [12].

1.4.3. Histopathology

The diagnosis of trichotillomania is usually made by clinical examination and patient history. However, occasionally especially in pediatric patient group both child and parents may deny the possibility of pulling or plucking as a cause of hair loss and especially in localized involved patients the diagnosis may be difficult. Histopathological examination may be necessary in these patients. Follicules of normal size, increased catagen and telogen hairs (up to 75%) which is a result of mechanical trauma to the hair frequently propelling anagen follicules into the catagen phase, pigmentary defects and casts, evidence of traumatized hair bulbs and trichomalacia (a complete but distorted, fully developed terminal hair in its bulb) are the most common findings in histological examination of trichotillomania [13, 14]. Catagen hairs may be present in areas that have recently been injured and telogen hairs may present after a few weeks from pulling. Some hair follicles in anagen phase may be present, but they are usually seen empty because of hair shaft avulsion. If the hair matrix and suprabulbar epithelium are injured, but not severely disrupted, the follicle may remain in the anagen phase which may produce a hair shaft. Follicles can show distortion of the bulbar epithelium and sometimes conspicuous hemorrhage.

Hair shaft avulsion may deposit melanin pigment in the hair papilla and peribulbar connective tissue [13, 14]. Frequently, chunks of pigmented hair matrix or cortex cells are torn from their moorings during the plucking process and come to rest in superficial portions of the follicles. These cells then shrink to form a dark black homogeneous clump called a pigment cast. Pigment casts which are very characteristic for trichotillomania simply occur as the by-product of fragmented, ectopic matrix or cortical epithelium and usually seen in the isthmus or infundibulum. Trichomalacia, which defines shaft abnormalities such as distorted in shape, smaller than normal and incompletely cornified, is very characteristic for trichotillomania.

These injuries of pulling or plucking to the bulbar portions of follicles do not induce inflammation but may cause follicular microhemorrhage within the lower portion of the follicle. A few eosinophils may be rarely seen around the lower portion of the traumatized follicule. Also miniaturization of follicules is usually not seen in trichotillomania and absence of inflammatory infiltrate and loss of miniaturization are usually serve to differentiate it from alopecia areata [14].

1.5. Differential diagnosis

Tinea capitis, alopecia areata, loose anagen hair, monilethrix, lichen planopilaris and secondary syphilis need to be considered in the differential diagnosis of trichotillomania. Trichoscopy, medical history and scalp biopsy can be used to distinguish trichotillomania from other diseases. Catagen and telogen hair numbers are found to be increased and usually there are no signs of inflammation unless there is an infection in histologic examination. The number of catagen hairs exceeds telogen hairs in chronic lesions. Perifollicular hemorrhage may be found at the circumference of the hair bumbs [1].

Potassium hydroxide examination, fungal culture and Wood's lamp examination may be performed to exclude tinea capitis. The hair is weak and may easily be pulled out in tinea capitis.

Alopecia areata plaques are oval and well-demarked. A hair pull test may be helpful as a diagnostic test for alopecia areata. Telogenic hairs may be pulled out easily in alopecia areata, which indicates the activity of the disease in contrast with trichotillomania. Shaving the involved area and waiting for the regrowth may also be useful for the diagnosis of trichotillomania. Alternatively, a small part of the hair is clipped near the scalp with scissors and the hairs in trichotillomania display uniform hair regrowth.

Trichoscopy may also be utilized for differential diagnosis. Exclamation mark hairs and yellow dots may be seen and white hairs are usually not involved in alopecia areata [11]. The trichotillomania plaque has broken and irregular coiled hair and the hair density is decreased. Black dots, follicular hemorrhages, v-sign may be seen [12].

1.6. Treatment

As mentioned above, trichotillomania is a psychiatric disorder with dermatological findings which is characterized by compulsive avulsion of hair shafts leading to thin, ragged, broken hairs on the affected region clinically [15]. The inability to control self-pulling of hair resulting in hair loss may progress into alopecia in long time.

Treatment procedure must be multidisciplinary including both dermatological but mainly psychiatric approach to increase the effectiveness of the therapy and prevent relapse.

Cognitive and behavioral therapies (CBT), antipsychotic agents, selective serotonin reuptake inhibitors (SSRI), tricyclic antidepressants are the main options of treatment [7, 16–18]. The most appropiate therapeutic approach must be chosen according to the patient's age, medical status and mental status.

Cognitive and behavioral therapies are the first steps of treatment and must be considered together with pharmacotherapeutics in treatment [16, 19]. In a randomized controlled trial with 7–8-year-olds, cognitive-behavioral therapies alone were found to decrease the symptoms in 75% of the participants [16].

The results about efficacy of SSRIs are conflicting. They were reported to be the safest and well-established medication choice. However, the clinical results show that medication, which is usually an SSRI, in addition to CBT, is more successful, if CBT alone fails.

In a meta-analysis which was reported in 2007, in which the efficacies of pharmacologic and behavioral treatments were evaluated in treatment of trichotillomania, it was found that SSRIs were not more effective than placebo. In two trials clomipramine was found to be more effective compared with placebo. In three trials, it was shown that there is a beneficial effect of habit reversal therapy compared with no intervention [20].

In another systematic review which was published in 2013, similar results were found. In two included trials, fluoxetine was not more effective than placebo in reducing the mean severity rating of hair pulling. Clomipramine was found to be more effective than placebo, although 3 of 10 participants receiving clomipramine dropped out because of drug-related adverse effects [21].

At last, in a recent meta-analysis of 11 randomized trials, the efficacy of behavioral therapy and SSRI for the treatment of trichotillomania; the outcome measure was the standardized mean difference of change in hair pulling [22]. This publication demonstrated a large effect for behavioral therapy and only a moderate effect for SSRI. A greater treatment effect was reported for clomipramine in two included trials [22].

The side effects and limited efficacy of pharmacological treatment, especially in pediatric population and difficulty in long-term maintenance of behavioral therapies require alternative options of treatment. The glutamatergic system dysregulation is involved in obsessive-compulsive disorders etiology and it has been reported that N-acetyl-cysteine (NAC) might have a therapeutic effect on these entities by acting on the glutamatergic system and reducing oxidative stress [23]. It was reported as a safe and effective treatment option given 1200 mg/d per os. The efficacy of the glutamate modulator NAC was evaluated in a small randomized trial including 50 adults with trichotillomania [24]. N-acetylcysteine was more effective than placebo in reducing hair-pulling symptoms as measured by the Massachusetts General Hospital Hair Pulling Scale. A subsequent trial in children and adolescents did not find any beneficial effect of NAC compared with placebo [24, 25].

2. Traction alopecia

2.1. Introduction

Traction alopecia (TA) is defined as loss of hair caused by repetitive or continuous and prolonged tension applied to the hair [26–28]. It was first described using the terminology *alopecia groenlandica* to refer to the hair loss attributed to tight ponytails which girls and women wear in Greenland [29]. Although TA is more prevalent among females of African ancestry, it has been described in a wide range of populations, including nurses, ballerinas, Sikh boys and men, to name a few [30–34]. Research has convincingly demonstrated that certain habitual practices of hairstyling are implicated in the pathogenesis of TA [35–39].

2.2. Epidemiology

Most of the population-based studies concerning the prevalence of TA originate from South Africa [35–37]. Overall, TA was found to be more common in females compared to males and in women compared to girls, presumably due to a longer history of hairdressing [37]. Importantly, in a large cohort of African adults in Cape Town, almost one-third of women had findings consistent with TA on scalp examination [35]. Of note, 17.1% of South African schoolgirls had TA, with increasing prevalence rates from the first year of school to the last year of high school [36]. A similar rate (18.4%) was observed in another study examining a population of 201 African American girls from the United States [38]. In males, TA seems to be considerably less prevalent, however, two notable exceptions are Sikh boys and men, who adhere to the religious practice of tightly knotting their scalp and/or beard hair and boys/men wearing dreadlocks or cornrows [32–35, 40].

2.3. Pathogenesis

Traction alopecia is typically noncicatricial and reversible in its early stages, whereas it may progressively result in permanent scarring in the long term [27, 28, 41]. It is well recognized that traction causes an inflammatory, sometimes subclinical, folliculitis. The exact pathomechanism leading from follicular inflammation to follicle damage and hair loss remains to be elucidated; however, follicular miniaturization is considered to play a possible role [28, 42–44].

2.4. Predisposing factors

The factors predisposing to the development of TA fall into two major categories: (1) traumatic hairstyling practices and (2) application of chemicals and/or heat to the hair [27]. It has been shown that the combination of both factors greatly increases the risk of TA, cautioning against the application of traction on chemically relaxed hair [36–38]. Importantly, hairdressing practices causing symptoms such as stinging, pain, or crusting are associated with an increased risk of TA [37, 39]. "Tenting" of the hair follicle, which manifests as elevation of the scalp skin due to tight pulling, has been interpreted as a sign of excessive tension [27, 39, 43]. A more recent literature review classified hairstyles into low risk, moderate risk and high-risk [39]. Accordingly, the excessive use of very tight buns or ponytails belongs to the category of high-risk hairstyles, as do dreadlocks, cornrows and braids [38, 39, 45]. Another well-recognized factor associated with TA is the use of hair extensions, especially if applied to relaxed hair [39, 46]. According to the aforementioned review, other hairstyles such as braids and/or weaves are considered high-risk if they are combined with chemical relaxation of the hair [39]. Moreover, hairpins used to fix the nurse's cap to the scalp may be related to hair loss [30]. Alopecia initially presenting with a traumatic ulcer was described in association with hairstyles requiring multiple hairpins [47].

2.5. Diagnosis

2.5.1. Clinical findings

Two main categories of TA have been recognized: marginal and nonmarginal [46]. The former is more common and typically presents as bandlike loss of hair along the temporoparietal margin or frontal hairline (**Figure 1**) [48]. Marginal TA is usually attributable to traumatic hairstyles, whereas nonmarginal TA may be caused by hairpins or buns [40, 47, 49]. A peculiar form of TA, termed "horseshoe pattern" by the authors, was described as a result of weft hair extensions [46]. Hair loss in nonmarginal localizations may sometimes present a diagnostic challenge and require more detailed history taking and/or histopathological examination [27, 48].

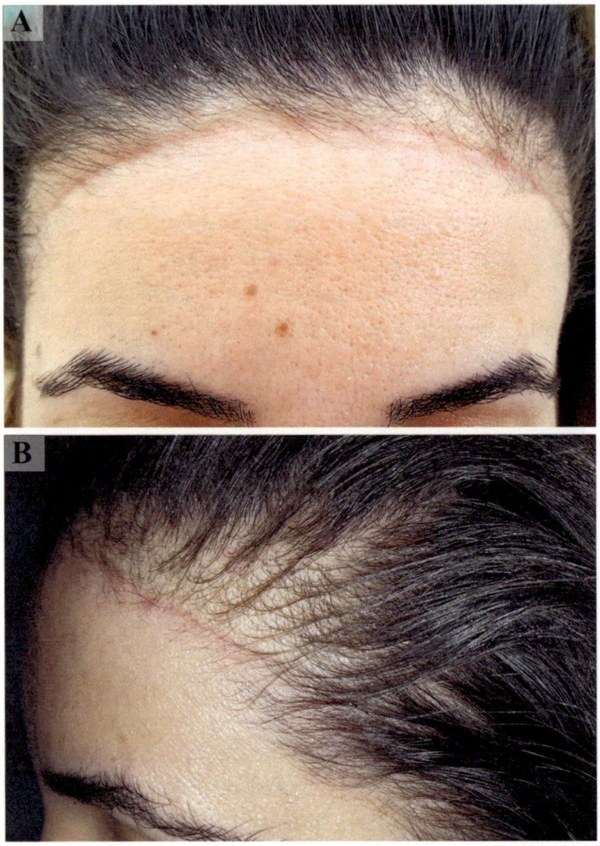

Figure 1. Marginal traction alopecia along the frontal hairline **(A)** and temporoparietal margin **(B)** in a woman who applied excessive traction to her hair.

The earliest clinical sign of TA is considered to be perifollicular erythema in the areas of the scalp exposed to maximum tension, which may progress to folliculocentric papules and pustules. However, these initial findings may be unrecognized by the patient and physician alike [22, 28, 31]. The presentation may be acute or more commonly, chronic and progressive. Patients may provide a history of symptoms such as stinging or tenderness during hairdressing practices [27]. As noted earlier, the alopecia is typically nonscarring in the early stages, but may become irreversible later during the disease course, following a "biphasic" course [27]. Correspondingly, follicular markings tend to be decreased in the late stages of TA [27, 31, 43]. An important clinical caveat in the diagnosis of TA is the "fringe sign," defined as the presence of retained hairs along the frontal and/or temporal margin. This useful finding was observed in early and late stages of TA alike (**Figure 2**) [43].

In general, TA is considered to have no systemic associations. Nonetheless, there is an anecdotal report of a 25-year-old woman with prolonged traction resulting in a combination of TA, cutis verticis gyrata and intractable headache. Her headache resolved as she was advised to change her habitual hairstyle, which also stopped further hair loss [50].

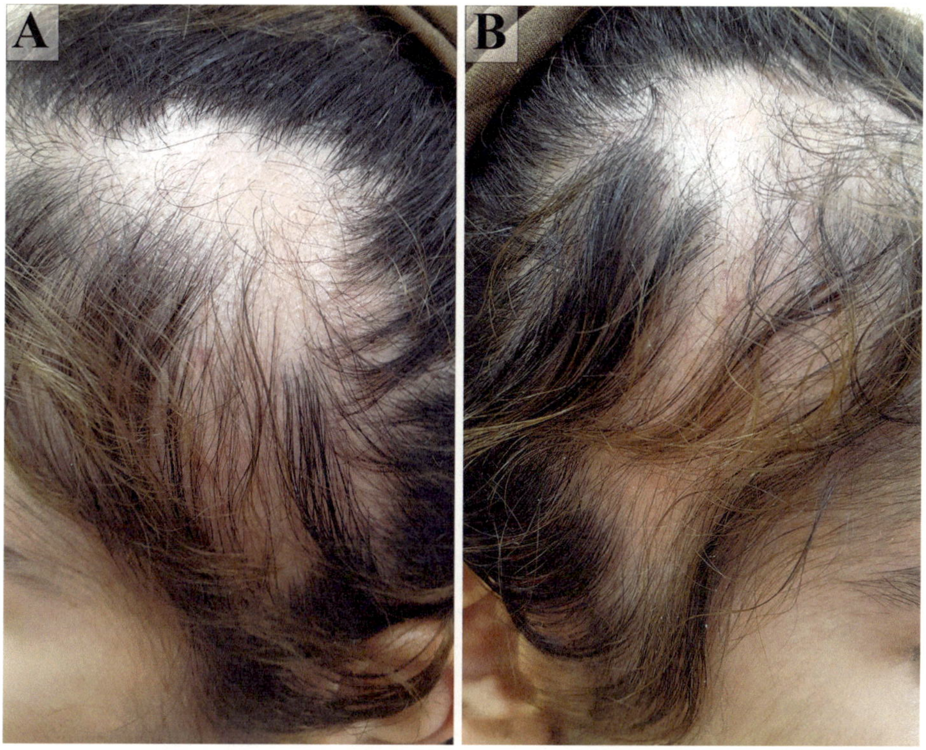

Figure 2. "Fringe sign" demonstrated in a woman with longstanding traction alopecia as a group of retained hairs along the temporoparietal hairlines and located in front of the alopecic patches bilaterally.

2.5.2. Dermoscopy

Dermoscopy may be utilized as a useful aid to confirm the clinical diagnosis of TA and/or differentiate it from other entities presenting with hair loss. In a cross-sectional study from Korea, broken hairs and black dots were observed in 100 and 92% of patients with TA, respectively. Of these findings, broken hairs were noted in all patients with trichotillomania, as well (**Figure 3**). Other dermoscopic findings associated with TA in this study were clustered short vellus hairs, yellow dots and atypical red vessels, with decreasing frequency [51]. The presence of hair casts has been emphasized as an important dermoscopic sign of TA, described as cylindrical structures encircling the proximal hair shafts [52]. It has been demonstrated that observation of hair casts on dermoscopic examination is an indicator of ongoing traction [53] and should be interpreted as a warning sign that hairstyle changes should be implemented to halt the progression of alopecia [52]. More recently, the trichoscopic finding of "flame hairs"was reviewed in a population of patients with various hair disorders. Of note, flame hairs were noted in slightly more than one half of the patients with trichotillomania, whereas they were observed in less than 5% of patients with TA. This disparity was attributed by the authors to the extent of the acute mechanical damage to the hair follicle being more prominent in trichotillomania compared to that in TA [54].

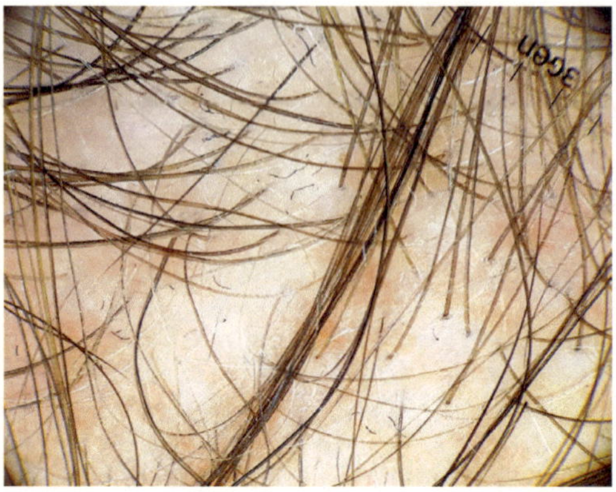

Figure 3. Broken and irregular coiled hairs, decreased hair density in dermoscopic examination.

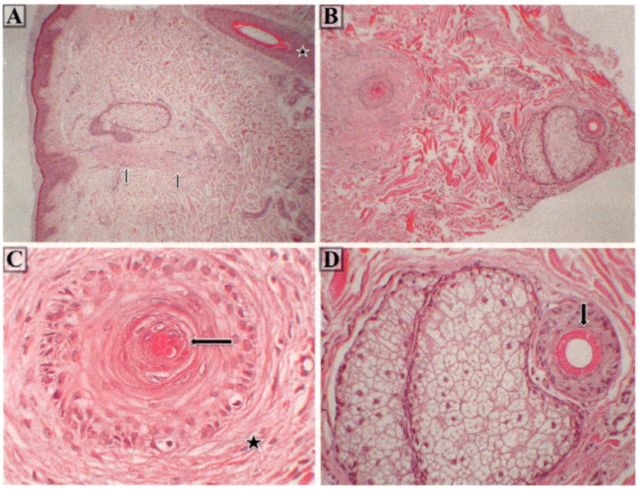

Figure 4. (A) Perifollicular fibrosis on superficial dermis ⬅ and an anagen follicule with hair shaft avulsion ★- H&Ex100, **(B)** catagen/telogen hair follicules- H&Ex40, **(C)** intrafollicular erythrocytes ⬅ and perifollicular fibrosis ★ H&Ex400 and **(D)** an empty follicule with hair shaft avulsion ⬅ H&E ×200.

2.5.3. *Histopathology*

Histologic findings of TA parallel the biphasic course of the disease mentioned previously [27]. Early stages of TA are considered to resemble trichotillomania, whereas more advanced stages of TA are similar to "burned-out" forms of cicatricial alopecia [55]. More specifically, early TA is characterized by increased numbers of telogen and catagen hairs and trichomalacia. In contrast to primary scarring alopecias, sebaceous glands are generally preserved in TA (**Figure 4**). With prolonged traction, terminal follicles tend to decrease in number and are progressively replaced by fibrous tracts [27, 28, 43]. Furthermore, vellus-sized hairs may be observed on histology which are thought to correspond to the aforementioned "fringe sign" noted on physical examination [27]. Differentiation of late-stage TA from primary scarring alopecias may be challenging and it has been demonstrated that transverse sections may be advantageous compared to vertical sections in differential diagnosis [56].

2.6. Differential diagnosis

The clinical differential diagnosis of TA depends on the distribution pattern of hair loss. For marginal type TA, the most important entities to be considered in the differential diagnosis are alopecia areata with an ophiasis pattern and frontal fibrosing alopecia [27, 43]. A noteworthy caveat is that TA only affects scalp hair exposed to traction, whereas body hair, eyebrows and/or nails may be involved in alopecia areata or frontal fibrosing alopecia [27]. Another important differential diagnosis is androgenetic alopecia. These two conditions may also coexist and in fact androgenetic alopecia is thought to predispose an individual to the development of TA due to the miniaturized hairs [30, 40, 43]. Nonmarginal TA, on the other hand, may be considered within the differential diagnosis of a broad range of conditions, including alopecia areata, trichotillomania, telogen effluvium and discoid lupus erythematosus [40, 48].

Central centrifugal cicatricial alopecia (CCCA) is another condition mainly seen in females of African descent [57]. The relationship between traction/TA and CCCA remains controversial [58]. Ackerman and coauthors categorized CCCA as a form of TA, [59] and a retrospective comparative study detected a strong association between CCCA and the use of tractional hairstyles with artificial hair extensions [60]. However, a more recent study failed to reveal an association between CCCA and tractional hairstyles. Interestingly, among more than 1000 female participants, not a single individual had a concomitant diagnosis of CCCA and TA in the same study, suggesting that CCCA and TA may not be closely related [58].

2.7. Prevention and treatment

Prevention is an integral part of management of TA, as appropriate measures to eliminate traction can stop hair loss before it becomes permanent [27, 28, 61]. It is important to recognize that TA most often originates during childhood and adolescence, suggesting that public education should primarily focus on these at-risk populations [27, 43, 44]. Prevention strategies have been detailed elsewhere [39, 44]. Briefly, management should rely on two main principles: preferring loose hairstyles and avoiding heat and chemicals [27, 39]. Patients may be encouraged to switch from high-risk hairstyles to low-risk hairstyles, such as loose buns and ponytails [39]. An important message is that pain during hairstyling be interpreted as a sign that excessive tension has been applied and that particular hairstyle should better be avoided [39, 44].

Medical or surgical treatment should only be considered after traction has been minimized [39]. There is a paucity of evidence-based literature data with regard to the medical treatment of TA. Topical or intralesional corticosteroids and topical or systemic antibiotics may be utilized to suppress the inflammation in the early stages of the disease [61].Topical minoxidil was described as effective in an anecdotal report [42] and recommended by some authors [27, 43, 61], although controlled trials are lacking. An interesting study demonstrated the protective effect of piloerection induced by topical phenylephrine against the development of TA, suggesting a potential role of α_1-adrenergic receptor agonists in the treatment of TA [41]. For extensive TA, surgical treatment has been described [45, 62]. Of note, a scoring system was developed ("M-TAS score") to evaluate the severity of marginal type TA and facilitate assessment of treatment effectiveness [63].

Author details

Tugba Kevser Uzuncakmak*, Melek Aslan Kayıran, Burak Tekin and Filiz Cebeci

*Address all correspondence to: drtugbakevser@gmail.com

Department of Dermatology, Medical Faculty, Goztepe Training and Research Hospital, Istanbul Medeniyet University Istanbul, Turkey

References

[1] Zimova J, Zimova P. Trichotillomania: bizarre pattern of hair loss at 11-year-old girl. Acta Dermatovenerol Croat. 2016; 24: 150–153.

[2] Woods DW, Houghton DC. Diagnosis, evaluation and management of trichotillomania. Psychiatry Clin North Am. 2014; 37: 301–317.

[3] Stein DJ, Kogan CS, Atmaca M, Fineberg NA, Fontenelle LF, Grant JE, Matsunaga H, Reddy YC, Simpson HB, Thomsen PH, van den Heuvel OA, Veale D, Woods DW, Reed GM. The classification of obsessive-compulsive and related disorders in the ICD-11. J Affect Disord. 2016; 190: 663–674. DOI: 10.1016/j.jad.2015.10.061.

[4] Yik YI, How AK. A 'Hairy' problem: trichotillomania, trichophagia and trichobezoars. Singapore Med J. 2016 Jul;57(7):411. DOI: 10.11622/smedj.2016125.

[5] Nisha SC, Jeroen N, Matilde I, Ramon G and Arnold PO. Trichotillomania in children. Skin Appendage Disord. 2015; 1: 18–24.

[6] Goyal D, Surya S, Elder J, McCall WV, Graham K. Sleep-isolated trichotillomania (SITTM): a case report. Innov Clin Neurosci. 2016; 13: 40–42.

[7] Keijsers GP, Maas J, van Opdorp A, van Minnen A. Addressing self-control cognitions in the treatment of trichotillomania: a randomized controlled trial comparing cognitive therapy to behaviour therapy. Cognit Ther Res. 2016; 40: 522–531.

[8] Carli Murphy, B.S., Rachel Redenius, Erin O'Neill, Sarah Zallek, M.D. Sleep-isolated trichotillomania: a survey of dermatologists. J Clin Sleep Med. 2007; 3: 719–721.

[9] Shoenfeld N, Rosenberg O, Kotler M, Dannon PN.Tricotillomania: pathopsychology theories and treatment possibilities. Isr Med Assoc J. 2012 Feb;14(2):125–9.

[10] Grillo E, Vano-Galvan S, Diaz-Ley B, Jaén P Patchy hair loss on the pubis—a case study. Aust Fam Physician. 2013; 42: 487–489.

[11] Finner AM Alopecia areata: Clinical presentation, diagnosis and unusual cases. Dermatol Ther. 2011; 24: 348–354. DOI: 10.1111/j.1529-8019.2011.01413.

[12] Ankad BS, Naidu MV, Beergouder SL, Sujana L. Trichoscopy in trichotillomania: a useful diagnostic tool. Int J Trichol. 2014 Oct;6(4):160–163. DOI: 10.4103/0974-7753.142856

[13] Muller SA. Trichotillomania: a histopathologic study in sixty-six patients. J Am Acad Dermatol. 1990; 23: 56–62.

[14] Elder DE, Elenitsas R, Johnson BL, Ioffreda MD, Miller J, Miller OF. Inflammatory and other benign disorders of skin appendages. In: Atlas and Synopsis of Lever's Histopathology of the Skin, 2nd Edition. China: Lippincott Williams & Wilkins, 2007. pp. 408–410.

[15] Basta-Juzbašić A, Bukvić Mokos Z. Skin changes in primary psychiatric disorders. Acta Dermatovenerol Croat. 2015; 23: 87–95.

[16] Landuyt G, Dierckx B, de Nijs PF, Dieleman GC. Treatment options for paediatric trichotillomania. Tijdschr Psychiatr. 2016; 58: 463–470.

[17] Sasaki T, Iyo M. Treatment of puberty trichotillomania with low-dose aripiprazole. Ann Gen Psychiatry. 2015;14: 18. DOI: 10,1186/s12991-015-0056-0.

[18] Rothbart R, Stein DJ. Pharmacotherapy of trichotillomania (hair pulling disorder) an updated systematic review. Expert Opin Pharmacother. 2014; 15: 2709–2719. DOI: 10.1517/14656566.2014.972936.

[19] Trainor K. Treating trichotillomania in children and adolescents: CBT versus medication. Am J Psychiatry. 2007; 164: 1610–1611.

[20] Bloch MH, Landeros-Weisenberger A, Dombrowski P, et al. Systematic review: pharmacological and behavioral treatment for trichotillomania. Biol Psychiatry 2007; 62: 839.

[21] Ninan PT, Rothbaum BO, Marsteller FA, et al. A placebo-controlled trial of cognitive-behavioral therapy and clomipramine in trichotillomania. J Clin Psychiatry 2000; 61: 47.

[22] McGuire JF, Ung D, Selles RR, et al. Treating trichotillomania: a meta-analysis of treatment effects and moderators for behavior therapy and serotonin reuptake inhibitors. J Psychiatr Res 2014; 58: 76.

[23] Grant JE, Odlaug BL, Kim SW. N-acetylcysteine, a glutamate modulator, in the treatment of trichotillomania: a double-blind, placebo-controlled study. Arch Gen Psychiatry 2009; 66: 756.

[24] Bloch MH, Panza KE, Grant JE, et al. N-Acetylcysteine in the treatment of pediatric trichotillomania: a randomized, double-blind, placebo-controlled add-on trial. J Am Acad Child Adolesc Psychiatry 2013; 52: 231.

[25] Smith L, Tracy DK, Giaroli G. What future role might N-acetyl-cysteine have in the treatment of obsessive compulsive and grooming disorders?: A systematic review. J Clin Psychopharmacol. 2016; 36: 57–62. DOI: 10.1097/JCP.0000000000000431.

[26] Whiting DA. Traumatic alopecia. Int J Dermatol. 1999; 38:34–44.

[27] Mirmirani P, Khumalo NP. Traction alopecia: how to translate study data for public education—closing the KAP gap? Dermatol Clin. 2014; 32:153–161. DOI: 10.1016/j.det.2013.12.003

[28] Khumalo NP, Callender VD. African hair. In: Blume-Peytavi U, Tosti A, Whiting DA, Trüeb RM, editors. Hair Growth and Disorders. 1st ed. Berlin: Springer; 2008. p. 483–507. DOI: 10.1007/978-3-540-46911-7

[29] Hjorth N. Traumatic marginal alopecia; a special type: alopecia groenlandica. Br J Dermatol. 1957; 69:319–322.

[30] Hwang SM, Lee WS, Choi EH, Lee SH, Ahn SK. Nurse's cap alopecia. Int J Dermatol. 1999; 38:187–191.

[31] Samrao A, Chen C, Zedek D, Price VH. Traction alopecia in a ballerina: clinicopathologic features. Arch Dermatol. 2010;146:930–931. DOI: 10.1001/archdermatol.2010.183.

[32] Kanwar AJ, Kaur S, Basak P, Sharma R. Traction alopecia in Sikh males. Arch Dermatol. 1989; 125:1587.

[33] James J, Saladi RN, Fox JL. Traction alopecia in Sikh male patients. J Am Board Fam. Med 2007; 20:497–498.

[34] Karimian-Teherani D, El Shabrawi-Caelen L, Tanew A. Traction alopecia in two adolescent Sikh brothers-an underrecognized problem unmasked by migration. Pediatr Dermatol. 2011; 28:336–338. DOI: 10.1111/j.1525-1470.2011.01241.x

[35] Khumalo NP, Jessop S, Gumedze F, Ehrlich R. Hairdressing and the prevalence of scalp disease in African adults. Br J Dermatol. 2007; 157:981–988. DOI: 10.1111/j.1365-2133.2007.08146.x

[36] Khumalo NP, Jessop S, Gumedze F, Ehrlich R. Hairdressing is associated with scalp disease in African schoolchildren. Br J Dermatol. 2007; 157:106–110. DOI: 10.1111/j.1365-2133.2007.07987.x

[37] Khumalo NP, Jessop S, Gumedze F, Ehrlich R. Determinants of marginal traction alopecia in African girls and women. J Am Acad Dermatol. 2008; 59:432–438. DOI: 10.1016/j.jaad.2008.05.036

[38] Rucker Wright D, Gathers R, Kapke A, Johnson D, Joseph CL. Hair care practices and their association with scalp and hair disorders in African American girls. J Am Acad Dermatol. 2011; 64:253–262. DOI: 10.1016/j.jaad.2010.05.037

[39] Haskin A, Aguh C. All hairstyles are not created equal: What the dermatologist needs to know about black hairstyling practices and the risk of traction alopecia (TA). J Am Acad Dermatol. DOI: 10.1016/j.jaad.2016.02.1162

[40] Hantash BM, Schwartz RA. Traction alopecia in children. Cutis. 2003; 71:18–20.

[41] Goren A, Shapiro J, Sinclair R, Kovacevic M, McCoy J. α1-AR agonist induced piloerection protects against the development of traction alopecia. Dermatol Ther. 2016; 29:160–163. DOI: 10.1111/dth.12324

[42] Khumalo NP, Ngwanya RM. Traction alopecia: 2% topical minoxidil shows promise. Report of two cases. J Eur Acad Dermatol Venereol. 2007; 21:433–434. DOI: 10.1111/j.1468-3083.2006.01933.x

[43] Samrao A, Price VH, Zedek D, Mirmirani P. The "Fringe Sign"—a useful clinical finding in traction alopecia of the marginal hair line. Dermatol Online J. 2011; 17:1.

[44] Khumalo NP. The "fringe sign" for public education on traction alopecia. Dermatol Online J. 2012; 18:16.

[45] Ozçelik D. Extensive traction alopecia attributable to ponytail hairstyle and its treatment with hair transplantation. Aesthetic Plast Surg. 2005; 29:325–327. DOI: 10.1007/s00266-005-0004-5

[46] Ahdout J, Mirmirani P. Weft hair extensions causing a distinctive horseshoe pattern of traction alopecia. J Am Acad Dermatol. 2012; 67:e294–295. DOI: 10.1016/j.jaad.2012.07.020

[47] Ntuen E, Stein SL. Hairpin-induced alopecia: case reports and a review of the literature. Cutis. 2010; 85:242–245.

[48] Barbosa AB, Donati A, Valente NS, Romiti R. Patchy traction alopecia mimicking areata. Int J Trichol. 2015; 7:184–186. DOI: 10.4103/0974-7753.171588

[49] Trüeb RM. "Chignon alopecia": a distinctive type of nonmarginal traction alopecia. Cutis. 1995; 55:178–179.

[50] Kanwar AJ, Ghosh S, Thami GP, Kaur S. Alopecia and cutis verticis gyrata due to traction presenting as headache. Int J Dermatol. 1992; 31:671–672.

[51] Shim WH, Jwa SW, Song M, Kim HS, Ko HC, Kim BS, Kim MB. Dermoscopic approach to a small round to oval hairless patch on the scalp. Ann Dermatol. 2014; 26:214–220. DOI: 10.5021/ad.2014.26.2.214.

[52] Tosti A, Miteva M, Torres F, Vincenzi C, Romanelli P. Hair casts are a dermoscopic clue for the diagnosis of traction alopecia. Br J Dermatol. 2010; 163:1353–1355. DOI: 10.1111/j.1365-2133.2010.09979.x

[53] Zhang W. Epidemiological and aetiological studies on hair casts. Clin Exp Dermatol. 1995; 20:202–207.

[54] Miteva M, Tosti A. Flame hair. Skin Appendage Disord. 2015; 1:105–109. DOI: 10.1159/000438995

[55] Sperling LC. Scarring alopecia and the dermatopathologist. J Cutan Pathol. 2001; 28: 333–342.

[56] Donovan JC, Mirmirani P. Transversely sectioned biopsies in the diagnosis of end-stage traction alopecia. Dermatol Online J. 2013; 19:11.

[57] Whiting DA, Olsen EA. Central centrifugal cicatricial alopecia. Dermatol Ther. 2008; 21: 268–278. DOI: 10.1111/j.1529-8019.2008.00209.x

[58] Khumalo NP, Gumedze F. Traction: risk factor or coincidence in central centrifugal cicatricial alopecia? Br J Dermatol. 2012; 167: 1191–1193. DOI: 10.1111/j.1365-2133.2012.11050.x

[59] Ackerman AB, Charissi C, Jones RE, Walton NW III. Hot comb alopecia/follicular degeneration syndrome in African American women is traction alopecia! Dermatopathol Pract Concept. 2000; 6: 320–336.

[60] Gathers RC, Jankowski M, Eide M, Lim HW. Hair grooming practices and central centrifugal cicatricial alopecia. J Am Acad Dermatol. 2009; 60:574–578. DOI: 10.1016/j.jaad.2008.10.064.

[61] Callender VD, McMichael AJ, Cohen GF. Medical and surgical therapies for alopecias in black women. Dermatol Ther. 2004; 17: 164–176. DOI: 10.1111/j.1396-0296.2004.04017.x

[62] Earles RM. Surgical correction of traumatic alopecia marginalis or traction alopecia in black women. J Dermatol Surg Oncol. 1986; 12: 78–82.

[63] Khumalo NP, Ngwanya RM, Jessop S, Gumedze F, Ehrlich R. Marginal traction alopecia severity score: development and test of reliability. J Cosmet Dermatol. 2007; 6:262–269. DOI: 10.1111/j.1473-2165.2007.00345.x

Chapter 13

Psychosocial Aspects of Hair Loss

Hilal Gokalp

Additional information is available at the end of the chapter

http://dx.doi.org/10.5772/66156

Abstract

Hair loss (alopecia) is a common dermatological condition that affects men and women of all ages. It can be due to a wide variety of causes including scarring and non-scarring diseases. Although alopecia is not a life-threatening condition, it has significant psychological impact on the quality of life. Mental disorders such as anxiety, depression, social phobia, posttraumatic stress disorder, and suicidal thoughts are increased among alopecia patients. On the other hand, alopecia frequency increases during the course of psychological disorders. In this chapter, psychosocial aspects of hair loss and the relationship between alopecia and psychological disorders are reviewed.

Keywords: alopecia, anxiety, depression, hair loss, psychiatric disorders, psychological disorders

1. Introduction

Studies have shown dermatologic diseases to be closely associated with psychological problems. Psychological diseases have even been suggested to occasionally cause dermatologic problems, while the reverse has also been suggested. Psychological/psychiatric disorders have been detected at rates up to 60% in dermatology patients treated as inpatients and 30% in those treated as outpatients [1]. Alopecia (hair loss) is an important dermatological condition due to its common psychological effects. The current role of healthy hair as regards to perception of power, good looks, charm, and beauty is an indisputable fact. Healthy hair is an important complement of physical well-being. Therefore, hair loss causes significant psychological problems, whatever its underlying pathophysiology.

Alopecia can affect women and men of all ages and has significant social and psychological results [2]. Although the hair loss itself does not cause a functional problem, it is visually an important part of the outer appearance in both women and men. The loss or disruption of this part can cause several psychological/psychiatric problems such as depression, anxiety, anger, fatigue, low self-esteem, embarrassment, discomfort with appearance, lower self-regard, self-consciousness, less sexual activity, decrease in school performance, social withdrawal, and suicidal ideation [3–5]. Recent studies have shown the stress level experienced by patients with alopecia to be at a level similar to many severe, chronic, and life-threatening diseases [2–6].

Several factors such as autoimmune and inflammatory diseases, infections, hormonal factors, physical or chemical factors, neoplasms, and congenital diseases can cause alopecia. Alopecia is divided into two as scarring and non-scarring alopecia [7]. The psychosocial aspect will be reviewed according to the common reasons causing hair loss in this section. The common reasons for hair loss are summarized in **Table 1**.

1. Non-scarring alopecia
• Androgenetic alopecia
• Telogen effluvium
• Anagen effluvium
• Chemotherapy-induced alopecia
• Alopecia areata
• Trichotillomania
• Psychogenic pseudoeffluvium
2. Scarring alopecia

Table 1. Common hair loss causes.

2. Psychosocial impact of non-scarring alopecia

Approximately 50% of women and men experience alopecia at some stage [8]. Most of these problems consist of (1) androgenetic alopecia (AGA), (2) telogen or anagen effluvium, and (3) alopecia areata (AA), which develop with different pathophysiologic mechanisms. Certain specific conditions (4) have also been described.

2.1. Androgenetic alopecia

Androgenetic alopecia is also known as male type hair loss and is seen more commonly in males. Genetic and hormonal factors play an important role in the development. It is most frequently observed in middle-aged white men. Roughly 30% of white men at the age of 30, 50% at the age of 50, and 80% at the age of 70 are affected by this condition [9]. Various results have been obtained in the studies conducted on the psychological effects of AGA, which in fact is considered a part of the natural aging process by many men. Men have stated that AGA disrupts the body image and causes stress without a significant loss of psychological functionality in a study conducted by Cash some decades ago [10]. The condition has been shown to lead to higher rates of psychological problems especially in men who are young, who do not have a romantic relationship, who think physical appearance is essential for self-esteem, and who were insecure even before the development of alopecia [4, 10–13]. These symptoms increase as the severity of AGA increases [11]. AGA starting early such as the early 20s has especially been reported to cause the individual to compare himself with his peers and gradually lead to lack of self-esteem. Such people can also become obsessed with AGA and spend much time and money on its treatment [3, 12, 14]. Normal subjects asked to evaluate bald (with advanced AGA) individuals with those with normal hair found the first group older, less masculine, and physically and socially less attractive [11]. Young individuals with AGA who are aware of such notions in the community suffer increased psychological stress, as reflected in the increased demands for treatment and hair transplantation. However, the AGA usually observed in males causes less severe psychological effects than other types of alopecia [15].

The psychological stress in women is usually more severe. Hair is one of the most important components of the physical appearance in women. A study reported 52% of females and 28% of males to be very/extremely unhappy with AGA when 96 female and 60 males AGA patients were compared. When female subjects with AGA were compared with females with another dermatologic disease, the first group was found to be more stressful, suffers more social anxiety and has less self-esteem. A significant decrease was recorded in their quality of life compared to the control group [16]. However, every woman with AGA is not psychologically affected equally. Female patients with diffuse pattern AGA were observed to be less social in particular [4, 9, 16].

2.2. Telogen effluvium/Anagen effluvium

Losses due to hair cycle disorders can be as telogen effluvium (TE) or anagen effluvium (AE), depending on the stage the hair is affected [17].

2.2.1. Telogen effluvium

Telogen effluvium develops mainly due to febrile disorders, surgery, accidents, giving birth, severe diets, thyroid disorders, eating disorders, vitamin and mineral deficiencies, severe emotional stress, and certain drugs [18, 19].

The ratio of loss in telogen effluvium cases is usually under 50% [19, 20]. Hair loss needs to be more than 50% to be visible [17]. Therefore, TE is often accepted as a benign process and usually continues for <6 months. However, the potential hair loss of over 300 hair follicles per day in these patients can cause emotional distress and significantly reduce the quality of life. Acute or chronic stress can cause TE development, while TE itself can cause secondary stress, leading to a vicious cycle [21]. Although the condition is common, studies on the psychosocial effect of TE are limited in number. However, the TE-stress-TE vicious cycle is thought to lead to anxiety and depressive symptoms, especially in women who are more concerned about their outer appearance [3, 4].

2.2.2. *Anagen effluvium*

The loss of hair at the anagen stage which is the growth phase is named AE. Unlike TE, intense loss is observed quickly. Since normally 80–90% of the hair on scalp is at the anagen stage, 10–20% of the hair remains [18, 22].

Alopecia developing due to chemotherapeutic agents can be TE but is commonly AE. In addition to chemotherapy, AE causes include radiotherapy, protein-energy malnutrition, heavy metal poisoning, connective tissue disease, pemphigus vulgaris, other drugs (L-dopa, cyclosporine, colchicine, bismuth), and systemic disorders causing peribulbar inflammation such as syphilis and systemic lupus erythematosus [17]. However, chemotherapy-induced alopecia (CIA) has been presented in more detail due to the significant psychosocial effect it creates.

2.2.3. *Chemotherapy-induced alopecia*

Chemotherapy-induced alopecia develops due to chemotherapy and has several psychosocial effects such as anxiety, depression, and low self-esteem affecting the quality of life. Although many improvements have been achieved in side effects related to chemotherapy, especially in the last three decades, CIA still appears to be an unresolved side effect. It is even possible for chemotherapy options that are less successful but do not cause CIA to be preferred to more successful treatments. Even the idea of the development of alopecia in patients after the diagnosis of cancer can cause traumatic fear and anxiety [23, 24]. CIA has been shown to be among the main three chemotherapy-related side effects causing distress and to be more significant in female patients [23–25]. Alopecia was found to be the most burdensome side effect in a study conducted on female patients with early stage breast cancer [26]. In fact, CIA was shown to cause more psychosocial effects than mastectomy in certain patients [27]. Loss of hair, which is another feminine characteristic, in females undergoing mastectomy was reported to cause more psychological effect than lung cancer chemotherapy-related alopecia [28]. Once CIA develops, 13% of patients with a gynecological malignancy feel that they are no longer wanted by their partners [29].

Chemotherapy-induced alopecia is one of the major stress resources because it is the most visible reminder of the disease, the need for treatment and death [23]. However, although generally being a major stress resource, CIA does not have the same psychosocial effect on every patient. There are also those who try to appear normal, make fun of alopecia, shave their hair without waiting for complete loss, share their baldness on social media, and try to hide the alopecia with a wig, although the number of people who choose to become asocial is considerable [23, 30]. Some patients even believe that CIA is a proof of a strong treatment and will lead to a better survival, perhaps as a defense mechanism. CIA can also cause psychosocial problems in the family in addition to the person receiving the chemotherapy. Shyness in engaging in social environments with the family was shown to develop in school-age children of patients with CIA [23, 24].

Chemotherapeutics can cause both AE and TE based on the drug used, dose and the patient's susceptibility [17]. Many current cytotoxic agents can cause severe alopecia. However, the degree of alopecia can vary depending on the cytotoxic agents used, and the half-life, dose and administration route of the agent. For example, taxanes used at more frequent intervals and at low doses cause less CIA than those used at longer intervals and higher doses. The CIA rates are lower with the new cytotoxic agents. However, when combined with other cytotoxic agents, these new treatment modalities have been reported to also cause CIA at a certain rate [24]. Taking various psychosocial measures against the unavoidable side effect of CIA in many patients, receiving chemotherapy has been suggested to possibly contribute to the person's well-being [23, 24, 31]. It is recommended that the patient is engaged in a conversation on the importance of hair and the reaction to alopecia before chemotherapy, and the patient told that the hair will usually grow again after chemotherapy, especially for female patients. It is also recommended to talk about whether they will cover the scalp after alopecia develops and what cover they would prefer. This approach may increase compliance with the treatment as well as the effects such as emotional stress, anxiety, and depression as the patient will prepare himself/herself for the alopecia [23, 32]. The patients can also be recommended to cut their hair short as it can minimize the hair loss appearance. However, long hair can be used to cover the alopecia area when chemotherapeutics that do not cause total alopecia.

2.3. Alopecia areata

Alopecia areata is a chronic disease with a lifetime incidence of 2.1%. It starts suddenly and causes circular hair loss with sharp borders [33]. Although the etiopathogenesis is unknown, genetic, immunological, environmental, infectious, and psychological factors are known to play a role in the development. AA has a significant effect on the quality of life and is actually the type of alopecia where the relationship to psychological factors has been studied in most detail. Psychological findings and consequences of AA are summarized in the **Table 2**.

Social and family problems have been reported to affect AA patients more commonly than other individuals and their capacity to cope with events tend to be less. They can therefore encounter psychological problems such as depression, anxiety, and paranoid disorders in long term. However, variable results have been obtained in the studies. In fact, while some studies report a significant psychological/psychiatric disease in 93% of AA patients, others have reported no role of psychological factors in the development [4–6, 34]. The predominant view at present is that AA is frequently associated with psychological/psychiatric disease [34, 35].

Alopecia areata is related to many psychological/psychiatric disorders as a result of the decrease in the quality of life. AA patients were diagnosed with one or multiple psychological/ psychiatric disorders at a lifelong rate of 74% in the study by Colon et al. The incidence of lifetime major depressive symptoms and anxiety disorders in AA patients was estimated as 39% in the same study [36]. Besides, antisocial personality disorder and posttraumatic stress disorder were observed at a high rate in those patients. AA patients have been reported to be depressed, anxious, hysterical, hypochondriac, introverted individuals who were unsuccessful

Findings of alopecia areata	Psychological consequences of alopecia areata
• Character and behavioral changes	• Antisocial personality disorder
• Lowered self-esteem	• Posttraumatic stress disorder
• Psychologically painful	• Generalized anxiety disorder
• Disturbed mood	• Major depression
• Self-evaluation	• Adjustment disorders
• Feels less attractive	• Obsessive-compulsive disorder
• Interpersonal sensitivity	• Panic disorder
• Talks frequently about alopecia	• Social phobia
• Compares own hair with others	
• Discomfort in front of others	
• Anger, hostility, stress	
• Obsessive, anxious, asocial, ashamed, and dependent personalities	
• Reduced social freedom and quality of life	
• Significant increased psychological distress in patient and the family	
• Suicidal intent	

Table 2. Psychological findings and consequences of alopecia areata.

in their social relationships in later studies [4–6, 34, 37–39]. The rate of suicide attempts has been reported to be higher and their characteristics to be more commonly associated with alexithymia [40, 41]. Alexithymia is a cognitive disorder of the identification and expression of emotions. Impairment of emotional awareness, social cohesion, and interpersonal relationships is among the main features. It has therefore been suggested that considering alexithymia could be useful while evaluating the psychological condition of AA patients [4]. AA was found to be less common in schizophrenia compared to other psychiatric disorders in a study conducted on 5117 patients and control group subjects. This has led to speculation on how schizophrenia provides some kind of protection against AA [42].

Alopecia areata has been shown to affect the quality of life at higher rates and also cause higher anxiety and depression scores in children, adolescents and women in evaluations conducted by age group and gender [37]. The rate of suffering from at least one psychiatric disorder was found to be 78%, the major depression rate to be 50%, and the obsessive-compulsive disorder (OCD) rate to be 35.7% in a study on the psychological/psychiatric effects of AA on children [43]. AA developing in the childhood period was observed to cause concentration difficulties and lead to a decrease in school success [35].

Although the prevalence of psychological/psychiatric disease is observed to have increased greatly in patients with AA, another point of view is that psychological/psychiatric diseases may actually trigger AA. It was shown in a case-control study that the psychological/psychiatric disorder rates in AA patients were higher but the psychological/psychiatric disorder had started before AA in 50% of these patients. Besides, one in four patients was reported to lead a stressful life before the start of the disease. Since AA and psychologic/psychiatric diseases are interrelated and the one that starts first can vary, it may be best for psychologists and psychiatrists to treat AA patients together with dermatologists [42].

2.4. Special considerations

2.4.1. Trichotillomania

Trichotillomania is an impulse control disorder characterized by chronic hair pulling and has a negative effect on the quality of the life of both the patients and the families. In addition to pulling scalp hair, patients can also pull hair in other body areas such as the eyebrows, eyelashes, beard, mustache, arms, and groin to a smaller extent. Trichotillomania is primarily included among psychiatric disorders in the obsessive-compulsive spectrum due to its similarity to OCD [44]. It mainly starts in childhood and adolescence with a mean age of onset of 12 years although it can be seen in adults even in elderly people. It can start in childhood and become chronic with fluctuating episodes. Trichotillomania is more common in females. It can be confused with AA, especially in adult patients and in the initial phase of the disease [45–47]. It has been reported that 40% of trichotillomania patients were never diagnosed and 58% never received treatment [48].

Trichotillomania is considered to occur mainly through a learning process similar to habit development [49]. It had been suggested to emerge as a major coping behavior in response to stress and to become solidified in time [47]. The main characteristic of trichotillomania is that the person pulls the hair at a level that can cause baldness. The patients mention a feeling of stress before pulling the hair and feeling relief afterward [4, 47]. However, this "stress-relief" feeling is not described by the majority of pediatric and adolescent patients. Certain rituals such as "pulling the hair with a special gesture, symmetrical pulling, putting the hair into the mouth after pulling" are usually present in these patients. One of these rituals, hair swallowing (trichophagy), has been reported in 5–18% of the patients [47]. Trichophagy can lead to serious complications such as vomiting, weight loss and ileus by causing trichobezoar formation [47, 50]. Association with nail biting, thumb sucking, nose picking, masturbation, bad friendships, and school problems can be especially present in pediatric patients [4]. Besides, at least one more psychiatric disorder such as anxiety disorder, attention deficit-hyperactivity disorder, depression and OCD have been found in more than a third of pediatric patients with trichotillomania [47]. The incidence of other psychiatric/psychological disorders and especially mood and personality disorders, anxiety, and substance use is increased in adult patients with trichotillomania compared to normal individuals. Avoiding daily activities is more common in adult patients, and avoiding social and sexual intimacy, negative mood, and decreased professional productivity can be present. Although the cases are often sporadic, familial cases have also been reported. Higher rates of anxiety disorder, alcoholism, drug addiction, antisocial personality disorder, attention deficit-hyperactivity disorder, OCD, depression, and suicidal behavior have also been found in the first-degree relatives of patients with trichotillomania compared to healthy individuals [45, 50, 51]. Psychological findings and disorders associated with trichotillomania are summarized in **Table 3**.

	Pediatric trichotillomania	Adult trichotillomania	First-degree relatives
Psychological findings	• Nail biting • Thumb sucking • Nose picking • Masturbation • Bad friendships • School problems	• Antisocial personality • Avoiding social and sexual intimacy • Negative mood • Substance use • Decreased professional productivity	• Antisocial personality • Alcoholism • Drug addiction • Suicidal behavior
Psychological disorders	• Anxiety disorder • Attention deficit-hyperactivity disorder • Depression • Obsessive-compulsive disorder	• Anxiety disorder • Mood and personality disorders	• Anxiety disorder • Attention deficit-hyperactivity disorder • Depression • Obsessive-compulsive disorder

Table 3. Psychological findings and disorders associated with trichotillomania.

Although the diagnosis can usually be made with the history and examination, patients may not report their problem due to shame, and fear of being mocked or being labeled as a lunatic. The physician should therefore not approach the behavior in an incriminating or condescending manner and should be careful while referring these patients to psychiatry.

2.4.2. Psychogenic pseudoeffluvium

A substantial number of patients with normal scalp hair and without any sign of alopecia complain of alopecia at dermatology outpatient departments. This condition is identified as *"imaginary hair loss"* or *"psychogenic pseudoeffluvium"* and can be a symptom of an underlying psychological disease. Depression and anxiety disorders are common in these patients. Problems about marriage and the prevalence of depression are believed to be increased in married female patients thought to be suffering from psychogenic pseudoeffluvium. One must also consider that *"body dysmorphic disorder"* or *"delusion of alopecia,"* which can be included among psychotic disorders, could be present in these patients. Obsessive-compulsive behavior such as looking at the mirror for hours to check the hair can be present in these patients [47, 52]. These patients are among the most grueling cases for dermatologists and should be directed to psychiatrists/psychologists in an appropriate manner.

3. Psychosocial effects of scarring alopecia

Scarring alopecia is a condition characterized by loss of hair as a result of replacement of the follicular structure by fibrous tissue [53]. Scarring alopecia is more common in women. It develops mainly due to lichen planopilaris, discoid lupus erythematosus, frontal fibrosing alopecia, dissecting cellulitis, folliculitis decalvans, central centrifugal alopecia, tufted folliculitis, perifolliculitis abscedens et suffodiens, and pseudopelade (Brocq) [54]. However, nonfollicular conditions (traumatic, burn-induced, inflammatory, infectious, neoplastic, and genetic conditions) can also affect the scalp and cause secondary scarring alopecia. Whatever the underlying reason, scarring alopecias usually create more psychosocial effect than nonscarring alopecias. Pradhan et al. have recently reported moderate-severe psychosocial stress in almost 75% of their patients with scarring alopecia. Although worry about the outer appearance is more prominent in female patients, the psychological effect of scarring alopecia has been reported to be equally severe in both genders. Aesthetic concerns have been found to be higher in younger patients with these patients feeling older due to scarring alopecia. The condition leads to feeling physically unattractive, loss of confidence, and embarrassment in this age group. However, the duration of the disease has been shown not to be proportional to the psychosocial effect it creates and the psychological stress not to decrease even if the disorder becomes chronic [53]. Although it was thought that individuals who were single would experience more stress with the disorder, no difference was found between married and single subjects. This could be related to the condition being more common in women and women receiving less psychological support from male spouses in a male-dominated world. Patients with more localized scarring alopecia were also found to experience less stress than patients with diffuse scarring alopecia because they can cover these areas with their normal hair [38, 53, 54].

The quality of life of female patients with scarring alopecia was shown to be more affected and consequently anxiety and depression to be more common in a study where female patients with and without scarring were compared [54].

It has also been suggested that patients spend a lot of time and effort to normalize their appearance leading to decreased success in friendship, work, and school life in scarring alopecia with a destructive and progressive course [53].

Early diagnosis with clinicopathological correlation and starting treatment at an early stage is essential to prevent irreversible hair loss in scarring alopecia. Starting psychological support from the early stage is also essential in terms of a holistic treatment approach.

4. Conclusion

Hair is the most visible and striking characteristic of the body. It is a very important component for the psychologically healthy development of the individual from childhood to adulthood and even till death. Mental disorders associated with hair loss present with many different psychological/psychiatric symptoms. However, many psychological/psychiatric disorders can also cause hair loss. These two interconnected groups are now identified as psychotrichological disorders. The psychosomatization basis of these patients who usually present to dermatology outpatient departments should be investigated and if necessary they should be referred to a psychiatrist and/or psychologist for proper psychopharmacotherapy with behavior therapy, depth psychology, and antidepressants or anxiolytics as required.

Author details

Hilal Gokalp

Address all correspondence to: hgokalp@kuh.ku.edu.tr

Department of Dermatology, Koç University School of Medicine, Istanbul, Turkey

References

[1] Gupta MA, Gupta AK. Psychiatric and psychological co-morbidity in patients with dermatologic disorders: epidemiology and management. Am J Clin Dermatol. 2003;4:833–842. PMID:14640776

[2] Springer K, Brown M, Stulberg DL. Common hair loss disorders. Am Fam Physician. 2003;68:93–102. PMID:12887115

[3] Cash TF. The psychology of hair loss and its implications for patient care. Clin Dermatol. 2001;19:161–166. doi:10.1016/S0738-081X(00)00127-9

[4] Yazıcı E, Erol A. Psychiatric approach to alopecia. Turkiye Klinikleri J Cosm Dermatol-Special Topics. 2015;8:73–78.

[5] Aghaei S, Saki N, Daneshmand E, Kardeh B. Prevalence of psychological disorders in patients with alopecia areata in comparison with normal subjects. ISRN Dermatol. 2014;2014:304370. doi:10.1155/2014/304370

[6] Cartwright T, Endean N, Porter A. Illness perceptions, coping and quality of life in patients with alopecia. Br J Dermatol. 2009;160:1034–1039. doi:10.1111/j.1365-2133.2008.09014.x

[7] Mounsey AL, Reed SW. Diagnosing and treating hair loss. Am Fam Physician. 2009;80:356–362. PMID:19678603

[8] Price VH. Treatment of hair loss. N Engl J Med. 1999;341:964–973. doi:10.1056/nejm199909233411307

[9] Ellis JA, Sinclair R, Harrap SB. Androgenetic alopecia: pathogenesis and potential for therapy. Expert Rev Mol Med. 2002;4:1–11. doi:10.1017/S1462399402005112

[10] Cash TF. The psychological effects of androgenetic alopecia in men. J Am Acad Dermatol. 1992;26:926–931. PMID:1607410

[11] Stough D, Stenn K, Haber R, Parsley WM, Vogel JE, Whiting DA, et al. Psychological effect, pathophysiology, and management of androgenetic alopecia in men. Mayo Clin Proc. 2005;80:1316–1322. doi:10.4065/80.10.1316

[12] Budd D, Himmelberger D, Rhodes T, Cash TE, Girman CJ. The effects of hair loss in European men: a survey in four countries. Eur J Dermatol. 2000;10:122–127. PMID: 10694311

[13] Kranz D. Young men's coping with androgenetic alopecia: acceptance counts when hair gets thinner. Body Image. 2011;8:343–348. doi:10.1016/j.bodyim.2011.06.006

[14] Girman CJ, Rhodes T, Lilly FRW, et al. Effects of self-perceived hair loss in a community sample of men. Dermatology. 1998;197:223–229. PMID: 9812025

[15] Cash TF. The psychosocial consequences of androgenetic alopecia: a review of the research literature. Br J Dermatol. 1999;141:398–405. doi:10.1046/j.1365-2133.1999.03030.x

[16] Cash TF, Price VH, Savin RC. Psychological effects of androgenetic alopecia on women: comparisons with balding men and with female controls. J Am Acad Dermatol. 1993;29:568–575. PMID: 8408792

[17] Aksoy G. Alopecias due to hair cycle abnormalities. Turkiye Klinikleri J Cosm Dermatol-Special Topics. 2015;8:10–14.

[18] Trueb RM. Diffuse hair loss. In: Blume-Peytavi U, Tosti A, Whiting DA, Trueb R, eds. Hair Growth and Disorders. Berlin: Springer; 2008. pp. 259–272.

[19] Jackson AJ, Price VH. How to diagnose hair loss. Dermatol Clin. 2013;31:21–28. doi: 10.1016/j.det.2012.08.007

[20] Han A, Mirmirani P. Clinical approach to the patient with alopecia. Semin Cutan Med Surg. 2006;25:11–23. doi:10.1016/j.sder.2006.01.003

[21] Hadshiew IM, Foitzik K, Arck PC, Paus R. Burden of hair loss: stress and the underestimated psychosocial impact of telogen effluvium and androgenetic alopecia. J Invest Dermatol. 2004;123:455–457. doi:10.1111/j.0022-202x.2004.23237.x

[22] Kanwar AJ, Narang T. Anagen effluvium. Indian J Dermatol Venereol Leprol. 2013;79:604–612. doi:10.4103/0378-6323.116728

[23] Hesketh PJ, Batchelor D, Golant M, Lyman GH, Rhodes N, Yardley D. Chemotherapy-induced alopecia: psychosocial impact and therapeutic approaches. Support Care Cancer. 2004;12:543–549. doi:10.1007/s00520-003-0562-5

[24] Dua P, Heiland MF, Kracen AC, Deshields TL. Cancer-related hair loss: a selective review of the alopecia research literature. Psychooncology. 2015. doi:10.1002/pon.4039

[25] Griffin AM, Butow PN, Coates AS, Childs AM, Ellis PM, Dunn SM, et al. On the receiving end. V: Patient perceptions of the side effects of cancer chemotherapy in 1993. Ann Oncol. 1996;7:189–195. PMID:8777177

[26] Kiebert GM, Hanneke J, de Haes CJ, Kievit J, van de Velde CJ. Effect of peri-operative chemotherapy on the quality of life of patients with early breast cancer. Eur J Cancer. 1990;26:1038–1042. PMID:2148877

[27] Tierney AJ. Preventing chemo- therapy-induced alopecia in cancer patients: is scalp cooling worthwhile? J Adv Nurs. 1987;12:303–310. doi:10.1111/j.1365-2648.1987.tb01336.x

[28] McGarvey EL, Baum LD, Pinkerton RC, Rogers LM. Psychological sequelae and alopecia among women with cancer. Cancer Pract. 2001;9:283–289. doi:10.1111/j.1523-5394.2001.96007.pp.x

[29] Munstedt K, Manthey N, Sachsse S, Vahrson H. Changes in self- concept and body image during alopecia induced cancer chemotherapy. Support Care Cancer. 1997;5:139–143. PMID:9069615

[30] Williams J, Wood C, Cunningham-Warburton P. A narrative study of chemotherapy-induced alopecia. Oncol Nurs Forum. 1999;26:1463–1468. PMID: 11064878

[31] Batchelor D. Hair and cancer chemotherapy: consequences and nursing care—a literature study. Eur J Cancer Care. 2001;10:147–163. doi:10.1046/j.1365-2354.2001.00272.x

[32] Whelan T, Rath D, Willan A, Neimanis M, Czukar D, Levine M. Evaluation of a patient file folder to improve the dissemination of written information materials for cancer patients. Cancer. 1998;83:1620–1625. PMID: 9781957

[33] Mirzoyev SA, Schrum AG, Davis MD, Torgerson RR. Lifetime incidence risk of alopecia areata estimated at 2.1% by Rochester Epidemiology Project, 1990–2009. J Invest Dermatol. 2014;134:1141–1142. doi:10.1038/jid.2013.464

[34] Güleç AT, Taşkıntuna N, Duru Ç, Saray Y, Akçalı C. The role of psychological factors in alopecia areata and the impact of the disease on quality of life. TURKDERM. 2002;36:178–181.

[35] Sellami R, Masmoudi J, Ouali U, Mnif L, Amouri M, Turki H, et al. The relationship between alopecia areata and alexithymia, anxiety and depression: a case-control study. Indian J Dermatol. 2014;59:421–430. doi:10.4103/0019-5154.135525

[36] Colon EA, Popkin MK, Callies AL, Dessert NJ, Hordinsky MK. Lifetime prevalence of psychiatric disorders in patients with alopecia areata. Compr Psychiatry. 1991;32:245–251. doi:10.1016/0010-440X(91)90045-E

[37] Bilgiç Ö, Bilgiç A, Bahalı K, Bahali AG, Gürkan A, Yılmaz S. Psychiatric symptomatology and health-related quality of life in children and adolescents with alopecia areata. J Eur Acad Dermatol Venereol. 2014;28:1463–1468. doi:10.1111/jdv.12315

[38] Hunt N, McHale S. The psychological impact of alopecia. BMJ. 2005;331:951–953. doi: 10.1136/bmj.331.7522.951

[39] Tucker P. Bald is beautiful? The psychosocial impact of alopecia areata. J Health Psychol. 2009;14:142–151. doi:10.1177/1359105308097954

[40] Cordan Yazici A, Başterzi A, Tot Acar S Üstünsoy D, Ikizoglu G, Demirseren D, et al. Alopecia areata and alexithymia. Turk Psikiyatri Dergisi. 2006;17:101–106.

[41] Layegh P, Arshadi H, Shahriari S, Pezeshkpour F, Nahidi Y. A comparative study on the prevalence of depression and suicidal ideation in dermatology patients suffering from Psoriasis, Acne, Alopecia areata and Vitiligo. Iran J Dermatol. 2010;13:106–111. doi:10.1155/2014/304370

[42] Chu SY, Chen YJ, Tseng WC, Lin MW, Chen TJ, Hwang CY, et al. Psychiatric comorbidities in patients with alopecia areata in Taiwan: a case-control study. Br J Dermatol. 2012;166:525–531. doi:10.1111/j.1365-2133.2011.10714.x

[43] Ghanizadeh A. Comorbidity of psychiatric disorders in children and adolescents with alopecia areata in a child and adolescent psychiatry clinical sample. Int J Dermatol. 2008;47:1118–1120. doi:10.1111/j.1365-4632.2008.03743.x

[44] Van Ameringen M, Patterson B, Simpson W. DSM-5 obsessive-compulsive and related disorders: clinical implications of new criteria. Depress Anxiety. 2014;31:487–493. doi: 10.1002/da.22259

[45] Papadopoulos AJ, Janniger CK, Chodynicki MP, Schwartz RA. Trichotillomania. Int J Dermatol. 2003;42:330–334. doi:10.1046/j.1365-4362.2003.01147.x

[46] Pacan P, Kantorska-Janiec M, Kiejna A. Trichotillomania. Psychiatr Pol. 1998;32:799–805. PMID:10216392

[47] Fettahoğlu EÇ. Hair loss related to primary psychiatric disorders. TURKDERM. 2014;48:52–55. doi:10.4274/turkderm.48.s12

[48] Cohen LJ, Stein DJ, Simeon D, Spadaccini E, Rosen J, Aronowitz B, et al. Clinical profile, comorbidity, and treatment history in 123 hair pullers: a survey study. J Clin Psychiatry. 1995;56:319–326. PMID:7615485

[49] Duke DC, Keeley ML, Geffken GR, Storch EA. Trichotillomania: a current review. Clin Pyschol Rev. 2010;30:181–193. doi:10.1016/j.cpr.2009.10.008

[50] Tolin DF, Franklin ME, Diefenbach GJ, Anderson E, Meunier SA. Pediatric trichotillomania: descriptive psychopathology and an open trial of cognitive behavioral therapy. Cogn Behav Ther. 2007;36:129–144. doi:10.1080/16506070701223230

[51] Flessner CA, Woods DW, Franklin ME, Keuthen NJ, Piacentini J. Cross sectional study of women with trichotillomania: a preliminary examination of pulling styles, severity, phenomenology, and functional impact. Child Psychiatry Hum Dev. 2009;40:153–167. doi:10.1007/s10578-008-0118-5

[52] Trüeb RM. Systematic approach to hair loss in women. J Dtsch Dermatol Ges. 2010;8:284–298. doi:10.1111/j.1610-0387.2010.07261

[53] Pradhan P, D'Souza M, Bade BA, Thappa DM, Chandrashekar L. Psychosocial impact of cicatricial alopecias. Indian J Dermatol. 2011;56:684–688. doi:10.4103/0019-5154.91829

[54] Katoulis AC, Christodoulou C, Liakou AI, Kouris A, Korkoliakou P, Kaloudi E, et al. Quality of life and psychosocial impact of scarring and non-scarring alopecia in women. J Dtsch Dermatol Ges. 2015;13:137–142. doi:10.1111/ddg.1254

Section 8

Hair Loss in Children

Chapter 14

Hair Loss in Children, Etiologies, and Treatment

Khitam Al-Refu

Additional information is available at the end of the chapter

http://dx.doi.org/10.5772/67379

Abstract

Hair loss in children is a common and important complaint in dermatology and pediatric clinics and can be considered as a difficult and challenging problem in some cases. Early management is needed as this has its effect on development of normal mental and physical growth of children. Alopecia or hair loss is of particular concern in pediatric group, as it is associated with more significant psychological consequences in this growing age group and has patterns that are different from that seen in adults. There are common and uncommon causes for this complaint, and this usually covers a broad differential diagnosis. This chapter has been written in an attempt to distinguish the types of hair loss (acquired and congenital, common and uncommon), to facilitate the diagnostic causes of this problem, and finally to reach a proper treatment.

Keywords: children, hair loss, etiology

1. Introduction

Hair loss in children is a common and important complaint in dermatology and pediatric clinics and can be considered as a difficult and challenging problem in some cases. This problem of irreversible hair loss can be a worrying one for parents and kids. In addition, the diagnosis may be a challenge for the doctors to reach a proper diagnosis and therapy for their patients. Early management is needed as this has its effect on development of normal mental and physical growth of children.

Alopecia or hair loss is of particular concern in a pediatric group, as it is associated with more significant psychological consequences in this growing age group and has patterns that are different from that seen in adults.

Similar to hair loss in adults [1], this problem can be caused by a number of conditions, but in patterns that are different in frequencies and presentations from those seen in adults. There are common and uncommon causes for this complaint, and this usually covers a broad differential diagnosis [2]. This chapter has been written in an attempt to distinguish the types of hair loss (acquired and congenital, common and uncommon), to facilitate the diagnostic causes of this problem, and finally to reach a proper treatment.

2. Normal hair growth

To fully understand hair loss during childhood, a basic comprehension of normal hair growth is necessary [3, 4]. Generally, at 22 weeks of intrauterine life, the developing fetus has all of its hair follicles formed. At this stage, there are nearly about one million of hair follicles on the head. Hair on the scalp grows about 0.3–0.4 mm/day or about 6 inches/year.

At any given time, a random number of hairs will be in one of three stages of growth and shedding: anagen, catagen, and telogen. Each phase has specific characteristics that determine the length of the hair. All three phases occur simultaneously; one strand of hair may be in the anagen phase, while another is in the telogen phase.

Essentially, there are three basic groups of hair based on hair follicle size [5].

(A) Lanugo hair is long, unpigmented, and very fine, and the very first hair fiber to be produced is by a hair follicle. As an embryo develops, the hair follicles form and begin to produce this type of hair. This first wave of growth is normally shed by the embryo at around 8 months gestation and replaced by terminal or vellus hair ready for birth. However, sometimes babies can be born with this coat of lanugo hair (called "congenital hypertrichosis lanuginosa").

(B) Vellus is short, fine, unpigmented hair. This type of hair is commonly seen on the nose and over the cheeks.

(C) Terminal, it is long, coarse, pigmented, and frequently contains a medulla. During puberty, many hair follicles around the genitals, armpits, beard, and chest in men transform from vellus hair to terminal hair under the direction of hormones. Equally, hormones can cause terminal hairs to revert to vellus hair production as in androgenetic alopecia.

3. Congenital causes of hair loss

Congenital hair loss is a loss of hair that is present at birth; the following conditions are some of possible causes of congenital hair loss.

3.1. Nevus sebaceous of Jadassohn

Nevus sebaceous of Jadassohn (**Figure 1**) (also known, as sebaceous nevus) is a yellow-orange, waxy, and hairless plaque that typically occurs on the scalp [6]. Such nevi are present

http://dx.doi.org/10.5772/67379

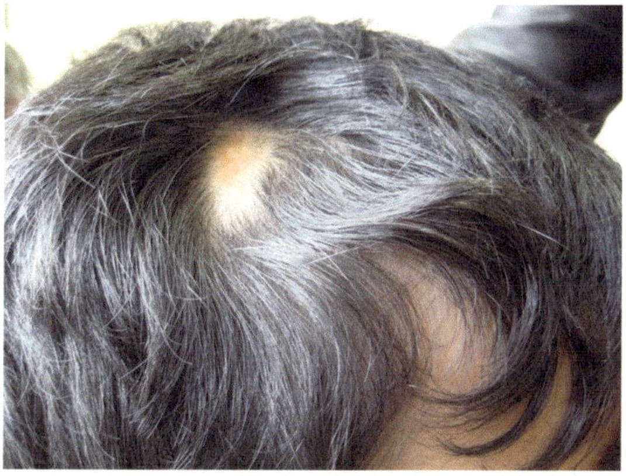

Figure 1. This is a 5-year-old male patient presented with yellow plaque, waxy on the scalp without hair growth. This plaque was since birth.

at birth or early childhood as a congenital plaque without hair but at the age of puberty show remarkable overgrowth (due to the activity of sebaceous glands at this age). Hair follicles are not present within the lesion itself, but lesions on the scalp may be covered over by surrounding hair, so careful examination is important. Skin growths such as benign tumors and basal cell carcinoma can arise in sebaceous nevi, usually in adulthood. Rarely, sebaceous nevi can give rise to sebaceous carcinoma.

3.2. Aplasia cutis congenita

Aplasia cutis congenita (also known as "Cutis aplasia," "Congenital absence of skin," and "Congenital scars") is a heterogeneous group of disorders characterized by the absence of a portion of skin in a localized or widespread area at birth [7, 8]. The defect may involve only the epidermis and upper dermis (localized and noninflammatory defect) resulting in minimal alopecia, or it may extend into the deep dermis, subcutaneous tissue, or rarely periosteum, skull, and dura (especially in the deeper and lager one). This deep and severe form of aplasia cutis can be associated with a neural cranial tube defect (encephalocoele or meningocoele), which can be demonstrated by an ultrasound scan showing misplaced brain tissue outside the skull. It is the most common congenital cicatricial alopecia and manifests as a solitary defect on the scalp in 70% of cases, but it may sometimes occur as multiple lesions. Most lesions of aplasia cutis congenita occur on the scalp vertex just lateral to the midline, but defects may also occur on the face, trunk, or limbs, sometimes symmetrically.

3.3. Ectodermal dysplasia

Ectodermal dysplasias are described as "heritable conditions in which there are abnormalities of two or more ectodermal structures such as hair, teeth, nails, or sweat gland function, in addition to another abnormality in a tissue of ectodermal origin, e.g., ears, eyes, lips, mucous membranes of the mouth, or nose, central nervous system" [9]. It is not a single disorder, but a group of syndromes. The signs and symptoms of ectodermal dysplasia differ markedly between the different types of the condition and depend on the structures that are affected. Signs and symptoms are not usually apparent in newborns and may not be picked up till infancy or childhood. The affected individuals have abnormalities of the hair follicles (the scalp and body hair may be thin, sparse, and very light in color). The hair may grow very slowly or sporadically, and it may be excessively fragile, curly, or even twisted (**Figure 2**).

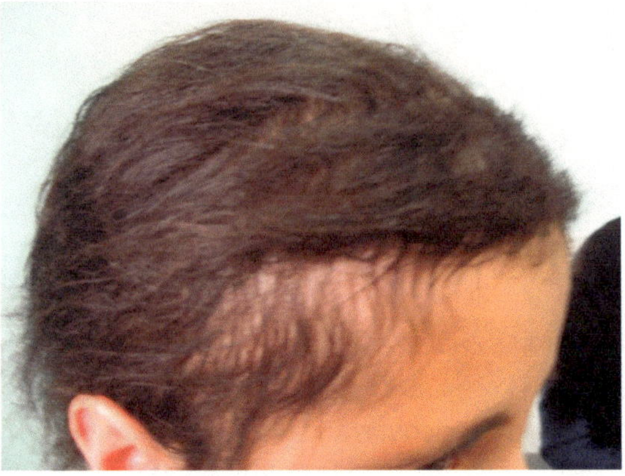

Figure 2. A child presented with fragile, curly hair since birth; the main complaint was persistent short and fragile hair. This child had also cone-shaped teeth and scanty eyebrows.

3.4. Hair shaft defects

Hair shaft abnormalities are characterized by changes in color, density, length, and structure [10]. Hair shaft alterations often result from structural changes within the hair fibers and cuticles, which may lead to brittle and uncombable hair.

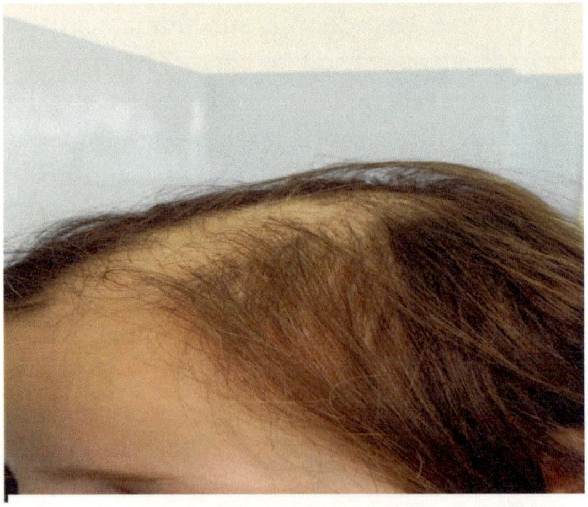

Figure 3. A female child with loose anagen hair syndrome. It is prominent that the hair was relatively sparse and does not grow long. Hair is of fair color, and hair shafts were of reduced caliber.

Hair shaft defects may result in dry and lusterless hair, coarse or fizzy hair, uncombable hair, and fragile hair. Hair shaft diseases may occur as localized or generalized disorders.

3.5. Loose anagen hair syndrome

Loose anagen syndrome is a benign, self-limiting condition where anagen hairs are easily and painlessly extracted and mainly reported in childhood [11]. It can be seen in normal population and in alopecia areata. The hair is relatively sparse and does not grow long. Hair is of fair color and hair shafts of reduced caliber, and an early age of onset are features. Usually, the hairs are not fragile, and there are no areas of breakage (**Figure 3**).

4. Acquired causes of hair loss

Common causes [12–15] of hair loss in children include telogen effluvium, tinea capitis, bacterial infections, traction alopecia, trichotillomania, and alopecia areata. In addition to the previous, other less common causes of hair loss can be seen including thyroid disorders and illnesses, such as systemic lupus erythematosus, diabetes mellitus, or iron deficiency anemia, malnutrition, structural abnormalities of the hair shaft that usually result in easy breakage and dry brittle hair. Hair types are influenced by ethnic groups that vary from region to region, and subsequently, this may reflect itself on the variation of common and uncommon causes of hair loss. This usually covers a broad differential diagnosis, and correct diagnosis, specific environmental and cultural factors may reflect itself on the prevalence of specific types of hair loss in children.

4.1. Common causes

There are five common types of hair loss in children: alopecia related to tinea capitis, alopecia areata, traction alopecia, telogen effluvium, and trichotillomania/trichotillosis.

4.1.1. Tinea capitis

Tinea capitis (ringworm of the scalp) is one of the more common causes of hair loss [16]. It is a disease caused by superficial fungal infection (superficial mycosis or dermatophytosis) of the skin of the scalp, with a propensity for attacking hair shafts and follicles. Tinea capitis is the most common pediatric dermatophyte infection worldwide [15].

Tinea capitis may present in several ways such as:

1. Dry scaling—resembling seborrheic dermatitis, but usually with moth-eaten hair loss (**Figure 4**).
2. Black dots—the hairs are broken off at the scalp surface, which is scaly, smooth areas of hair loss (**Figure 5**).

3. Kerion—severely inflamed deep abscesses.

4. Favus—yellow crusts and matted hair.

5. Carrier state with no symptoms and only mild scaling (*Trichophyton tonsurans*).

The potential of scarring and permanent alopecia is common in tinea capitis if left untreated (**Figure 6**).

Regarding the in vivo hair invasion in tinea capitis, there are three recognized types:

1. Ectothrix invasion is characterized by the development of arthroconidia on the exterior of the hair shaft and usually fluoresces a bright greenish-yellow color under a Wood lamp ultraviolet light. Common agents include *Microsporum canis, Microsporum gypseum, Trichophyton equinum,* and *Trichophyton verrucosum*.

2. Endothrix invasion results from infection with *T. tonsurans, Trichophyton violaceum* and *Trichophyton soudanense*. The hair shaft is filled with fungal branches (hyphae) and spores and usually does not fluoresce with Woods light. All endothrix-producing agents are anthropophilic (e.g., *T. tonsurans, T. violaceum*).

3. Favus, usually caused by *Trichophyton schoenleinii,* produces favus-like crusts or scutula and corresponding hair loss.

4.1.2. Alopecia areata

It is an autoimmune disease in which hair is lost from the scalp (**Figure 7**) or other hairy areas such as eyebrows, eyelashes, and other hairy areas in the body. It often results in bald spots on the scalp, especially in the first stages [17]. Rarely, the condition can spread to the entire scalp (alopecia totalis) or to the entire skin (alopecia universalis) (**Figure 8**). This type of alopecia is characterized by nonscarring alopecia (no fibrosis or inflammation), where the hair shafts are gone, but the hair follicles are preserved, making this type of alopecia reversible. Typically,

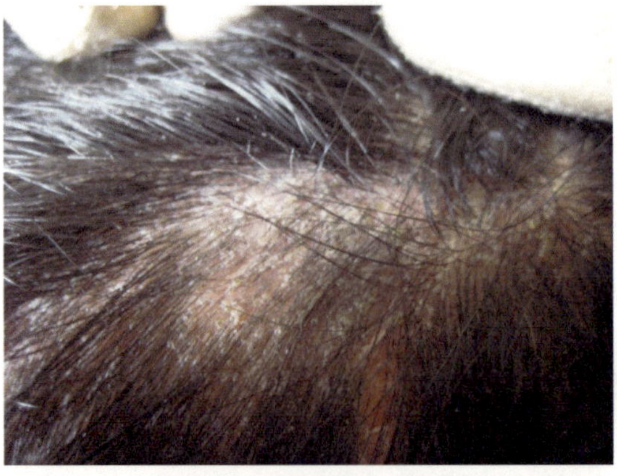

Figure 4. Tinea capitis in child presented as seborrheic dermatitis.

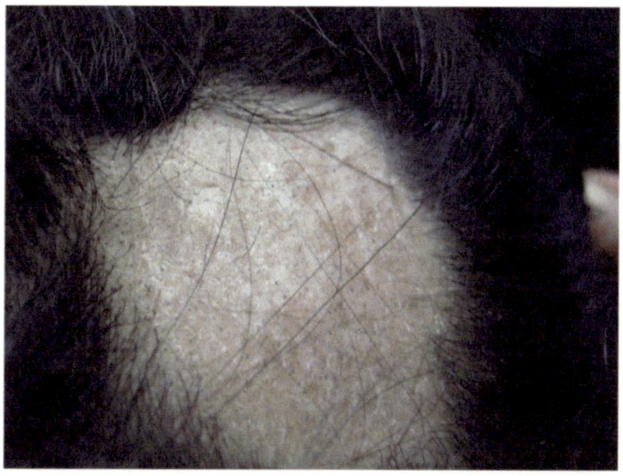

Figure 5. Tinea capitis in child with black dots presentation. There is no inflammation or no scales.

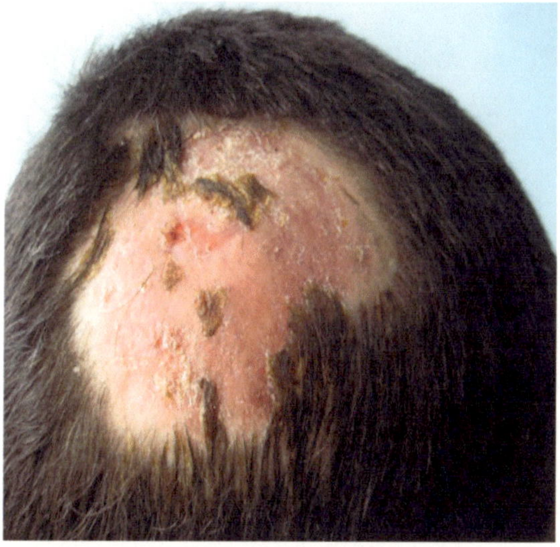

Figure 6. A child with scarring alopecia secondary to untreatable tinea capitis.

the patient first presented with small bald patches. The underlying skin is unscarred and looks superficially normal. These patches can take many shapes but are most usually round or oval. The disease may also go into remission for a time or may be permanent. It is common in children. Exclamation point hairs, narrower along the length of the strand closer to the base, may present and represent an activity of the disease.

4.1.3. Traction alopecia

Traction alopecia is a gradual hair loss, caused primarily by frequent and chronic hair pulling (**Figure 9**), and this is usually due to habit of hair styling [18]. It is also seen occasionally in longhaired people who use barrettes to keep hair out of their faces. There is a large variation

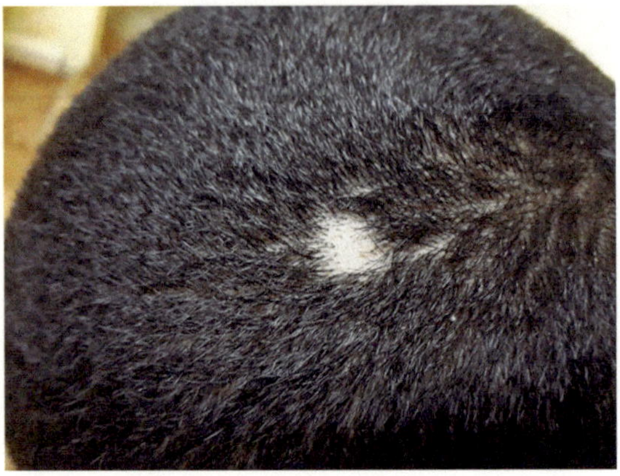

Figure 7. Small patch of alopecia areata; the skin is normal with no scales or no erythema.

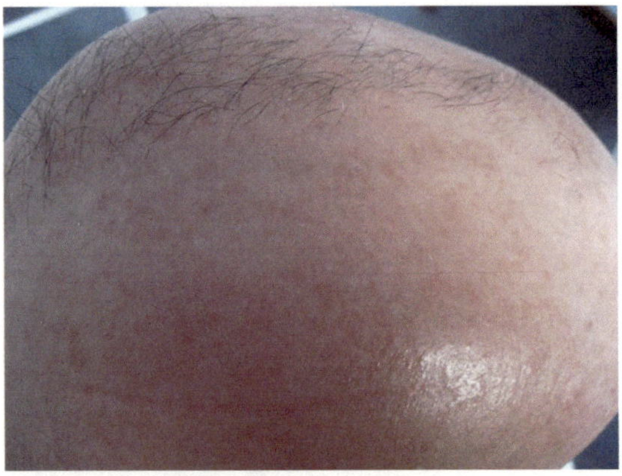

Figure 8. Alopecia totalis with prominent exclamation marks.

in the pattern of clinical presentation of traction alopecia. If there is no suspicion of traction, it can be difficult to diagnose. Patients may present with (itching, redness, scaling, folliculitis or pustules, multiple short broken hairs, thinning, and hair loss). At a later stage, vellus hairs (fine short hairs) develop and terminal hair follicles reduce and are replaced by fibrotic fibrous tracts (scars).

4.1.4. Telogen effluvium

This is not an uncommon cause of hair loss in children; it refers to an abnormality of the normal hair cycle leading to excessive loss of telogen hair [19]. In telogen effluvium, many factors happen to interrupt the normal life cycle of hair and to throw many or all of the hairs into the telogen phase. After few weeks of the insult, partial or complete baldness appears. Frequent

http://dx.doi.org/10.5772/67379

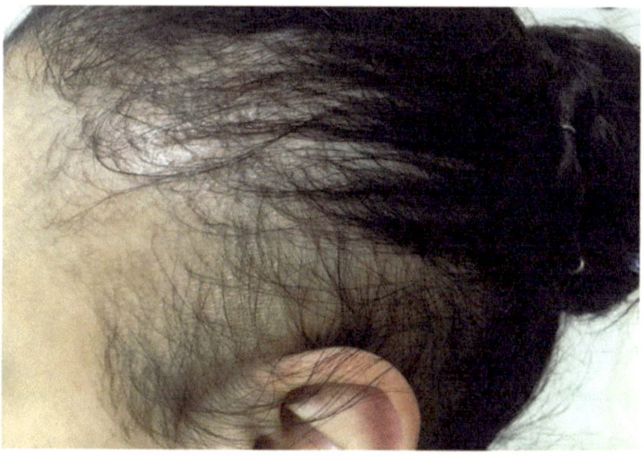

Figure 9. Traction alopecia.

triggers include physiologic effluvium of the newborn, in this type; babies often lose their hair during the first 6 months. Similar to adult type of telogen effluvium, many different events can cause telogen effluvium, including extremely high fevers, severe previous illnesses, surgery under general anesthesia, severe prolonged emotional stress, severe injuries, and the use of certain prescription medication.

4.1.5. Trichotollimenia

Trichotollimenia (**Figure 10**) is defined as a child or a teen that compulsively pulls out her hair and is thought to be related to obsessive-compulsive disorder [20]. These children have noticeable hair loss and often need treatment from a child psychiatrist and/or a child psychologist who specializes in trichotillomania. The hair loss is patchy and characterized by broken hairs of varying length. Patches are typically seen on the side of the child's dominant hand.

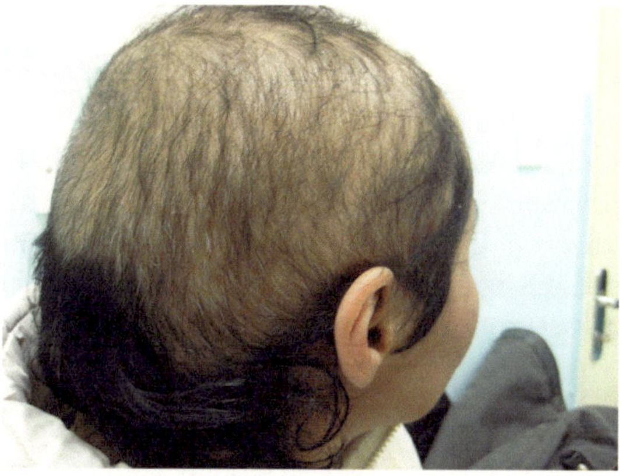

Figure 10. Trichotollimenia. The hair loss is patchy and characterized by broken hairs of varying length.

4.2. Uncommon causes

Rarer reasons for alopecia in children include pressure-induced alopecia, alopecia related to nutritional deficiency or toxic ingestion, and androgenetic alopecia. Other causes such as lichen planopliaris, chronic skin inflammation, universal pruritus, and severe dehydration.

5. Diagnosis of hair loss in children

In an attempt to facilitate the diagnosis of hair loss in children, it is helpful to have a proper history from the parents; the key points in patient's history are age of onset of the patient; onset of hair loss: sudden or gradual; extent of alopecia: patchy or diffuse; associated symptoms; mental development; emotional triggers in the previous few months; and any accompanying complaints (e.g., fatigue, weight changes, and nail or skin abnormalities); past medical history (including chronic illnesses, surgeries, medication, autoimmune); family history of alopecia, autoimmune disease, dermatologic or psychiatric disorders; hair-grooming practices (chemicals, tight braiding) [21, 22]. Thorough examination of scalp as well as other hair-bearing areas of the body is another key factor in diagnosis of hair loss. The examination should have the following components: type of hair loss: localized or diffuse; scarring or nonscarring; any hair shaft abnormalities; exclamation marks; hair texture and fragility; presence of pustules, scales, and erythema. Clinical examination of the entire body is necessary to evaluate hair loss, including teeth, skin, and mucous membranes.

The activity of hair shedding can be evaluated by hair pull test in which approximately 20 hairs are grasped and firmly tugged away from the scalp and then the number of extracted hairs is counted. Normally, fewer than three hairs per area should come out with each pull. If more than 10 hairs are obtained, the pull test is considered positive. The root of the plucked hair can be examined under a microscope to determine the phase of growth and is used to diagnose a defect of telogen, anagen, or systemic disease. Telogen hairs have tiny bulbs without sheaths at their roots. When the diagnosis of hair loss is unsure; a biopsy allows for differing between scarring and nonscarring forms. Skin biopsies are taken from areas of inflammation, usually around the border of the bald patch.

Further investigations are needed according to the suspected cases of tinea capitis, alopecia areata, or telogen effluvium. In tinea capitis, the diagnosis should be confirmed by microscopy and culture of skin scrapings (a potassium hydroxide preparation); woods lamp examination: as screening to detect flourescing species. When telogen effluvium is suspected, and there is no obvious trigger of telogen effluvium, blood tests are needed and include complete blood count; serum ferritin; serum zinc, antinuclear antibody; and thyroid function test.

Newly, dermoscope (trichoscope) [23, 24] is a noninvasive method of examining hair and scalp. It allows differential diagnosis of hair loss in most cases, especially in cases of hereditary hair shaft abnormalities. In the last few years, many studies have been published in this field. It may be performed with a manual dermoscope (×10 magnification) or a videodermoscope (up to ×1000 magnification). In particular, trichoscopy enhances the diagnosis of androgenetic alopecia, alopecia areata, telogen effluvium, trichotillomania, and congenital triangular alopecia, scarring alopecia, tinea capitis, and hair shaft disorders.

6. Treatment

For the majority of the cases of hair loss in children, a dermatologist would be able to diagnose these conditions and prescribe the appropriate treatment. But some hair disturbances have no effective treatment, and for others, no single treatment is 100% successful. Congenital and hereditary hypotrichosis and hair shaft abnormalities often have no effective treatment.

For tinea capitis, treatment usually involves systemic antifungal therapy, such as griseofulvin, which is taken by mouth for 8 weeks. Tinea capitis is also treated with antifungal shampoo to decrease shedding of fungus, which is used to wash the scalp 2–3 times a week. It is very important to continue the use of the oral medication and shampoo for the entire 8 weeks. Children who have tinea capitis are not required to leave school if treatment is used as directed but should be careful not to share any objects that touch the heads such as hats and pillows. Most children are not contagious when using the oral medication and shampoo.

Alopecia areata is an unpredictable disease, and even with complete remission, it is possible for it to occur again throughout your child's lifetime. While there is no cure, and unfortunately since there is no FDA-approved drugs specifically designed to treat the disease in some children. Many have their hair back within a year, although regrowth is unpredictable and many will lose hair again. The treatment of alopecia areata [25] depends on the severity of involvement. If the disorder is mild and does not cause the patient very much distress, waiting for a spontaneous remission is a sensible option. Treatment with zinc as a putative immunemodulator generally has no side effects and is, therefore, suitable for use in children. Topical and systemic immunomodulators are currently being employed for treating alopecia areata, but their efficacy against alopecia areata has not been established. Children with permanent hair loss can be offered surgical hair transplantation or camouflage devices, such as wigs.

In trichotillominea [26], counseling and psychotropic drugs such as clomipramine or sertraline, N-acetyl cysteine, and behavior modification techniques (e.g., habit-reversal therapy) are effective treatment options. These are novel therapeutic agents found to be effective in trichotillomania.

Traction alopecia [27] is a reversible alopecia and cessation of the offending hair practice is the treatment. But if the traction is continued over years, mechanical damage to hair follicles may result in permanent hair loss.

In telogen effluvium, assuming there is no intervening pathological process, the loss is usually replaced in 6–12 months. Treatment revolves around addressing the underlying cause

Author details

Khitam Al-Refu

Address all correspondence to: alrefukhi@yahoo.com

School of medicine Muta University, Jordan

References

[1] Banka N, Bunagan MJ, Shapiro J: Pattern hair loss in men: Diagnosis and medical treatment. Dermatol Clin. 2013; **31**: 129-40.

[2] Hamm H: Acquired alopecia in childhood. Hautarzt. 2013; **64**: 371-9; quiz 380-1.

[3] Barth JH: Normal hair growth in children. Pediatr Dermatol. 1987; **4(3)**: 173-84.

[4] Dawber RP: The embryology and development of human scalp hair. Clin Dermatol. 1988; **6(4)**: 1-6.

[5] Fenske NA, Lober CW: Structural and functional changes of normal aging skin. J Am Acad Dermatol. 1986; **15(4 Pt 1)**: 571-85.

[6] Kovich O: Hale E. "Nevus sebaceus". Dermatol Online J. 2005; **11(4)**: 16.

[7] Caksen H, Kurtoglu S: Our experience with aplasia cutis congenita. J Dermatol. 2002; **29(6)**: 376-9.

[8] Frieden IJ: Aplasia cutis congenita: A clinical review and proposal for classification. J Am Acad Dermatol 1986; **14(4)**: 646-60.

[9] Chee SY, Wanga CH, Lina WD, Tsaia FJ. Ectodermal dysplasia (ED) syndrome. Biomedicine (Taipei). 2014; **4**: 27. Epub 2014 Nov 26.

[10] Itina PH, Fistarol SK: Hair shaft abnormalities—clues to diagnosis and treatment. Dermatology. 2005; **211**: 63-71.

[11] Dhurat RP, Deshpande DJ: Loose anagen hair syndrome. Int J Trichol. 2010; **2(2)**: 96-100.

[12] Nnoruka EN, Obiagboso I, Maduechesi C: Hair loss in children in South-East Nigeria: Common and uncommon cases. Int J Dermatol. 2007; **46**: 18-22.

[13] Sarifakioglu E, Yilmaz AE, Gorpelioglu C, Orun E: Prevalence of scalp disorders and hair loss in children. Cutis. 2012; **90**: 225-9.

[14] Al-Refu K: Hair loss in children: Common and uncommon causes—clinical and epidemiological study in Jordan. Int J Trichol. 2013; **5(4)**: 185-9.

[15] Mandt N, Vogt A, Blume-Peytavi U: Differential diagnosis of hair loss in children. J Dtsch Dermatol Ges. 2004; **2**: 399-411.

[16] Chokoeva AA, Zisova L, Sotiriou E, Miteva-Katrandzhieva T: Tinea capitis: A retrospective epidemiological comparative study. Wien Med Wochenschr. 2016; **10**. [Epub ahead of print].

[17] Freyschmidt-Paul P, Happle R, Hoffmann R: Alopecia areata. Klinik, Pathogenese und rationale Therapie einer T-Zell-vermittelten Autoimmunerkrankung. Hautarzt 2003; **54**: 713-22.

[18] Urbina F, Sudy E, Barrios M: Traction folliculitis: 6 cases caused by different types of hairstyle that pull on the hair. Actas Dermosifiliogr. 2009; **100(6)**: 503-6.

[19] Alves R, Grimalt R: Hair loss in children. Curr Probl Dermatol. 2015; **47**: 55-66.

[20] Grant JE, Odlaug BL: Update on pathological skin picking. Curr Psychiatry Rep. 2009; **11(4)**: 283-8.

[21] Castelo-Soccio L: Diagnosis and management of alopecia in children. Pediatr Clin North Am. 2014; **61(2)**: 427-42.

[22] Odom RB, Davidsohn I, James WD, Henry JB, Berger TG, Clinical diagnosis by laboratory methods. Dirk M. Elston. Andrews' Diseases of the Skin: Clinical Dermatology. Saunders Elsevier. 2006. ISBN 0-7216-2921-0.

[23] Rudnicka L, Rakowska A, Kerzeja M, Olszewska M: Hair shafts in trichoscopy: Clues for diagnosis of hair and scalp diseases. Dermatol Clin. 2013; **31(4)**: 695-708.

[24] Lencastre A, Tosti A: Role of trichoscopy in children's scalp and hair disorders. Pediatr Dermatol. 2013; **30**: 674-82.

[25] Messenger AG, McKillop J, Farrant P, McDonagh AJ, Sladden M: British Association of Dermatologists' guidelines for the management of alopecia areata 2012. Br J Dermatol. 2012; **166**: 916–26.

[26] Rahman O, Toufexis M, Murphy TK, Storch EA: Behavioral treatment of trichotillomania and trichophagia in a 29-month-old girl. Clin Pediatr. (Phila.). 2009; **48:** 951-3.

[27] Khumalo NP, Jessop S, Gumedze F, Ehrlich R: Determinants of marginal traction alopecia in African girls and women. J Am Acad Dermatol. 2008; **59(3)**: 432-8.

Section 9

Surgical Treatment of Hair Loss

Chapter 15

Follicular Unit Extraction (FUE) Hair Transplantation

Safvet Ors

Additional information is available at the end of the chapter

http://dx.doi.org/10.5772/66837

Abstract

Throughout the world, over 60% of men and 50% of women suffer from androgenetic alopecia and irreversible hair loss. This type of hair loss is a seminatural process, and medication can only temporarily inhibit it. At the moment, the solution for either androgenetic alopecia or other irreversible hair loss problems is the hair transplantation. Besides androgenetic alopecia, the many irreversible hair losses are being applied successfully by hair transplantation. In the past 10–15 years, a new hair restoration technique was introduced. This method is called follicular unit extraction (FUE) technique. FUE is an alternative which allows for quick extraction of follicular unit grafts. The hair transplantation can be used in various problems such as alopecia areata, congenital alopecia, burn sequelae, eyelash-eyebrow loss, beard loss, and mustache loss. In addition, it can camouflage the scars. The main objective of hair transplantation is to restore hair loss. We may not be able to recreate the appearance that the patients had in their early twenties; however, realistic expectations can be met with the help of technology. Based on our experience, FUE is the method that gives us the opportunity to best meet all patients' hair transplantation expectations.

Keywords: hair loss, baldness, hair transplantation, hair loss treatment, fue, fut, alopecia

1. Introduction

In recent years, hair loss has progressively increased because of the use of various chemical agents, environmental conditions, drugs, and inorganic foods [1, 2]. Androgenetic alopecia affects nearly half of the women and men around the world [3–5]. Hair loss at an early age can be quite traumatic, particularly among young men and women. Baldness can be also problematic in advanced ages, even over 50 years of age. Although there are many causes of hair loss, the most common is androgenetic alopecia. Patients and physicians primarily prefer medical treatment. However, medical treatment reveals successful results in a limited number of patients. In many cases of hair loss, particularly in androgenetic alopecia, hair transplantation may be the single method to solve this problem. Hair transplantation is also successfully applied for the treatment of many types of hair losses other than the androgenetic alopecia. The hair transplant can be used in cases such as various cicatricial alopecias, alopecia areata, congenital alopecias, postburn sequelae and to camouflage various skin marks [6, 7]. Both inherent and acquired losses of the beard, mustache, and eyebrow can also be successfully treated with hair transplantation [6, 7]. As hair loss has progressively become a great problem in all populations, patients truly desire to regain their hair and therefore, they may be abused by individuals who are not physicians and who use paramedical methods, particularly topical and herbal treatments.

2. Hair transplantation

Hair transplantation has been applied for many years, and it has gained great progress within the past decade. The duration of operation has shortened, and the number of grafts transferred in one session has substantially increased. Consequently, it is currently possible to obtain excellent outcomes by transferring tremendous amounts of grafts in one session (**Figures 1–5**).

2.1. FUT (follicular unit transfer)

Nearly a decade ago, skin patches were obtained from the occipital region, manually separating it to grafts and then transferring them to the recipient area. This method is called follicular unit transfer (FUT), although it is not the most proper definition. In this method, a linear scar remained at the occipital region (**Figure 6a**), healing duration was prolonged, and the patients felt pain, particularly while lying on the side of the donor area [8, 9]. Moreover, with the FUT method, approximately 1000–1500 graft transplantations were able to be done at one session, which is insufficient for satisfactory outcomes in most patients. The main disadvantages of the FUT method were eliminated with the wide application of the follicular unit extraction (FUE) method within the past one decade [10].

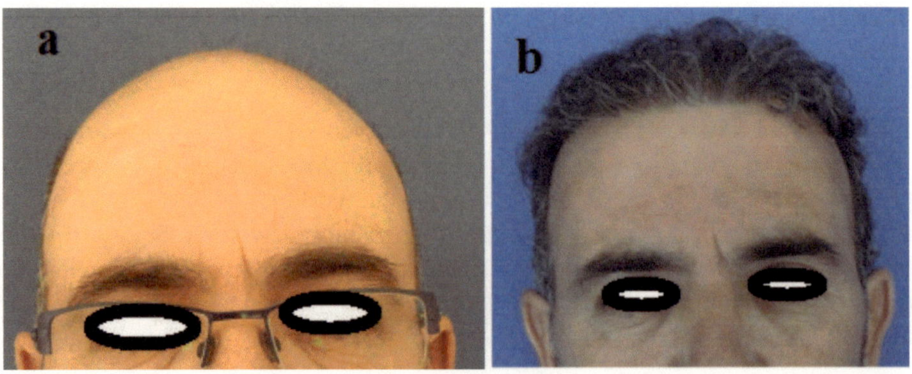

Figure 1. (a) Preoperative photos of androgenetic alopecia, (b) Postoperative photos.

http://dx.doi.org/10.5772/66837

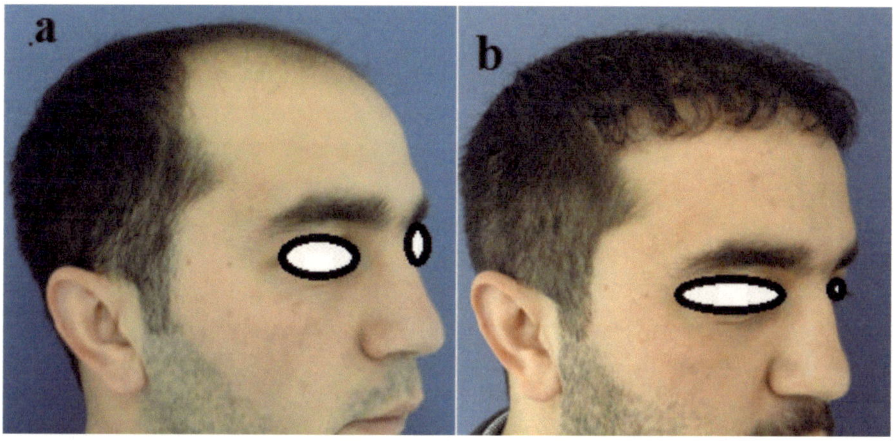

Figure 2. (a) Preoperative photos of androgenetic alopecia, (b) Postoperative photos.

2.2. Follicular unit extraction (FUE)

With the current frequent use of the FUE method, almost none of the patients receive the FUT method for hair transplantation. In particular, the use of a micromotor (**Figure 7**) for graft extraction within the past 5–6 years has made a breakthrough in hair transplantation [8, 9]. Before micromotor use, the grafts were only extracted by manual punches. Approximately 2000 grafts could be extracted in 3–4 h with the manual method, and the extraction of grafts greater than this number was difficult to achieve for the operators. With the wide application of the micromotor method, the number of transplanted grafts in 1 h has increased up to 5000–6000 [6]. The micromotor method has made the application of hair transplantation quite easy for the operators [6]. The ideal age is 30–35 years for hair transplantation. Nevertheless, in patients with hair loss at younger ages, hair concentrating transplantation procedures can be applied before the development of complete baldness. We consider that waiting for total hair loss is not absolutely essential, since individuals do not desire several radical changes to their image. In young men, frontal hair transplantation, particularly in the range of 20–25 years of age, is quite important for the patient's psychology. If the remaining hair is lost in

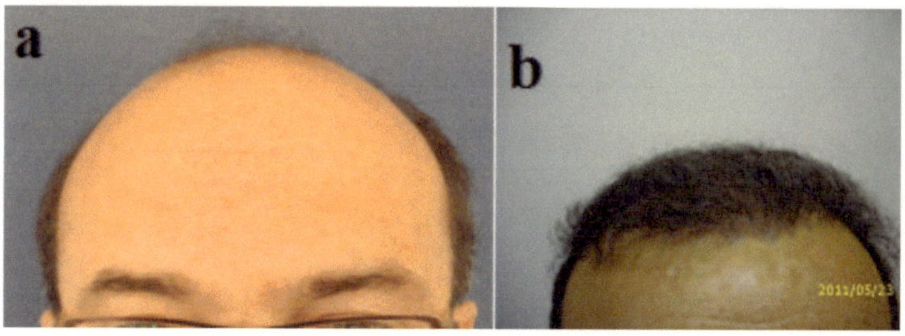

Figure 3. (a) Preoperative photos of androgenetic alopecia, (b) Postoperative photos.

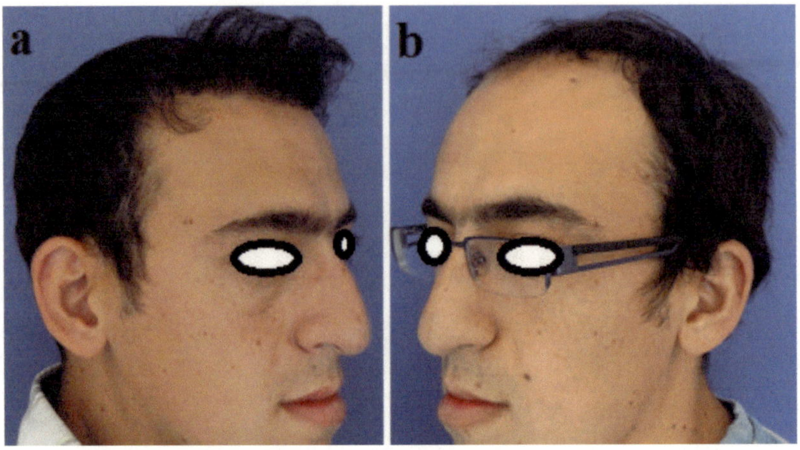

Figure 4. (a), Preoperative photos of androgenetic alopecia. (b), Postoperative photos.

the following years, transplantations can be applied in second and third sessions. It is not essential to wait for the advanced ages under these circumstances. It would also be useful to mention the surgical technique.

2.3. Surgical technique

Except for some unusual situations, the hair transplantation is applied under local anesthesia. It can also be performed under general anesthesia in children and in patients not accepting local anesthesia. Since the duration of the transplantation procedure is long, the patient must rest prior to the operation, must not drink alcoholic beverages several days prior to the procedure, must quit smoking if possible, and must not fast the morning before the operation, which are all important points. The hemoglobin analysis, and PT, PTT, INR, and ELISA tests, and other biochemical tests must absolutely be conducted preoperatively. In particular, local anesthetics may lead to hypotension and syncope in fasting state [11]. Lidocaine including adrenaline is used as a local anesthetic. A special care must be taken in the application of large numbers of graft transplantations with wide donor and recipient areas, since toxic doses of lidocaine can be reached in these situations. The dose must not exceed 5 mg/kg in the

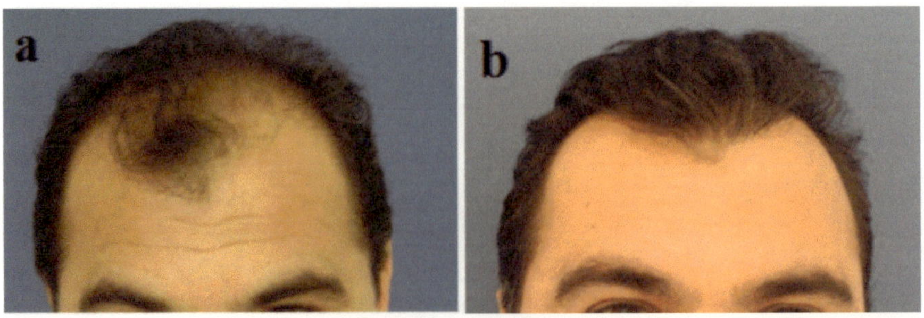

Figure 5. (a) Preoperative photos of androgenetic alopecia, (b) Postoperative photos.

http://dx.doi.org/10.5772/66837

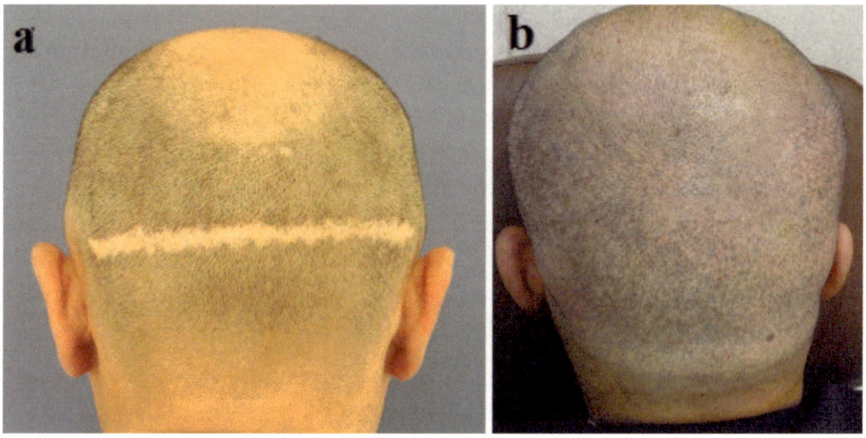

Figure 6. (a) After FUT hair transplant donor area seen, (b) After FUE hair transplant donor area seen.

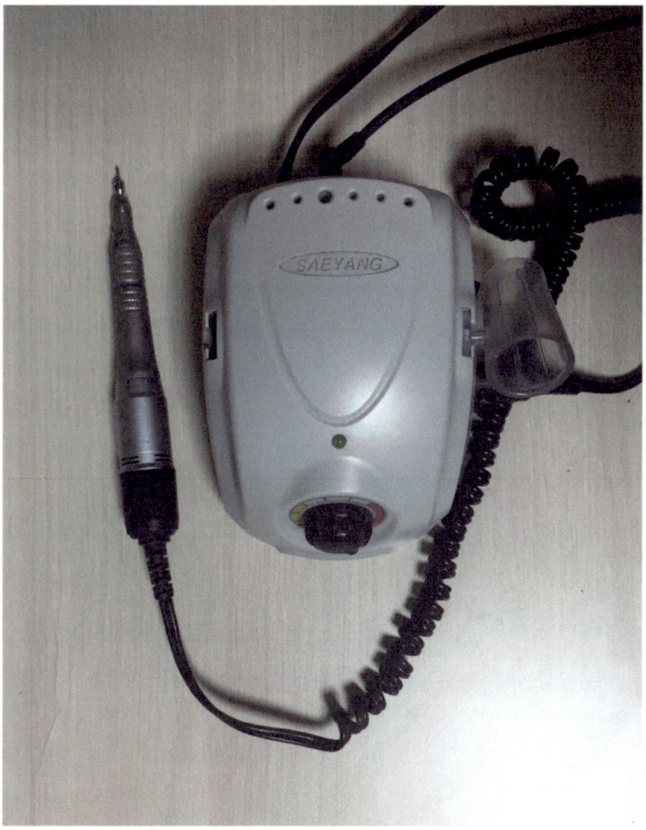

Figure 7. Micromotor for hair transplant.

administration of preparations including adrenaline. The most serious side effect of lidocaine is confusion due to central nervous system toxicity [11–13]. Moreover, hypotension, nausea, vomiting, dizziness, and tinnitus are among the common side effects. The risk of toxicity would be decreased, if the grafts are extracted by initially anesthetizing the donor area, and when the graft extraction is completed, by administering local anesthetic to the recipient area after waiting for a certain time period. If the signs of toxicity appear despite this application, the administration of a 100 cl feeding solution (a solution of 10% lipid + 20% glucose + 5.5% amino acids) by IV pouch, followed by the infusion of the same solution for a certain duration, would eliminate the signs of toxicity immediately. The risks of hypotension and syncope would be lower, if all administrations of local anesthetics are done on the supine position.

The grafts are extracted with punches measuring approximately 0.8–0.9 mm in width. The punches are 5–6 mm in length. These punches are disposable materials assembled at the tip of the micromotor. The velocity of the micromotor is 5000/min. The punches used must always be sharp, since the blunt punches damage the tissue. The number one haircut would make the application quite easy. The hairs at the donor area must be visible at a length of 1 mm on the scalp. The punches internalize the hair over the scalp in a proper slope with the angle of hair growth, cut respectively the skin, connective tissue, and aponeurosis, and stop when the distance to the follicle is 1 mm. They are inserted into the skin in a depth of about 3–3.5 mm, as

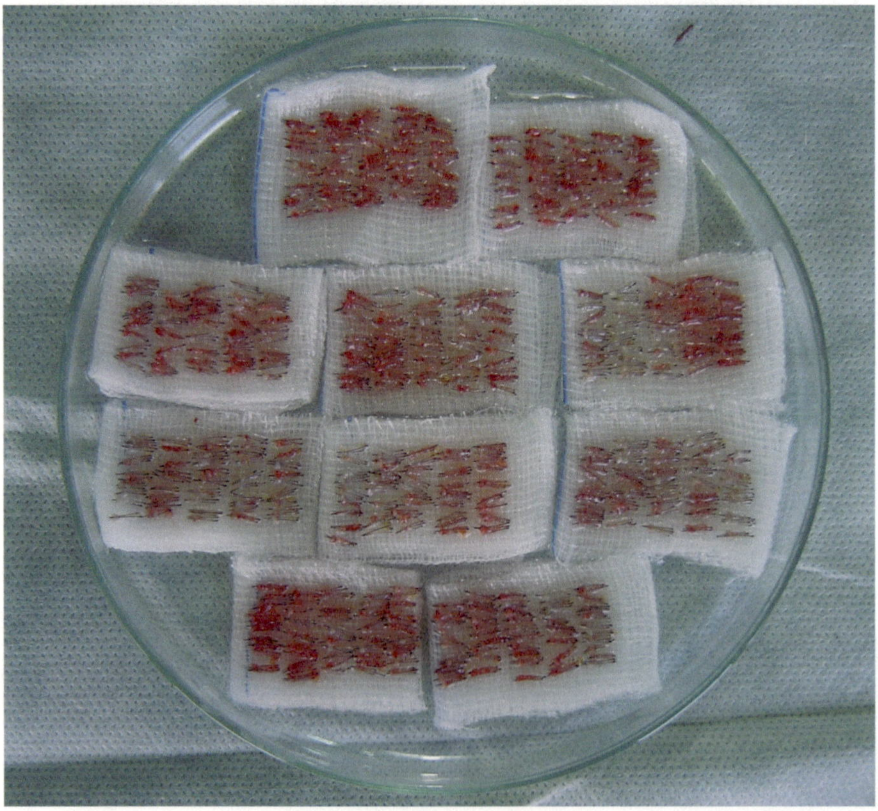

Figure 8. In FUE method, 500 hair graft ready for transplant.

deeper insertions may cause follicular damage. After the grafts are freed, they are collected by the aid of special collets. The collected grafts must be kept in isotonic saline solution (**Figure 8**).

The first extracted graft must initially be placed in the recipient area, and the last extracted graft must be transplanted at the final stage (**Figure 9**). Although it is reported that the grafts can be kept for longer times under suitable conditions, they should not be kept for longer than 4–5 h, if possible, as it would increase the possibility of their viabilities [6]. The depth of the follicles from the skin surface varies between 3.5 and 7 mm. The length of a graft is approximately 5 mm. Grafts shorter than 4 mm and those longer than 6 mm are both difficult to extract and to transplant [6]. The graft extraction is applied in prone position, while the transplantation has to be applied in a semi-seated position. This would lead to a lesser amount of bleeding, and the patient would also feel more comfortable.

Although it varies according to the patients and the number of hairs being transplanted, nearly 1–1.5 units of blood is lost during hair transplantation. Therefore, essential fluid support must be provided. Supratrochlear and supraorbital blocks must be done initially, after the patient is kept in the semi-seated position, and then, all the recipient area must be infiltrated with local anesthetic. Swelling the scalp slightly with a certain amount of physiological saline, after the local anesthetic infiltration, will decrease bleeding and would also make it easy to recognize the opened channels. For the procedure to open channels in the recipient area, razor blades of 1 mm in width and 5–6 mm in length are prepared by cutting. Opening a channel with a sharp razor blade is more advantageous compared to a scalpel blade No. 11. For a natural appearance, some degree of angulation must be formed, particularly when opening channels in the frontal and temporal regions. The grafts are placed at the recipient area one by one after channel opening. The epidermis must be kept outside during graft placement, in order to prevent a reaction. The graft should not be completely inserted into the channel. It takes 48 h for the grafts to be stabilized at the recipient area, by adhesion to the fibrin. Thus, the grafts may be removed from their places within the first 48 h, and therefore, they have to be protected carefully in this period. Since the hair transplantation is a composite tissue transfer, the duration of holding (penetration) is approximately days. After penetration, the grafts begin to grow soon, thereafter. The tissue growth usually takes place over 3–4 weeks; following the third week, the follicles remain within the skin, and the hair tips would be lost. Hair loss may

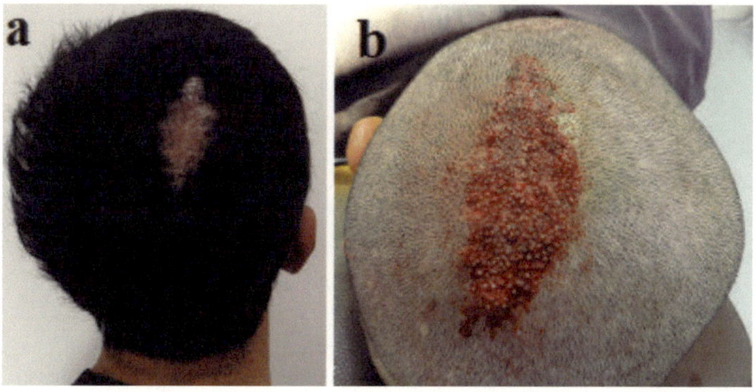

Figure 9. (a) photo of 14 years old boy Preoperative scatricial alopesia, (b) intraoperative photo after transplant.

never occur in a very small number of patients. Even when there is no hair loss, 4–6 months are required for hair elongation. The transplanted hairs grow in approximately 6 months, and they gain volume within the following 1 year. The number of growing hairs in the frontal region is equal to the number of graft transplants, while only the 70% of transplanted hairs grow in the vertex. A great number of transplanted hairs do not grow sometimes, at a rate of one in 200 patients, and the cause is unknown. The grafts are very easily extracted in some patients, while this procedure is quite difficult in some cases. These patients are considered as not appropriate for the FUE method; nevertheless, a meticulous operation might reveal the extraction of a required number of grafts. What is the optimal number of graft transplants in one session? Our experiences reveal that the patients tolerate this operation well within the first 5–6 h; after 6 h, complaints frequently arise such as boredom, fatigue, dizziness, and nausea. Consequently, the hair transplantation procedure should be completed within 6 h, if possible. In other words, the number of graft transplants is based on the number that can be achieved in 6 h.

2.4. Hair transplantation in women

Androgenetic alopecia cases have been progressively increasing particularly in women [3]. Hormonal analyses usually reveal no pathological results. Hair transplantation within an area of 8–10 cm from the frontal hairline toward the vertex yields an excellent outcome in female patients with androgenetic alopecia (**Figure 10**). The main problem of hair transplantation in women is the obligatory "number one haircut." Women can more easily camouflage it with the aid of accessories such as hair bands and toupees. The ratio of women to men is nearly 3/100 in hair transplantation [6].

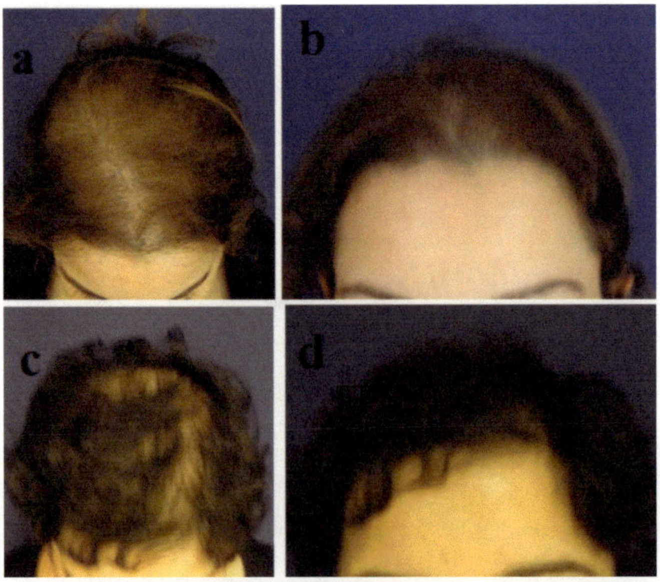

Figure 10. (a) frontal view; Preoperative photo of 35 years old woman has androgenetic alopecia, (b) top of head view Preoperative photo of 35 yeasr old woman has androgenetic alopecia, (c) postoperative 1 year later, (d) postoperative 1 year later.

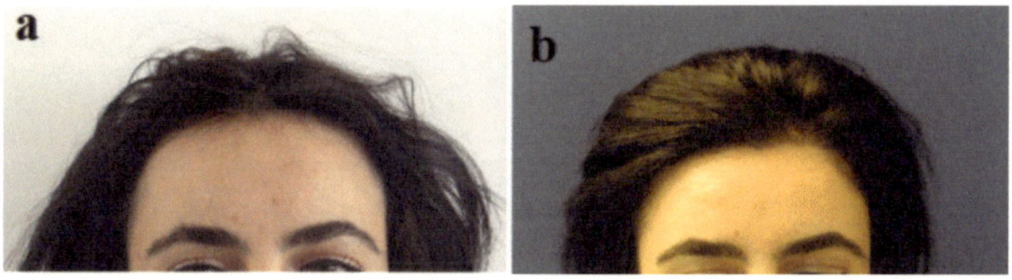

Figure 11. (a) Preoperative 30 years old women has large forehead, (b) 1 year later after hair transplant.

In women with genetically wide foreheads, the forehead can be narrowed with hair transplantation procedure (**Figure 11**). Deformities of the frontal bone and burn sequelae near the hairline can also be masked with hair transplantation (**Figure 12**). Since the women inherently have thinner hair, hair transplantation in women yields more natural outcomes than that in men [6].

2.5. Hair transplantation in adolescents

Hair loss due to alopecia areata and cicatricial alopecia is common at the ages of 14–15 years (**Figure 9**). Patchy areas of multiple alopecia exist as a result of burn sequelae, particularly in developing countries. The hair transplantation yields considerably successful results in these patients [6]. The subdermal soft tissue is quite insufficient in some of these patients. Despite this fact, the rate of graft penetration is substantially high. Expanders were previously used in these patients [14], while recently hair transplantation has become much more advantageous [6]. Although there is an insufficient number of studies about hair transplantation in children, this procedure can also be successfully applied in children, as in adults. The phases of hair transplantation, which are the penetration (holding) and hair growth, and their durations, are similar to those in adults [6]. Since the scalp is thin and the follicles are more superficial, hair transplantation in children requires a more meticulous operation.

2.6. Beard transplantation

Most patients admitted for beard transplantation often complain about a sparse beard. The burn sequelae rarely exist. Whatever the cause may be, the method in beard transplantation is similar to that of hair transplantation. The duration of beard growth is 6 months, as it is for hair. Due to the properties of subdermal soft tissue, the placement of grafts in beard transplantation is more difficult compared to that in hair transplantation (**Figures 15** and **16**).

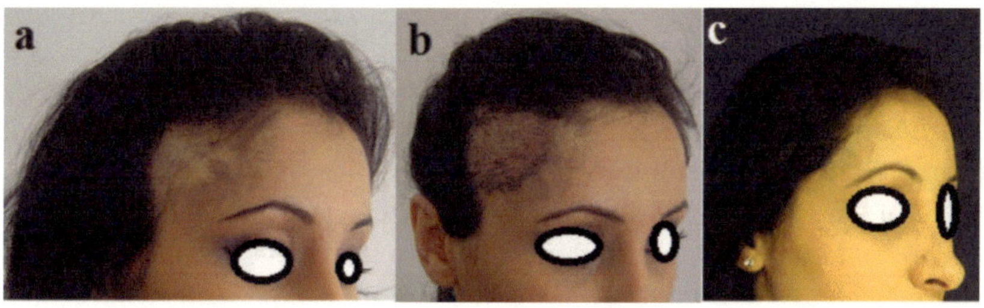

Figure 12. (a) 30 years old women; insufficient subcutan tissue due to burn Preoperative photos, (b) 2 years later hair transplant, (c) 2 years after hair transplantation.

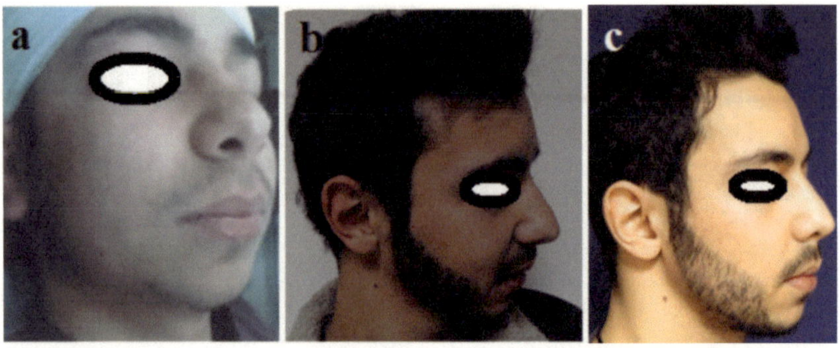

Figure 13. (a) Preoperative photo beard transplant, (b) Postoperative 1 year later, (c) postoperative 2 years later.

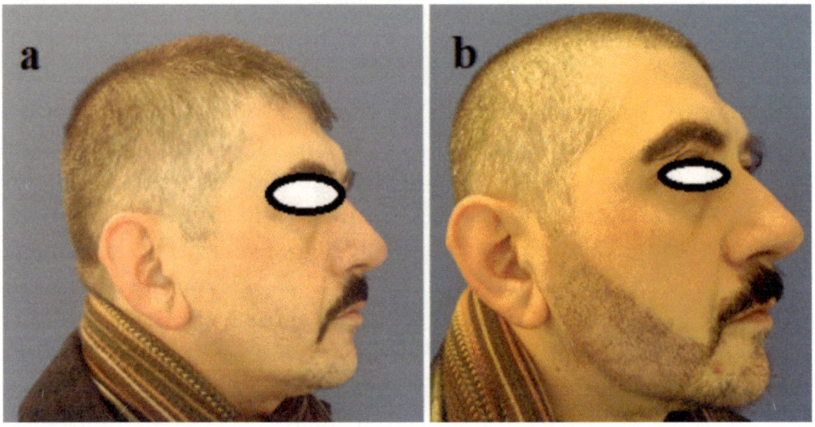

Figure 14. (a) Preoperative photo beard transplant, (b) 2 weeks later beard transplant.

2.7. Mustache transplantation

Mustache transplantation is sometimes applied in combination with beard transplantation, while it is also performed as an isolated mustache transplantation in some cases Hair transplantation is also the almost single treatment of cicatricial alopecias characterized by burn-induced multiple patches (**Figure 17**). The general procedural principles are identical.

2.8. Eyebrow transplantation

Eyebrow transplantation was previously applied due to eyebrow losses resulting from burns and cicatricial tissue. Hair transplantation is also the almost single treatment of cicatricial alopecias characterized by burn-induced multiple patches (**Figures 18** and **19**), while it is mostly preferred today by women desiring more thick, wide, and bushy eyebrows. The outcomes of hair transplantation are more natural in women, while those of the eyebrow transplantation are more natural in men. Eyebrow intensifying transplants may require a second session in women. The problems in eyebrow transplantation are as follows: the rapidly growing eyebrows hairs, difficulty in producing a sufficient eyebrow slope, and rarely, a sparse eyebrow.

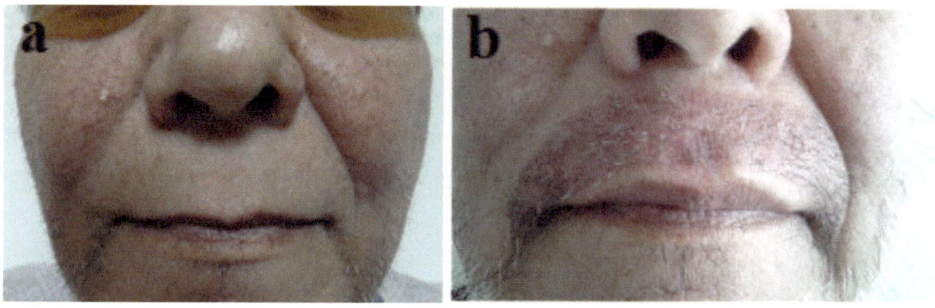

Figure 15. (a) 55 years old man Preoperative photo, (b) 10 days later after mustache transplant.

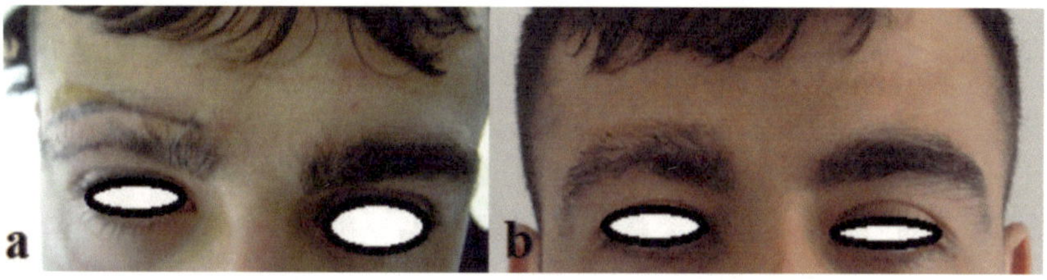

Figure 16. (a) Preoperative photo brow loss, (b) Postoperative photo brow transplant.

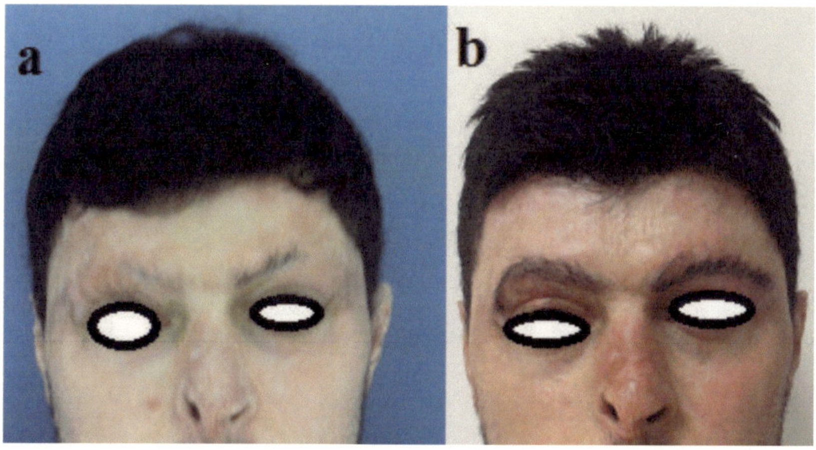

Figure 17. (a) Preoperative photo brow loss, (b) 2 years later brow transplant.

2.9. Cicatricial alopecias

Hair transplantation is also the almost single treatment of cicatricial alopecias characterized by burn-induced multiple patches (**Figures 9**, **12**, **13**, and **14**). The hair transplant can be used in cases such as various cicatricial alopecias, alopecia areata, congenital alopecias, postburn sequelae, and in the camouflage of various skin marks [6, 7]. Hair transplantation is also the almost single treatment of cicatricial alopecias characterized by burn-induced multiple patches (**Figure 18**). Radiation-induced hair loss can be treated by hair transplantation (**Figure 19**).

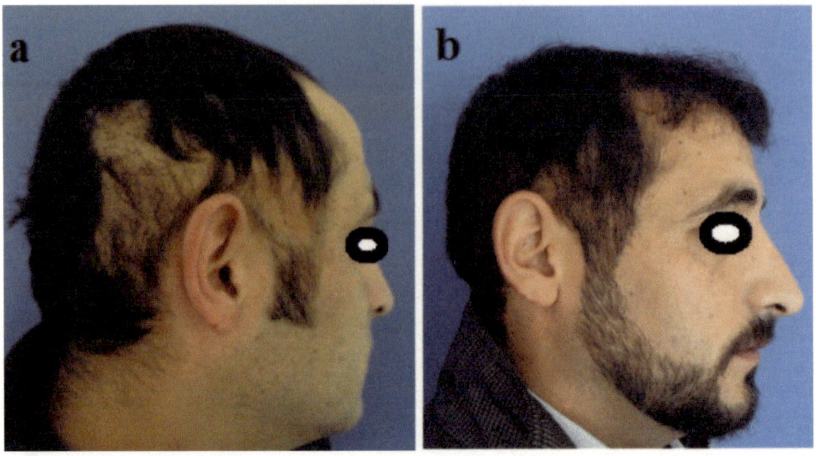

Figure 18. (a) Preoperative photo of burn scar patient, (b) 2 years later hair transplant.

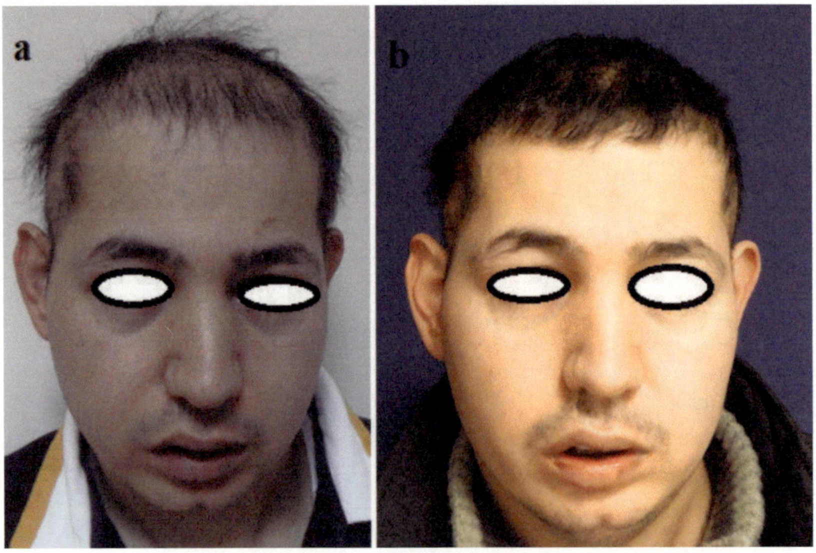

Figure 19. (a) Preoperative photo: 25 years old man, Radiation induced hair loss, (b) 1 year later hair transplant.

2.10. Unknown benefits of hair transplantation

Hair transplantation may be replaced with gene therapies and stem cell therapies in the future. However, the most effective method for treating irreversible hair losses is currently hair transplantation. Hair transplantation has many positive effects compared to the treatment of hair loss. Among these, one of the most important is the marked improvement of forehead wrinkles in the patients undergoing hair transplantation. The hair transplantation produces the effect of Botox on the forehead. Hair transplantation is also the almost single treatment of cicatricial alopecias characterized by burn-induced multiple patches (**Figure 13**).

In the patients with migraines undergoing hair transplantation, the migraine attacks improve markedly and the patients almost stop the use medications. Many unknown useful effects of hair transplantation will be discovered in the future. Better results can be obtained with the application of various supportive treatments, such as the mesotherapy following hair transplantation.

As a result, hair transplantation is perhaps the method that alters the image the most among all esthetic applications. Patients with baldness appear to be 10–15 years older than their real ages. Therefore, hair transplantation provides a type of psychotherapy by causing the patients to regain the images corresponding to their real ages. The positive attitudes of the patients after transplantation lead to an apparent optimism in their professional and private lives. In the patients without a sufficient donor area for hair transplantation, even hair transplantation in only the frontal region is sufficient to make them satisfied.

Acknowledgements

None of the authors has a financial interest in any of the products, devices, or drugs mentioned in this manuscript.

Author details

Safvet Ors

Address all correspondence to: saffetors@gmail.com

SO-EP Aesthetic and Plastic Surgery Clinic, Kayseri, Turkey

References

[1] Gan DC, Sinclair RD: Prevalence of male and female pattern hair loss in Maryborough. J Investig Dermatol Symp Proc 2005;10:184–189.

[2] Otberg N, Finner AM, Shapiro J: Androgenetic alopecia. Endocrinol Metab Clin North Am 2007;36:379–398.

[3] Varothai S, Bergfeld WF: Androgenetic alopecia: an evidence-based treatment update. Am J Clin Dermatol 2014;15(3):217–230.

[4] Bienova M, Kucerova R, Fiura skova M, Hajdu ch M, Kolar Z: Androgenetic alopecia and current methods of treatment. Acta Dermatovenerol Alp Panonica Adriat 2005;14(1):5–8

[5] Baumann LS, Kelso EB: Selections from current literature: androgenetic alopecia: the science behind a new oral treatment. Fam Pract 1998;15(5):493–496

[6] Ors S, Ozkose M, Ors S: Follicular unit extraction hair transplantation with micromotor: eight years experience. Aesthetic Plast Surg 2015;39(4):589–96.

[7] Orentreich N: Autografts in alopecia and other selected dermatological conditions. Ann N Y Acad Sci 1959;83:463–479.

[8] Bisaccia E, Scarborough D: Hair transplant by incisional strip harvesting. J Dermatol Surg Oncol 1994;20:443–448.

[9] Bernstein RM, Rassman WR: Follicular transplantation: patient evaluation and surgical planning. Dermatol Surg 1997;23:771–784.

[10] Rassman WR, Bernstein RM, McClellan R, Jones R, Worton E, Uyttendaele H: Follicular unit extraction: minimally invasive surgery for hair transplantation. Dermatol Surg 2002;28:720.

[11] Dutton WA: Convulsions following pudendal block by lignocaine. Lancet 1955;269(6905):1368–9.

[12] Deacock AR: The toxicity of lignocaine 2 percent. A case report. Anaesthesia 1961;16:363–5.

[13] Wigand FT: Untoward reaction to lidocaine; report of case. J Oral Surg (Chic) 1958;16(4):334–6.

[14] Guzey S, Alhan D, Şahin I, Aykan A, Eski M, Nişancı M: Our experiences on the reconstruction of lateral scalp burn alopecia with tissue expanders. Burns 2015;41(3):631–7.

Chapter 16

Complications of Hair Transplantation

Murat Küçüktaş

Additional information is available at the end of the chapter

http://dx.doi.org/10.5772/66838

Abstract

Recently, hair transplantation has been frequently commonly applied for aesthetic surgical procedures. Hair transplantation has a low complication rate compared to other aesthetic surgical procedures. However, it can cause serious complications if proper attention is not given. But there are a wide range of possible complications that are less severe and manageable. Common postoperative complications include pain, edema, asymmetry, bleeding, visible scarring, folliculitis, crusting, graft dislodgement, hiccups, effluvium, pruritus, and hypoesthesia. Other less common postoperative complications include hypertrophic scarring and keloid, arteriovenous fistula, infection, cobblestoning, syncope, pigment alteration, necrosis, granulomatous reaction, pyogenic granuloma, and Kaposi's varicelliform eruptions. The most serious complication of hair transplantation is necrosis.

Keywords: complications of hair transplantation, necrosis, hair surgery

1. Introduction

Recently, hair transplantation has been frequently commonly applied for aesthetic surgical procedures. Hair transplantation has a low complication rate according to other aesthetic surgical procedures. However, it can lead to serious complications if proper attention is not given. But there are a wide range of possible complications that are less severe and manageable. Common postoperative complications of hair transplantation are listed in **Table 1**.

Common postoperative complications
Pain
Edema
Asymmetry
Bleeding
Visible scarring
Folliculitis
Crusting
Graft dislodgement
Hiccups
Effluvium
Pruritus
Hypoesthesia

Table 1. Common postoperative complications of hair transplantation.

2. Pain

Postoperative pain in most of the patients occurs after hair transplantation surgery. This pain occurs especially in hair transplantation performed with FUT (follicular unit transplant). Because due to the transection of peripheral nerves during strip harvesting. In FUE (follicular unit extraction) method, an average of 3000 graft transplantation procedures lasts for 6–8 h. Muscle pain can occur depending on the lying position during this period. Small breaks need to be given during the process, intraoperative analgesic injection and postoperative NSAID (nonsteroidal anti-inflmmatory drugs) use to prevent and reduce pain [1].

3. Edema

Postoperative edema is the most common complication in hair transplantation. The average incidence of postoperative edema in hair transplantations varies from 40 to 50%. Edema can develop due to tumescent anesthesia and trauma during processing. Tissue edema begins at the time of surgery, but it is only evident 3–5 days later when it descends over the forehead. Occasionally, edematous fluid travels into the periorbital tissues and causes periorbital ecchymosis. Additionally, in some cases, this edema is so severe that patients cannot open his/her eyes.

To prevent and minimize edema, patients should be explained in the lying position during the postoperative period. The use of massage, cold pack, systemic steroids, infiltrative steroids, and NSAID can reduce edema.

4. Asymmetry

Attentive planning and marking of the recipient site will minimize the risk of asymmetry. Causes of asymmetry include the design of false frontal hairline, density difference between the right and left frequency, and previously deformed head. Always check your design markings in a mirror, viewed from behind the patient's head and at his eye level and get his approval as well. You will frequently be surprised how different it looks in the mirror than when you are standing in front and 2 m away [2].

5. Hemorrhage bleeding

The scalp, whether hair bearing or bald, has an abundant blood supply, but the incidence of hemorrhage is surprisingly small. Less often, bleeding occurs after the patient leaves the clinic. Applying pressure for 15 minutes with a clean gauze is very effective for reducing the risk of hemorrhage.

During the preoperative evaluation, patients should be screened for history of bleeding diathesis, for intake of aspirin, nonsteroidal anti-inflammatory agents, vitamin E, alcohol, anabolic steroids, or other anticoagulative agents. Topical minoxidil and smoking must be stopped at least 2 weeks prior to the surgery. Intraoperative recipient-site bleeding is not uncommon and can, usually, be minimized by injection with epinephrine-containing tumescent solutions [3–5].

6. Visible scarring

Visible scarring in the donor area is the most common patient complication encountered in hair transplantation. Hair transplant performed with FUT can leave linear scar at donor region. In the hair transplantation with FUE, visible scarring may occur due to the frequent and abreast entrance of the punch. To avoid this situation, frequent and side-by-side entered punch should not be performed. The treatment for patients with scar includes visible scar revision, hair transplantation, and micro-pigmentations.

7. Folliculitis

Folliculitis is the term used to describe hair follicle inflammation in response to infection, physical injury, or chemical exposure. The reported incidence of postoperative folliculitis in hair transplantations varies from 1.1 to 20% and the severity ranges from a mild, superficial inflammation with mild erythema, and scattered pustules. The infection can occur in either the recipient or the donor area. The treatment of folliculitis depends on the underlying cause. When a mild folliculitis begins 2–3 months postoperatively, hair growth is the probable cause. In such cases, the initial treatment includes warm compresses for 15 min three times daily, and a topical antibiotic ointment such as mupirocin [6].

8. Crusting

Crusting occurs on dry to superficial epidermis of the surrounding graft and bleeding after 24–48 h of hair transplant. Crusting disappears after an average of 7–10 days.

The crusts do not affect the graft survival or the healing process unless they persist for a long period. A first washing is recommended after 48 h to dissolve early crusts. Applying a moisturizer or an emollient is recommended before 30–45 min of washing for softening of crusts. If crusts are still present after postoperative 9–10 days, wet compress or vapor is applied.

9. Graft dislodgement

Graft dislodgement usually occurs in the initial 3 days after hair transplant operation. Direct trauma is the main cause of graft dislodgement. Grafts do not survive long time in the external environment. When trauma or similar reasons occur, graft dislodgement should be replaced as quickly as possible. Patients can store graft dislodgement for a short period in lens solution, saline, or brackish liquid, thereby preventing drying of grafts.

10. Hiccups

Hiccups are an uncommon complication of hair transplantation. The reported incidence of hiccups in hair transplantations is 4.11%. Hiccups are found intraoperatively or shortly after the operation. Usually, it lasts for 2–3 days in the absence of treatment. They can also result from excessive air aspiration consequent to the stimulation of diaphragmatic muscle movements by very excited or vocal patients [7].

11. Postoperative effluvium/shock loss

Postoperative effluvium of preexisting recipient area hair occurs after near transplant, but significant effluvium is far less common. Postoperative effluvium causes recipient site creation, vascular disruption, or edema. It usually presents 2–4 weeks after surgery. However, the majority of the affected hairs begin to regrow after 2–3 months. To reduce postoperative effluvium, protection of existing hair during the recipient site creation should be noted, limiting recipient site size and density to prevent excessive vascular disruption and reducing postoperative edema. Postoperative minoxidil may reduce the incidence of this problem [8].

12. Donor hair effluvium

Hair effluvium is a relatively common occurrence in recipients, especially in females, whereas in donors, it is significantly less common. It usually presents within 6 weeks of surgery as temporary hair loss along the inferior and superior margins of linear wounds, or as diffuse hair loss in the case of FUE. Most likely, it is a consequence of anagen effluvium, in response to interrupted blood supply. Patients should be reassured that the problem spontaneously resolves within 3–4 months, but minoxidil can hasten hair regrowth.

13. Pruritus

Pruritus can be seen after hair transplantation in the donor and the recipient areas. Wound healing process may be the cause. Other reasons may be the use of minoxidil after hair transplantation. Scalp irritation can be caused depending on the frequency of use and the concentration of minoxidil. Topical steroids or and antihistamines are recommended for the treatment of many patients.

14. Loss of sensation

Temporary loss of sensation nearly always occurs in the donor and recipient areas, and is the result of the severing of nerves by the punch as it bores out donor and recipient sites. Patients usually notice this, but rarely complain about it. Sensation returns over a period of 6–12 months after the procedure is completed [9]. Less common complications of hair transplantation are listed in **Table 2**.

Less common postoperative complications
Hypertrophic scarring and keloid
Arteriovenous fistula
Infection
Cobblestoning
Syncope
Pigment alteration
Necrosis
Granulomatous reaction
Pyogenic granuloma
Kaposi's varicelliform eruption

Table 2. Less common complications of hair transplantation.

15. Hypertrophic scar or keloid

Keloid and hypertrophic scarring are rare occurrences in hair transplant complications. The reported incidence of keloid and hypertrophic scarring in hair transplantations is 0.1%. They represent an abnormal response to dermal injury, characterized by exuberant collagen deposition. Keloid scaring usually develops months or years after surgery and persists indefinitely. Individuals with a history of keloid scarring are not candidates for hair restoration surgery. Those with a high risk of developing keloids, due to ethnicity and age, or with a personal history of hypertrophic scarring, should be informed of the potential for abnormal scarring [9, 10].

16. Arteriovenous fistula

The postoperative complication of arteriovenous fistula is a rare complication of punch-graft hair transplantation. This complication has been observed after large punch-graft hair transplantation is done especially to the temporal region in the 1970s.

A pulsatile subcutaneous mass with an associated thrill or bruit and symptoms including pain or headache is a common presentation. Angiography is required for complete diagnostic evaluation.

Clinical findings usually resolve spontaneously within 6 months, but superficial vessels can be ligated if the surgeon is concerned about vessel rupture or cosmetic appearance [11–13].

17. Infections

Infections of the scalp are very rare because it is well vascularized. Serious infections occur in less than 1% of cases and are, usually, associated with poor hygiene, excessive crust formation, or preexisting medical risk factors. There are several measures to be followed for prevention and infection control after hair transplantation: clean and decontaminated operating room, use of sterilized material, donor area asepsis, use of disposable instruments, and antibiotic prophylaxis [14, 15].

18. Cobblestone appearance

The cobblestoning occurs when follicular units are implanted into hole or slits that are too small or implanted at the incorrect depth.

19. Syncope

Occasionally, very nervous patients faint or feel faint during the procedure, but this can be managed by simple measures such as lowering the head between the knees or laying the patient in a prone position [16].

20. Pigment alteration

Pigment alterations of the skin can appear after a hair transplant. The transplanted area should not be subjected to the sun for at least 1 month after hair transplant procedure. A hat (men) or a scarf (for women) is recommended.

21. Necrosis

Recipient area necrosis is a rare but dangerous complication that arises when an increased number of recipient grafts are utilized and de-vascularization of the scalp occurs as a result of dense splitting of the recipient skin that results in large wound areas.

Predisposing factors of skin necrosis: Recipient-site necrosis is a result of vascular compromise. Predisposing influences composed of patient's factors and technical factors are as follows:

- Patient's factors: Smoking, atrophic skin damage, diabetes mellitus, scarring of the recipient site, or a history of scalp surgery.
- Technical factors: Dense packing, megasessions, large openings, use of anesthetic or tumescent solutions with high epinephrine concentration, and deep recipient incisions.

The treatment of central recipient area necrosis focuses on wound debridement and the cultivation of a viable wound base. Extensive sharp debridement is not recommended, and limited sharp debridement of the hyperkeratotic edge of the wound will stimulate reepithelialization. The application of mupirocin ointment is recommended twice daily. Occasionally, for extensive areas of necrosis, scalp expansion may be required for repair. In the treatment of tissue necrosis, hair transplantation can be performed after recovering tissue necrosis [16].

Other less common postoperative complications include granulomatous reaction [17], pyogenic granuloma [18], epidermoid cysts or cysts, and Kaposi's varicelliform eruption [19].

Author details

Murat Küçüktaş

Address all correspondence to: drmuratkucuktas@hotmail.com

Doruk Yıldırım Hospital, Ankara, Turkey

References

[1] Parsley WM, Waldman MA. Postoperative phase. In: Unger WP, Shapiro R, Unger R, Unger M, eds. Hair Transplantation, 5th edn. New York, NY: Informa Healthcare, 2011: 416–27.

[2] Shiffman MA, Shiell RC, Lam SM. Managing complications in hair restoration. In: Lam S, eds. Hair Transplant 360 Advances, Techniques, Business Development Global Perspectives, Vol 3. New Delhi: Jaypee, 2014: 357–74.

[3] Unger WP. Hair transplantation in male-pattern alopecia. Can Med Assoc J. 1971; 105: 177–81.

[4] Lam SM. Complications in hair restoration. Facial Plast Surg Clin North Am. 2013; 21: 675–80. DOI: 10.1016/j.fsc.2013.07.010.

[5] Coleman WP, Klein JA. Use of the tumescent technique for scalp surgery, dermabrasion, and soft tissue reconstruction. J Dermatol Surg Oncol. 1992; 18: 130–5.

[6] Sandro S, Gonçalves AJ, Américo HJ, Flavia HJ. Surgical complications in hair transplantation a series of 533 procedures. Aesthet Surg J. 2009; 29: 72–6. DOI: 10.1016/j.asj.2008.11.005

[7] Loganathan E, Sarvajnamurthy S, Gorur D, Suresh DH, Siddaraju MN, Narasimhan RT. Complications of hair restoration surgery: a retrospective analysis. Int J Trichology. 2014; 6: 168–72. DOI: 10.4103/0974-7753.142861

[8] True RH, Dorin RJ. A protocol to prevent shock loss. Hair Transplant Forum Int. 2005; 15: 197.

[9] Juckett G. Management of keloids and hypertrophic scars. Am Fam Physician. 2009; 80: 253–60.

[10] Brown MD, Johnson T, Swanson NA. Extensive keloids following hair transplantation. J Dermatol Surg Oncol. 1990; 16: 867–9.

[11] Barros d'Sa AA, Heard CE. Arteriovenous fistula after hair transplantation. Br Med J. 1978; 11: 340–1.

[12] Semashko DC, Schwartz ME, Kaynan A, Harrington EB. Arteriovenous fistula following punch-graft hair transplantation. J Dermatol Surg Oncol. 1989; 15: 754–5.

[13] Davis AJ, Nelson PK. Arteriovenous fistula of the scalp secondary to punch autograft hair transplantation: angioarchitecture, histopathology, and endovascular and surgical therapy. Plast Reconstr Surg. 1997; 100: 242–9.

[14] Farjo N. Infection control and policy development in hair restoration. Hair Transplant Forum Int. 2008; 18: 141–4.

[15] David PM. Complications in hair restoration surgery. Oral Maxillofac Surg Clin North Am. 2009; 21: 119–48. DOI: 10.1016/j.coms.2008.10.010

[16] Feily A, Moeineddin F. Feily's method as new mode of hair grafting in prevention of scalp necrosis even in dense hair transplantation. Dermatol Pract Concept. 2015; 5: 41–6. DOI: 10.5826/dpc.0503a10

[17] Altchek DD, Pearlstein HH. Granulomatous reaction to autologous hairs incarcerated during hair transplantation. J Dermatol Surg Oncol. 1978; 4: 928–9.

[18] Sarnoff DS, Goldberg DJ, Greenspan AH, Albom MJ. Multiple pyogenic granuloma-like lesions following hair transplantation. J Dermatol Surg Oncol. 1985; 11: 32–4.

[19] Mansur AT, Demirci GT, Uzunismail MA, Yildiz S. A rare complication of follicular hair unit extraction: Kaposi's varicelliform eruption. Dermatol Pract Concept. 2016; 6: 15–7. DOI: 10.5826/dpc.0601a05

Section 10

Non-Surgical Treatment of Hair Loss

Chapter 17

New Modalities in the Treatment of Refractory Alopecia Areata

Arzu Kılıç

Additional information is available at the end of the chapter

http://dx.doi.org/10.5772/66591

Abstract

Alopecia areata (AA) is a common and complex T-cell–mediated inflammatory disorder. It may be patchy (localized), involve the entire scalp (alopecia totalis) or entire body (alopecia universalis). Alopecia totalis and universalis are often difficult to treat. Although many therapeutic options currently exist in alopecia areata, none of them are curative or preventive. Besides, none of them are approved by Food and Drug Administration (FDA). The disease unfortunately has an unpredictable course. The factors indicating a poor prognosis are the extent of hair loss at the presentation, long duration of the disease, and ophiasis pattern of hair loss. There are only a few randomized controlled studies conducted on recalcitrant AA. Recent research on immunology of hair follicle and recent developments in immunopathogenesis, together with the shared pathways of the disease with other autoimmune disorders, led investigators to focus on novel therapies that target specific immunological pathways. Herein, we will review shortly the current treatment options in recalcitrant alopecia areata based on recently published studies and then will focus on the recently developed broad-spectrum and targeted therapeutics.

Keywords: alopecia areata, refractory, treatment, new, biological treatment

1. Introduction

Alopecia areata (AA) is a common immune-mediated disorder [1]. It affects 0.1–0.2% of the general population and accounts for 0.7% to 3.8% of all patients attending to dermatology clinics [1, 2]. It affects both genders equally. Although onset may occur at any age, 60% of new cases had their first diagnosis before 20 years age [1, 2].

Despite its high prevalence, the exact cause and triggering factors of AA are still unknown [1–3]. It is considered to be a complex genetic, immune-mediated disease [1–5]. It targets primarily hair follicles and characterized by dense peribulbar lymphocytic infiltrate [4, 6]. Hair follicle is a dynamic immune privileged "miniorgan" with unique immune and hormone microenvironments. This means that hair follicles are immune-protected sites With deficient major histocompability complex (MHC) expression [7, 8]. Evidence suggests that AA results from the loss of immune privilege with presentation of autoantigens, triggered by environmental factors in genetically susceptible individuals [1, 3, 7–9]. Many genes that are found to be associated with AA are also related to the immune system [3, 9]. Cytotoxic CD8+ NKG2D+ T cells are key players in the pathogenesis of AA that produce interferon-γ (IFN-γ) [5, 10]. Interleukin (IL)-2 and IL-15 are well known drivers of cytotoxic activity by IFN-γ-producing CD8+ Tcells and natural killer (NK) cells [10]. Besides, recently published studies investigating the cytokine profile in lesional AA scalp indicates concurrent activation of Th1 and Th2 immune axes, as well as interleukin (IL)-23 and IL-32 cytokine pathways [11–13]. Also, in another recent study, it was supported that Th1-type cytokine profile is related to disease activity of AA, whereas Th2-type cytokines may be associated with the persistence of AA [14]. It is significant to understand both the pathomechanism of AA and responsible cytokines in order to develop new treatments for recalcitrant AA [3, 6, 7, 13].

In AA, most commonly affected area is the scalp [1, 2]. On scalp, it usually presents with well demarcated, one or more hairless patches with preserved follicular ostia and without erythema [1]. If 100% of the scalp hair is lost, it is named as alopecia totalis (AT). Any hair-bearing area such as beard, eyebrows, eyelashes, body, armpits, and pubic region may also be affected in AA, as well as the entire body, alopecia universalis (AU) [1, 2, 15]. Depending on the extent of involvement, AA can be associated with a dramatic reduction of quality of life [1, 2, 16, 17].

The association with other autoimmune diseases such as thyroid diseases, vitiligo, diabetes mellitus, pernicious anemia, rheumatoid arthritis may be seen with AA [2, 6, 17–19]. Atopy is twice as common in AA patients as it is in the general population [2, 16]. Other diseases and genetic disorders reported to be associated with AA include Down syndrome, Addison's disease, autosomal recessive autoimmune polyglandular syndrome, psoriasis, lupus, ulcerative colitis, and multiple sclerosis. These less common disorders are more likely to be associated with AT and AU [2].

AA has an unpredictable outcome [1, 2, 16]. Up to 50% of patients with limited patchy AA will recover within 1 year even without treatment [16, 17]; while 7–10% of patients can eventually develop the severe chronic form of the condition, which is refractory to most of the treatments [20]. The factors indicating a poor prognosis are the extent of hair loss presentation (extensive AA/AT/AU), an ophiasis pattern of hair loss, onset in childhood, a long duration of hair loss, associated atopy or autoimmune disease [1, 16, 17, 19]. The chance of full recovery is less than 10% in AT/AU [2].

2. Treatment

2.1. Conventional therapies

For the disease of AA, there exists currently neither a universally proven therapy that induces and sustains remission, nor a cure [21]. Various treatments are available; however, only a few randomized controlled studies in AA have been published [22]. Current treatment options include a variety of topical, intralesional, and systemic agents with the choice and recommendation based on the disease extent, duration of disease, associated disorders, and age of the patient [15, 23–25].

For recalcitrant AA, and particularly the AT and AU forms, finding appropriate therapeutics among currently available options is very challenging [13]. Current systemic treatment options mostly show limited efficacy and are often associated with major adverse effects in these cases [15, 24].

In this chapter, different treatment modalities in AA will be reviewed. As discussion of all the treatment modalities for AA is beyond the scope of this chapter, instead we rather focused our attention on current treatment regimens for recalcitrant and extensive AA, and on novel treatment modalities, which are still being under investigation.

2.1.1. Corticosteroids

2.1.1.1. Topical corticosteroids

Midpotent and potent topical corticosteroids (CSs) are usually used to treat AA, especially patchy type AA, but the evidence for their effectiveness is limited in recalcitrant AA [23–26]. CSs are thought to affect peribulbar lymphocytes and decrease inflammation around the bulb region, thereby allowing follicles to enter a normal hair cycle [25, 26].

2.1.1.2. Intralesional corticosteroids

For adult patients characterized with limited scalp involvement or in cases with involvement of eyebrows, intralesional corticosteroids (ILCSs) are considered as a first-line therapy [15, 21, 23]. Although, ILCSs have been used for about 50 years, no published randomized controlled trials have been found about this treatment in AA [22, 27].

2.1.1.3. Systemic corticosteroids

Systemic CSs are the most useful immunosuppressive therapy for patients with active AA [21, 23]. The suggested dosages for AA in adults are 1 mg/kg/day and 0.1–1 mg/kg/day for children. The dosages necessary to maintain hair regrowth in AA are daily between 30 mg and 150 mg [15]. However, there is little information available on the role of long-term use of systemic corticosteroids in chronic refractory AA [16, 24]. Combination with methotrexate (MTX) in the treatment of severe long-term AA might be more effective [28].

2.1.1.4. Systemic pulse corticosteroids

Systemic pulse corticosteroid therapy (PCT) is another choice in the treatment of recalcitrant and extensive AA [17, 23, 29]. The use of PCT was introduced to minimize the side effects associated with prolonged systemic corticosteroid therapy. However, placebo-controlled randomized studies with varying dosage schedules are required to standardize the treatment regimen, optimize the therapeutic efficacy, and evaluate the long-term outcomes [22, 24].

2.1.2. *Topical anthralin (dithranol)*

Although the mechanism of anthralin (dithranol) is unknown, the interaction of the drug with different cytokines such as IFNs, tumor necrosis factor (TNF), IL-1, and IL-10 points to a nonspecific immunomodulatory effect, which is responsible for regrowth [30]. There are a small number of uncontrolled case series [22, 30], in which, no randomized controlled study was found in recalcitrant AA.

2.1.3. *Topical immunotherapy (topical sensitizers)*

Topical immunotherapy (TI) with diphenylcyclopropenone (DPCP) or squaric acid dibutylester (SADBE) is recommended as a first-line therapy in adult patients with AA having more than 50% scalp involvement [23, 30]. No randomized controlled trials have been found to evaluate the effectiveness of TI in recalcitrant AA [22, 31]. A review of all articles published on TI concluded that 50–60% of the patients experienced worthwhile regrowth, although the range of response was very broad (9–87%) [31–34].

2.1.4. *Topical minoxidil*

Minoxidil is a topical preparation, of which the mechanism of action is not fully understood. Vasodilatation, angiogenesis, enhanced cell proliferation at the base of the bulb and differentiation above the dermal papilla, and potassium channel opening have all been proposed [23]. It was confirmed that topical minoxidil may induce new hair growth in AA but less likely to do so in more severe and extensive diseases [23, 24, 35].

2.1.5. *Topical prostaglandin analogues*

Prostaglandin (PG) F2α and its analogues have been shown to have stimulatory effects on murine hair follicles and follicular melanocytes in both telogen and anagen phases and also on the stimulation of conversion from telogen to anagen phase [24].

Although reports about effective clinical response have been found [36], two randomized controlled studies demonstrated an efficacy of topical latanoprost in the AA [37–39].

2.1.6. *Topical bexarotene*

Bexarotene is a retinoid X receptor agonist that induces T-cell apoptosis and effects as an immunomodulator [23]. In a randomized half-head trial study including patients of recalcitrant AA treated with topical bexarotene, no difference was demonstrated between the two sides [40].

2.1.7. *Calcineurin inhibitors*

2.1.7.1. *Cyclosporine*

Cyclosporine (Cyc) is an immunosuppressive agent that inhibits helper T-cell activity and suppresses the IFN-γ production. The treatment with Cyc alone or in combination with systemic steroids demonstrated variable clinical results with a response rate between 25% and 88.4% [17, 41–43].

http://dx.doi.org/10.5772/66591

Despite these effective results, side effects of Cyc make this therapy not appropriate for the long-term use [21]. Neither pimecrolimus nor tacrolimus was shown to be effective in AA [44–46].

2.1.8. Methotrexate

Methotrexate (MTX) is an immunosuppressive agent and a folic acid antagonist, which exerts its effect by inhibiting DNA synthesis and has anti-inflammatory properties [23].

Although no randomized controlled study has been found, MTX and low doses of oral corticosteroids might be an effective treatment for resistant AA, which should be evaluated in larger series [28, 47, 48].

2.1.9. Azathioprine

Azathioprine (AZT) is a cytotoxic and immunosuppressive drug and has selective effects on T lymphocytes [17, 23]. An open-label uncontrolled study and a recently published prospective study suggested that AZT Might be an alternative [49, 50].

2.1.10. Sulfasalazine

Sulfasalazine is an immunomodulatory and anti-inflammatory drug that inhibits the release of IL-2 and PGE2 and reduces the inflammatory cell chemotaxis and antibody production [51]. Several uncontrolled studies have interrogated the efficiency of the drug [51–53]. Although there are conflicting results and there is no randomized controlled study, sulfasalazine may be a hope for resistant and extensive cases. Additional larger studies should be conducted on this subject.

2.1.11. Simvastatin/ezetimibe

Statins are lipid-lowering drugs that also inhibit T-lymphocyte activation, downregulate expression of adhesion molecules, and have immunomodulatory effects [54]. Case series were reported demonstrating the efficiency of daily dosage of simvastatin 40 mg and ezetimibe 10 mg in AA [55–57]. Contrarily, Loi et al. reported a study of 20 patients (17 patients were evaluated) with recalcitrant AA, in which 14 of 17 were unresponsive [58]. All of these reports suggest that simvastatin/ezetimibe might be a promising agent in AA. Further randomized controlled studies are needed in recalcitrant AA.

2.1.12. Phototherapy

Having effects on Langerhans cells, cytokine profile, inducing apoptosis and promotion of immunosuppression make phototherapy a choice of treatment in AA [59]. There are several uncontrolled studies of psoralen plus ultraviolet A (PUVA) light with either oral or topical psoralens and either with local or whole body irradiation with response rates up to 60% in AA [60–62]. However, two retrospective reviews reported that PUVA is not an effective treatment method in AA [63, 64]. No randomized controlled trials for neither PUVA nor narrow band ultraviolet B (nbUVB) treatments have been found. A recent study suggested that the combination therapy with topical Cyc and PUVA may be an additional choice for severe and recalcitrant AA [65]. Four patients were reported responding by both clinically and histopathologically to UVA1 therapy [66].

2.1.13. Laser therapy

Recently, there has been a great interest in the potential treating role of laser and light-based therapies in various disorders including AA [67–69]. A study which investigated the efficacy of pulsed diode laser (904 nm) in the treatment of resistant patchy AA reported a regrowth rate in 94% of the patients, while no response was shown in control patches [68].

The efficacy of excimer laser was investigated in various reports with a failure of regrowth [69–72].

2.1.14. Miscellaneous treatments

Inosiplex (Isoprinosine): Inosiplex, an immunomodulator, was tried in a randomized controlled study with recalcitrant AA and significant regrowth was observed in the group treated with inosiplex [73].

Platelet-rich plasma (PRP): There are reports showing the efficacy of PRP in extensive AA [74–76]. A case with ophiasis type AA was reported to be treated successfully with PRP [74]. A recently published randomized controlled study suggested that PRP might be a safe and effective treatment for AA [75].

2.2. Targeted therapies

In recent years, various biological agents that target pathogenesis have been introduced for the treatment of various diseases. Understanding the pathomechanism of AA has led investigators to do research about the efficacy of new biological treatments in AA. There are still multiple possible therapeutic targets being explored. After going through the above mentioned current treatments, the below section will focus on the recent broad-spectrum and targeted therapeutics, centering upon suggested AA immune pathways.

2.2.1. Tumor necrosis factor (TNF)-α inhibitors

TNF-α is a proinflammatory cytokine that mediates inflammation and has a role in cell proliferation and differentiation [77]. TNF-α was shown to be elevated in the serum of patients with AA [78] and in lesional AA skin than nonlesional skin [12]. Although this evidence suggests that blocking TNF activity may improve AA, a clinical trial of 17 individuals was performed to investigate the effect of etanercept in AA. As a result of the study, it was found as ineffective [79]. Several reports have been published indicating the development of AA during a treatment of anti-TNF-α for another disease [80–86]. Gorcey et al. reported a patient with AU, refractory to various treatment modalities, who was successfully treated with adalimumab, while being treated for the flare of atopic dermatitis [87].

Pharmacogenetics and the inherent physiologic levels of TNF may explain why TNF inhibitors cause AA in some individuals, while treating AA in others. These conclusions warrant further investigation on this subject.

2.2.2. *IL-23 pathway antagonism*

2.2.2.1. *Ustekinumab*

Ustekinumab is a human monoclonal IgG1 antibody that binds with the p40 subunit of IL-12 and IL-23 and inhibits their activity [88].

The Th17 immunologic pathway and associated cytokines including IL23 and IL17 are important in the pathophysiology of psoriasis, psoriatic arthritis, and other spondyloarthropathies [13, 89].

Many studies have demonstrated that IL-23 has an important role by driving the expansion and functional maintenance of Th17 development [90].

Suárez-Fariñas et al. performed a study on microarray and RT-PCR profile of 27 lesional and 17 nonlesional scalp samples from patients with AA and compared them with normal scalp samples (n=6). Genes associated with T-cell migration/activation were found to be significantly induced in lesional vs. nonlesional AA tissues. IL-12/23p40 showed the highest increase in mRNA expression of all measured inflammatory markers in lesional scalp of AA compared with normal scalp from healthy subjects [12]. As increased Th1 serum cytokine levels have been associated with extensive AA, IL-12 inhibitors (ustekinumab) would be expected to treat or at least to prevent hair loss [11, 91].

Guttman-Yassky et al. demonstrated hair regrowth in three extensive AA patients (one had AU) treated with 90 mg subcutaneously. At the 20th week, all patients exhibited varying degrees of hair regrowth. The patient with AU, with the highest baseline inflammation and lowest expression of hair keratins, exhibited the highest regrowth [92].

On the other hand, case reports of AA developing during treatment with ustekinumab for psoriasis have also been published [93–95].

Future clinical trials including larger samples are needed to clarify the clinical efficacy of usteukinumab in AA.

2.2.3. *Th17/IL-17 antagonism*

2.2.3.1. *Secukinumab*

Secukinumab is a recombinant, high-affinity, fully human IgG1κ monoclonal antibody that selectively inhibits IL-17A [12, 96, 97].

IL-17A is known to induce the expression of T-cell and dendritic cell chemokines, which lead to the migration of memory T cells and dendritic cells to the inflammation area [97].

Tanemura et al. found the infiltration of CD4(+)IL-17A(+) Th17 cells in the dermis, particularly around hair follicles, in all 4 cases in their study [98].

A recent study by Atwa et al. examined IL-17, IL-21, IL-22, IL-6, and TNF-α levels in the serum of patients with AA and studied their association with the clinical type and severity of AA. All of these cytokines were found to be significantly higher in the AA group than in the control group. Significant positive correlations between the serum IL-17 and disease severity, between the serum TNF-α and disease severity were detected. Also significant positive correlation between serum IL-22 and duration of AA was detected [99].

Lew et al. conducted a case-control association study of 238 AA patients, in which, IL17A and IL17RA (IL-17A receptor) gene polymorphisms were detected [100].

These studies support a possible role for an anti-IL-17 treatment in AA. Secukinumab is being tested in a double-blind, randomized, placebo-controlled clinical trial for AA (ClinicalTrials.gov NTC02599129).

2.2.4. Broad T-cell inhibition

2.2.4.1. Apremilast

Apremilast is an orally available molecule that inhibits phosphodiesterase 4 (PDE4) [13, 101]. It is approved in the treatment of psoriasis, psoriatic arthritis, and currently tested in trials for atopic dermatitis, and other inflammatory and dermatological conditions [102].

Inhibition of PDE4 leads to reduced production of proinflammatory mediators, such as TNF, IFN-γ, IL-12/23p40, IL-17A, and IL-22 [101, 102]. On the other hand, apremilast has been reported to increase the production of IL-6 and IL-10 [101–104]. This is of interest, since IL-10 is a cytokine with potent anti-inflammatory properties, while IL-6 is a cytokine with pro- and anti-inflammatory features [101]. Apremilast also exerts its effects by hydrolyzing cyclic adenosine monophosphate (cAMP) and thus affects various inflammatory mediators. PDE4 antagonism results in elevated intracellular cAMP [101–103].

In a study by Keren et al. PDE4 was found highly elevated in the lesions of AA in a mouse model of AA; apremilast was shown to be effective with almost complete preservation of hair folliclues and resulted significant in reductions in inflammatory cytokines, such as PDEe, IFN-γ, and TNF-α [105]. Suárez-Fariñas et al. reported a highly increase of PDE4 in human AA lesions in their study [12]. In a furher study by Guttman-Yassky et al., levels of PDE4 were found to decrease after treatment with IL-12/IL-23 antagonist [92].

Apremilast might be an appropriate therapeutical option for AA and is under being investigation as a clinical trial (ClinicalTrials.com NCT02684123).

2.2.4.2. Janus kinase inhibitors

Janus kinase (JAK) inhibitors are potent antiinflammatory and antiproliferative agents [13, 106]. Tofacitinib is a pan-JAK inhibitor that is approved by the FDA for the treatment of rheumatoid arthritis and ruxolitinib is a JAK1/2 inhibitor that is approved for the treatment of polycythemia vera and myelofibrosis [107].

JAK family of protein-tyrosine kinases is made of four members: JAK1, JAK2, JAK3 and TYR2 (Tyrosine kinase2). The JAK/STAT pathway transduces extracellular signals from a variety of cytokines, growth factors and hormones to the nucleus and is responsible for the expression of thousands of protein-encoding genes [107, 108]. Targeting JAK1 or JAK2 was thought to be helpful for interfering with the signaling pathways implicated in the generation of pathogenic Th1 and Th17 cells in autoimmunity [106].

The possibility of reversal of AA by JAK inhibitors was successfully shown in murine model by blocking IFN-γ and interleukin-2 (IL-2) or IL-15 receptor β and by reducing the accumulation of CD8 + T cells [10, 109, 110]. Both JAK1 and JAK2 (ruxolitinib, baricitinib) and JAK3 (tofacitinib) inhibitors have been reported to effectively treat AA in various case reports [109–112].

Craiglow and King reported a patient with psoriasis who also had long standing AU. After 8 months of treatment with tofacitinib, the patient had full regrowth of hair on scalp along with significant regrowth on eyelashes, eyebrows and other body sides [111].

Jabbari et al. studied the effect of tofacitinib by clinically and by the changes in expression of AA- associated genes in skin as well as circulating CXCL10 levels with result sof significant hair growth along with change in skin and biochemical markers [109].

Gupta et al. reported two cases of recalcitrant AU treated with tofacitinib. Both cases showed full regrowth of hair on the body at the end of 8 months of treatment [112].

A case with AU treated with tofacitinib with a transient efficacy has also been reported [113].

Today, there are ongoing clinical trials for tofacitinib (ClinicalTrials.gov NCT02312882, NCT02197455, NCT02299297 and NCT02812342), ruxolitinib (NCT01950780), and baricitinib in the treatment of AA and in various inflammatory diseases, which will make us understand the exact effect of these treatments [13].

Topical JAK inhibitors have also been shown as effective in AD, psoriasis, dry eye disease and in allergic contact dermatitis model [114–117]. Topical JAK inhibitors may offer a good treatment option for especially for limited AA [13].

JAK inhibitors may replace some immunosuppressive treatments. Further clinical trials are warranted to clarify the exact effects of JAK inhibitors in AA.

2.2.4.3. *Abatacept*

Abatacept is a fusion protein of cytotoxic T-lymphocyte-associated antigen 4 (CTLA-4) with a portion of IgG1 (CTLA-4Ig) that selectively modulates T-cell co-stimulation. It binds to CD80/CD86 receptors on antigen-presenting cells and by this way blocks the interaction of CD80/86 with CD28 which is found on T-cells and inhibits full T-cell activation [118, 119]. In vitro, abatacept decreases T-cell proliferation, the production of inflammatory cytokines such as IFN-γ, TNF-α and IL-2 and B-cell immunological response [118]. Also, it was found to increase Treg cells, which was linked to downregulation of activation-associated marker molecules [120]. Abatacept is currently being used in rheumatoid arthritis with FDA approvement [13]. Since T-cell activation is crucial in the development of AA [9], there is a potential chance for abatacept in the treatment of AA. There is an ongoing study for abatacept (ClinicalTrials.gov NCT02018042).

2.2.5. *IL-2 modulation as a modifier of regulatory function*

2.2.5.1. *Aldesleukin*

Aldesleukin is a recombinant interleukin-2 (IL-2) molecule and a biological response modifier having various immunomodulatory properties [121]. Aldesleukin is currently approved only for treatment of renal cell carcinoma and metastatic melanoma and is usually used in high doses in these indications [122, 123]. It can be applied via intravenous or subcutaneous administration. In high intravenous bolus regimen, it has been reported to be highly toxic [121]. IL-2 is a key cytokine for T regulatory (reg) cell differentiation, homeostasis and functions [124]. In AA, an imbalance in the immune state of patients has been detected with altered T-helper cell and Treg cell functions [125, 126]. A study by Shin et al. revealed impaired function of CD4 T reg cells [127]. A study by Castela et al. evaluated the efficacy of low dose recombinant IL-2 treatment on five AA patients. Four of five patients had partial regrowth and the improvement continued up to 6 months after drug cessation. Pre and posttreatment biopsies were taken to compare the level of T reg cells and an increase was detected in posttreatment group [128]. Aldesleukin is now being under investigation and clinical studies with larger samples are needed to assess the exact efficacy of the drug (ClinicalTrials.gov NCT01840046).

2.2.6. Th2 pathway inhibition

2.2.6.1. Dupilumab

Dupilumab is a fully human monoclonal antibody directed against the α subunit of IL-4 receptor. It blocks the signaling of IL-4 and IL-13, both of which are the key cytokines in Th2-mediated pathways [13, 129]. The efficacy of dupilumab has been studied in atopic dermatitis (AD) and asthma with a rapid, significant clinical improvement [129–133]. Also, decreasing in the levels of serum and skin Th2 markers and Th17/IL-23 associated markers have been demonstrated [129].

Several studies support a shared genetic background between AA and AD, besides both diseases were shown to have upregulation of Th2 component and an IL-23 [12, 134, 135]. The history of atopy and autoimmune disease was also found to be associated with an increased risk of AA [2, 16, 136].

Suarez-Farinas et al. reported a study of 22 patients who also had AD. They sought a detailed molecular profile of the lesional and nonlesional AA transcriptomes with AA. A significant upregulation of Th2 cytokine IL-13 was found similar to AD lesions. A possible pathogenic role of Th2 axis in patients with AA was supported as a result of this study [12].

Fuentes-Duculan et al. studied pre- and posttreatment lesional biopsies of 6 patients with patchy AA and performed immunohistochemistry and gene expression analysis. They found a significant expression of inflammatory markers of IL-2, IL-15, Th1 and Th2 (IL-13, CCL17 and CCL18), IL-12/IL-23p40 before treatment. After treatment with intralesional corticosteroid injection, a significant downregulation was observed in IL-12/IL-23p40, CCL18 [11].

Sharing possible common pathways both in AA and AD make dupilumab also worth triable in AA.

2.2.6.2. Tralokinumab

Tralokinumab is an IgG4 humanized monoclonal antibody that targets neutralising IL-13 [13, 137]. IL-13 is a Th2 cell cytokine and has an important role in atopy [137]. Tralokinumab is under investigation for asthma and AD (ClinicalTrials.gov NC). As mentioned above,

Suárez-Fariñas et al. found the highest levels of IL-13 and IL23p40 mRNA expressions in lesional vs. nonlesional AA and in lesional AA vs. healthy subjects [12]. Tembhre et al. found significant high levels of IL-13 and IL-17A which suggested altered Th cell function [125].

These findings support a possible role of tralokinumab in AA which is now being under investigation (ClinicalTrais.gov NCT02684097).

3. Conclusions

Currently, many therapies are available and the treatment depends on many factors, such as the severity, extent, duration of the disease, and age of the patient.

Although many treatments are shown to be effective in extensive recalcitrant AA, the most important problems of the present studies include the limited number of randomized controlled studies, lack of evaluating the long-term efficacy and follow-up, small number of participants, and significant disease heterogeneity in patient selection.

Better understandings of the immunopathological mechanisms responsible in AA have led the clinical researches to develop better therapeutic options for AA. However, future larger studies are needed to clarify the immunological pathways responsible in AA, which will lead to further therapeutic developments.

Author details

Arzu Kılıç*

*Address all correspondence to: kilicarzu@gmail.com

Department of Dermatology, Balikesir University School of Medicine, Cagis Yerleskesi, Balikesir, Turkey

References

[1] Perera E, Yip L, Sinclair R. Alopecia areata. Curr Probl Dermatol. 2015; **47**: 67–75. DOI: 10.1159/000369406

[2] Alkhalifah A, Alsantali A, Wang E, McElwee KJ, Shapiro J. Alopecia areata update. Part I. Clinical picture, histopathology, and pathogenesis. J Am Acad Dermatol. 2010; **62**: 177–88. DOI: 10.1016/j.jaad.2009.10.032

[3] Biran R, Zlotogorski A, Ramot Y. The genetics of alopecia areata: new approaches, new findings, new treatments. J Dermatol Sci. 2015; **78**: 11–20. DOI: 10.1016/j.jdermsci.2015.01.004

[4] McElwee KJ, Tobin DJ, Bystryn JC, King LE Jr, Sundberg JP. Alopecia areata: an autoimmune disease? Exp Dermatol. 1999; **8**:371–9.

[5] McElwee KJ, Gilhar A, Tobin DJ, Ramot Y, Sundberg JP, Nakamura M, Bertolini M, Inui S, Tokura Y, King LE Jr, Duque-Estrada B, Tosti A, Keren A, Itami S, Shoenfeld Y, Zlotogorski A, Paus R. What causes alopecia areata? Exp Dermatol. 2013; **22**: 609–26.

[6] Hordinsky MK. Overview of alopecia areata. Investig Dermatol Symp Proc. 2013; **16**: S13-5. DOI: 10.1038/jidsymp.2013.4

[7] Ito T. Recent advances in the pathogenesis of autoimmune hair loss disease alopecia areata. Clin Dev Immunol. 2013; **2013**: 348546.

[8] Ito T. Hair follicle is a target of stress hormone and autoimmune reactions. J Dermatol Sci. 2010; **60**: 67–73. DOI: 10.1016/j.jdermsci.2010.09.006

[9] Gilhar A, Kalish RS. Alopecia areata: a tissue specific autoimmune disease of the hair follicle. Autoimmun Rev. 2006; **5**: 64-9. DOI: 10.1016/j.autrev.2005.07.001

[10] Xing L, Dai Z, Jabbari A, Cerise JE, Higgins CA, Gong W, de Jong A, Harel S, De Stefano GM, Rothman L, Singh P, Petukhova L, Mackay-Wiggan J, Christiano AM, Clynes R. Alopecia areata is driven by cytotoxic T lymphocytes and is reversed by JAK inhibition. Nat Med. 2014; **20**: 1043–9. DOI: 10.1038/nm.3645

[11] Fuentes-Duculan J, Gulati N, Bonifacio KM, Kunjravia N, Zheng X, Suárez-Fariñaz M, Shemer A, Guttman-Yassky E, Krueger JG. Biomarkers of alopecia areata disease activity and response to corticosteroid treatment. Exp Dermatol. 2016; **25**: 282–6.

[12] Suárez-Fariñas M, Ungar B, Noda S, Shroff A, Mansouri Y, Fuentes-Duculan J, Czernik A, Zheng X, Estrada YD, Xu H, Peng X, Shemer A, Krueger JG, Lebwohl MG, Guttman-Yassky E. Alopecia areata profiling shows TH1, TH2, and IL-23 cytokine activation without parallel TH17/TH22 skewing. J Allergy Clin Immunol. 2015; **136**:1277–87. DOI: 10.1016/j.jaci.2015.06.032

[13] Renert-Yuval Y, Guttman-Yassky E. A novel therapeutic paradigm for patients with extensive alopecia areata. Expert Opin Biol Ther. 2016; **16**: 1005–14. DOI: 10.1080/14712598.2016.1188076

[14] Zhang X, Zhao Y, Ye Y, Li S, Qi S, Yang Y, Cao H, Yang J, Zhang X. Lesional infiltration of mast cells, Langerhans cells, T cells and local cytokine profiles in alopecia areata. Arch Dermatol Res. 2015; **307**: 319-31. DOI: 10.1007/s00403-015-1539–1

[15] Wasserman D, Guzman-Sanchez DA, Scott K, McMichael A. Alopecia areata. Int J Dermatol. 2007; **46**: 121-31. DOI: 10.1111/j.1365–4632.2007.03193.x

[16] Finner AM. Alopecia areata: clinical presentation, diagnosis, and unusual cases. Dermatol Ther. 2011; **24**: 348-54. DOI: 10.1111/j.1529–8019.2011.01413.x

[17] Alkhalifah A. Alopecia areata update. Dermatol Clin. 2013; **31**: 93–108. DOI: 10.1016/j.det.2012.08.010

[18] Goh C, Finkel M, Christos PJ, Sinha AA. Profile of 513 patients with alopecia areata: associations of disease subtypes with atopy, autoimmune disease and positive family history. J Eur Acad Dermatol Venereol. 2006; **20**: 1055–60. DOI: 10.1111/j.1468-3083.2006.01676.x

[19] Tosti A, Bellavista S, Iorizzo M. Alopecia areata: a long term follow-up study of 191 patients. J Am Acad Dermatol. 2006; **55**: 438–41. DOI: 10.1016/j.jaad.2006.05.008

[20] Madani S, Shapiro J. Alopecia areata update. J Am Acad Dermatol. 2000; **42**: 549–66

[21] Shapiro J. Current treatment of alopecia areata. J Investig Dermatol Symp Proc. 2013; **16**: S42-4. DOI: 10.1038/jidsymp.2013.14

[22] Delamere FM, Sladden MM, Dobbins HM, Leonardi-Bee J. Interventions for alopecia areata. Cochrane Database Syst Rev. 2008; **2**: CD004413. DOI: 10.1002/14651858.CD004413.pub2

[23] Alkhalifah A, Alsantali A, Wang E, McElwee KJ, Shapiro J. Alopecia areata update: part II. Treatment. J Am Acad Dermatol. 2010; **62**: 191-202. DOI: 10.1016/j.jaad.2009.10.031

[24] Messenger AG, McKillop J, Farrant P, McDonagh AJ, Sladden M. British association of dermatologists' guidelines for the management of alopecia areata 2012. Br J Dermatol. 2012; **166**: 916–26. DOI: 10.1111/j.1365-2133.2012.10955.x

[25] Hordinsky M, Donati A. Alopecia areata: an evidence-based treatment update. Am J Clin Dermatol. 2014; **15**: 231–46. DOI: 10.1007/s40257-014-0086-4

[26] Inui S, Itami S. Contact immunotherapy-resistant alopecia areata totalis/universalis reactive to topical corticosteroid. J Dermatol. 2015; **42**: 937–9. DOI: 10.1111/1346–8138.12938

[27] Kassim JM, Shipman AR, Szczecinska W, Siah TW, Lam M, Chalmers J, Macbeth AE. How effective is intralesional injection of triamcinolone acetonide compared with topical treatments in inducing and maintaining hair growth in patients with alopecia areata? A Critically Appraised Topic. Br J Dermatol. 2014; **170**: 766–71. DOI: 10.1111/bjd.12863

[28] Joly P. The use of methotrexate alone or in combination with low doses of oral corticosteroids in the treatment of alopecia totalis or universalis. J Am Acad Dermatol. 2006;**55** :632-6.

[29] Seo J, Lee YI, Hwang S, Zheng Z, Kim DY. Intramuscular triamcinolone acetonide: an undervalued option for refractory alopecia areata. J Dermatol. 2016 Jul 23. DOI: 10.1111/1346–8138.13533

[30] Fiedler-Weiss VC, Buys CM. Evaluation of anthralin in the treatment of alopecia areata. Arch Dermatol. 1987; **123**: 1491–3.

[31] Hill ND, Bunata K, Hebert AA. Treatment of alopecia areata with squaric acid dibutylester. Clin Dermatol. 2015; **33**: 300–4. DOI: 10.1016/j.clindermatol.2014.12.001

[32] Wiseman MC, Shapiro J, MacDonald N, Lui H. Predictive model for immunotherapy of alopecia areata with diphencyprone. Arch Dermatol. 2001; **137**: 1063–8.

[33] Avgerinou G, Gregoriou S, Rigopoulos D, Stratigos A, Kalogeromitros D, Katsambas A. Alopecia areata: topical immunotherapy treatment with diphencyprone. J Eur Acad Dermatol Venereol. 2008; **22**: 320–3. DOI: 10.1111/j.1468-3083.2007.02411.x

[34] Durdu M, Özcan D, Baba M, Seçkin D. Efficacy and safety of diphenylcyclopropenone alone or in combination with anthralin in the treatment of chronic extensive alopecia areata: a retrospective case series. J Am Acad Dermatol. 2015; **72**: 640–50. DOI:10.1016/j.jaad.2015.01.008

[35] Fransway AF, Muller SA. 3 percent topical minoxidil compared with placebo for the treatment of chronic severe alopecia areata. Cutis. 1988; **41**: 431–5.

[36] Coronel-Pérez IM, Rodríguez-Rey EM, Camacho-Martínez FM. Latanoprost in the treatment of eyelash alopecia in alopecia areata universalis. J Eur Acad Dermatol Venereol. 2010; **24**: 481–5. DOI: 10.1111/j.1468-3083.2009.03543.x

[37] Ross EK, Bolduc C, Lui H, Shapiro J. Lack of efficacy of topical latanoprost in the treatment of eyebrow alopecia areata. J Am Acad Dermatol. 2005; **53**: 1095–6. DOI: 10.1016/j.jaad.2005.06.031

[38] Roseborough I, Lee H, Chwalek J, Stamper RL, Price VH. Lack of efficacy of topical latanoprost and bimatoprost ophthalmic solutions in promoting eyelash growth in patients with alopecia areata. J Am Acad Dermatol. 2009; **60**: 705–6. DOI: 10.1016/j.jaad.2008.08.029

[39] Ahsan MK, Urano Y, Kato S, Oura H, Arase S. Immunohistochemical localization of thyroid hormone nuclear receptors in human hair follicles and in vitro effect of L-triiodothyronine on cultured cells of hair follicles and skin. J Med Invest. 1998; **44**: 179–84.

[40] Talpur R, Vu J, Bassett R, Stevens V, Duvic M. Phase I/II randomized bilateral half-head comparison of topical bexarotene 1% gel for alopecia areata. J Am Acad Dermatol. 2009; **61**: 592.e1-9. DOI: 10.1016/j.jaad.2009.02.037

[41] Gupta AK, Ellis CN, Cooper KD, Nickoloff BJ, Ho VC, Chan LS, Hamilton TA, Tellner DC, Griffiths CE, Voorhees JJ. Oral cyclosporine for the treatment of alopecia areata. A clinical and immunohistochemical analysis. J Am Acad Dermatol. 1990; **22**: 242–50.

[42] Kim BJ, Min SU, Park KY, Choi JW, Park SW, Youn SW, Park KC, Huh CH. Combination therapy of cyclosporine and methylprednisolone on severe alopecia areata. J Dermatolog Treat. 2008; **19**: 216–20. DOI: 10.1080/09546630701846095

[43] Açıkgöz G, Calışkan E, Tunca M, Yeniay Y, Akar A. The effect of oral cyclosporine in the treatment of severe alopecia areata. Cutan Ocul Toxicol. 2014; **33**: 247-52. DOI: 10.3109/15569527.2013.839997

[44] Ucak H, Kandi B, Cicek D, Halisdemir N, Dertlioglu SB. The comparison of treatment with clobetasol propionate 0.05% and topical pimecrolimus 1% treatment in the treatment of alopecia areata. J Dermatolog Treat. 2012; **23**: 410–20. DOI: 10.3109/09546634.2011.590788

[45] Rigopoulos D, Gregoriou S, Korfitis C, Gintzou C, Vergou T, Katrinaki A, Kalogeromitros D. Lack of response of alopecia areata to pimecrolimus cream. Clin Exp Dermatol. 2007; **32**: 456–7. DOI: 10.1111/j.1365-2230.2007.02367.x

[46] Hunter N, Shaker O, Marei N. Diphencyprone and topical tacrolimus as two topical immunotherapeutic modalities. Are they effective in the treatment of alopecia areata among Egyptian patients? A study using CD4, CD8 and MHC II as markers. J Dermatolog Treat. 2011; **22**: 2–10. DOI: 10.3109/09546630903410182

[47] Anuset D, Perceau G, Bernard P, Reguiai Z. Efficacy and safety of methotrexate combined with low- to moderate-dose corticosteroids for severe alopecia areata. Dermatology. 2016; **232**: 242–8. DOI: 10.1159/000441250

[48] Droitcourt C, Milpied B, Ezzedine K, Hubiche T, Belin E, Akpadjan F, Taïeb A, Seneschal J. Interest of high-dose pulse corticosteroid therapy combined with methotrexate for severe alopecia areata: a retrospective case series. Dermatology. 2012; **224**: 369–73. DOI: 10.1159/000339341

[49] Farshi S, Mansouri P, Safar F, Khiabanloo SR. Could azathioprine be considered as a therapeutic alternative in the treatment of alopecia areata? A pilot study. Int J Dermatol. 2010; **49**: 1188–93. DOI: 10.1111/j.1365-4632.2010.04576.x

[50] Vañó-Galván S, Hermosa-Gelbard Á, Sánchez-Neila N, Miguel-Gómez L, Saceda-Corralo D, Rodrigues-Barata R, Jaén P. Treatment of recalcitrant adult alopecia areata universalis with oral azathioprine. J Am Acad Dermatol. 2016; **74**: 1007–8. DOI: 10.1016/j.jaad.2015.12.055

[51] Rashidi T, Mahd AA. Treatment of persistent alopecia areata with sulfasalazine. Int J Dermatol. 2008; **47**: 850–2. DOI: 10.1111/j.1365-4632.2008.03700.x

[52] Rashid S, Ahsan U, Saeed W. Efficacy and safety of sulphasalazine in treatment of alopecia areata. J Pakistan Assoc Dermatol. 2015; **25**: 298–302.

[53] Bakar O, Gurbuz O. Is there a role for sulfasalazine in the treatment of alopecia areata? J Am Acad Dermatol. 2007; **57**: 703–6.

[54] Namazi MR. Statins: novel additions to the dermatologic arsenal? Exp Dermatol. 2004; **13**: 337–9.

[55] Robins DN. Case reports: alopecia universalis: hair growth following initiation of simvastatin and ezetimibe therapy. J Drugs Dermatol. 2007; **6**: 946–7.

[56] Ali A, Martin JM 4th. Hair growth in patients alopecia areata totalis after treatment with simvastatin and ezetimibe. J Drugs Dermatol. 2010; **9**: 62–4.

[57] Lattouf C, Jimenez JJ, Tosti A, Miteva M, Wikramanayake TC, Kittles C, Herskovitz I, Handler MZ, Fabbrocini G, Schachner LA. Treatment of alopecia areata with simvastatin/ezetimibe. J Am Acad Dermatol. 2015; **72**: 359–61. DOI: 10.1016/j.jaad.2014.11.006

[58] Loi C, Starace M, Piraccini BM. Alopecia areata (AA) and treatment with simvastatin/ezetimibe: experience of 20 patients. J Am Acad Dermatol. 2016; **74**: e99-e100. DOI: 10.1016/j.jaad.2015.09.071

[59] Walker D, Jacobe H. Phototherapy in the age of biologics. Semin Cutan Med Surg. 2011; **30**: 190–8. DOI: 10.1016/j.sder.2011.08.004

[60] Lassus A, Eskelinen A, Johansson E. Treatment of alopecia areata with three different PUVA modalities. Photodermatol. 1984; **1**: 141–4.

[61] Behrens-Williams SC, Leiter U, Schiener R, Weidmann M, Peter RU, Kerscher M. The PUVA-turban as a new option of applying a dilute psoralen solution selectively to the scalp of patients with alopecia areata. J Am Acad Dermatol. 2001; **44**: 248–52. DOI: 10.1067/mjd.2001.110060

[62] Claudy AL, Gagnaire D. PUVA treatment of alopecia areata. Arch Dermatol. 1983; **119**: 975–8.

[63] Taylor CR, Hawk JL. PUVA treatment of alopecia areata partialis, totalis and universalis: audit of 10 years' experience at St John's Institute of Dermatology. Br J Dermatol. 1995; **133**: 914–8.

[64] Healy E, Rogers S. PUVA treatment for alopecia areata—does it work? A retrospective review of 102 cases. Br J Dermatol. 1993; **129**: 42–4.

[65] Park KY, Jang WS, Son IP, Choi SY, Lee MY, Kim BJ, Kim MN, Ro BI. Combination therapy with cyclosporine and psoralen plus ultraviolet a in the patients with severe alopecia areata: a retrospective study with a self-controlled design. Ann Dermatol. 2013; **25**: 12–6. DOI: 10.5021/ad.2013.25.1.12

[66] Herz-Ruelas ME, Welsh O, Gomez-Flores M, Welsh E, Miranda-Maldonado I, Ocampo-Candiani J. Ultraviolet A-1 phototherapy as an alternative for resistant alopecia areata. Int J Dermatol. 2015;**54**: e445-7. DOI: 10.1111/ijd.13054

[67] Tzung TY, Chen CY, Tzung TY, Kao FJ, Chen WC. Infrared irradiation as an adjuvant therapy in recalcitrant alopecia areata. Dermatol Surg. 2009; **35**: 721–3. DOI: 10.1111/j.1524-4725.2009.01120.x

[68] Waiz M, Saleh AZ, Hayani R, Jubory SO. Use of the pulsed infrared diode laser (904 nm) in the treatment of alopecia areata. J Cosmet Laser Ther. 2006; **8**: 27–30. DOI: 10.1080/14764170600607368

[69] Zakaria W, Passeron T, Ostovari N, Lacour JP, Ortonne JP. 308-nm excimer laser therapy in alopecia areata. J Am Acad Dermatol. 2004; **51**: 837–8. DOI: 10.1016/j.jaad.2004.05.026

[70] Gundogan C, Greve B, Raulin C. Treatment of alopecia areata with the 308-nm xenon chloride excimer laser: case report of two successful treatments with the excimer laser. Lasers Surg Med. 2004; **34**: 86–90. DOI: 10.1002/lsm.20002

[71] Al-Mutairi N. 308-nm excimer laser for the treatment of alopecia areata. Dermatol Surg. 2007; 33: 1483–7. DOI: 10.1111/j.1524-4725.2007.33320.x

[72] Al-Mutairi N. 308-nm excimer laser for the treatment of alopecia areata in children. Pediatr Dermatol. 2009; **26**: 547–50. DOI: 10.1111/j.1525-1470.2009.00980.x

[73] Georgala S, Katoulis AC, Befon A, Georgala K, Stavropoulos PG. Inosiplex for treatment of alopecia areata: a randomized placebo-controlled study. Acta Derm Venereol. 2006; **86**: 422–4. DOI: 10.2340/00015555-0138

[74] Donovan J. Successful treatment of corticosteroid-resistant ophiasis-type alopecia areata (AA) with platelet-rich plasma (PRP). JAAD Case Rep. 2015; **1**: 305–7. DOI: 10.1016/j.jdcr.2015.07.004

[75] Trink A, Sorbellini E, Bezzola P, Rodella L, Rezzani R, Ramot Y, Rinaldi F. A randomized, double-blind, placebo- and active-controlled, half-head study to evaluate the effects of platelet-rich plasma on alopecia areata. Br J Dermatol. 2013; **169**: 690–4. DOI: 10.1111/bjd.12397

[76] Singh S. Role of platelet-rich plasma in chronic alopecia areata: our centre experience. Indian J Plast Surg. 2015; **48**: 57–9. DOI: 10.4103/0970-0358.155271

[77] Zaba LC, Suarez-Farinaz M, Fuentes-Duculan J, Nograles KE, Guttman-Yassky E, Cardinale I, Lowes MA, Krueger JG. Effective treatment of psoriasis with etanercept is linked to suppression of IL-17 signaling, not immediate response TNF genes. J Allergy Clin Immunol. 2009; **124**: 1022–10. DOI: 10.1016/j.jaci.2009.08.046

[78] Kasumagic-Halilovic E, Prohic A, Cavaljuga S. Tumor necrosis factor-alpha in patients with alopecia areata. Indian J Dermatol. 2011; **56**: 494–6. DOI: 10.4103/0019-5154.87124

[79] Strober BE, Siu K, Alexis AF, Kim G, Washenik K, Sinha A, Shupack JL. Etanercept does not effectively treat moderate to severe alopecia areata: an open-label study. J Am Acad Dermatol. 2005; **52**: 1082–4. DOI: 10.1016/j.jaad.2005.03.039

[80] Garcia Bartels N, Lee HH, Worm M, Burmester GR, Sterry W, Blume-Peytavi U. Development of alopecia areata universalis in a patient receiving adalimumab. Arch Dermatol. 2006; **142**: 1654–5. DOI: 10.1001/archderm.142.12.1654

[81] Chaves Y, Duarte G, Ben-Said B, Tebib J, Berard F, Nicolas JF. Alopecia areata universalis during treatment of rheumatoid arthritis with anti-TNF-alpha antibody (adalimumab). Dermatology. 2008; **217**: 380. DOI: 10.1159/000162180

[82] Le Bidre, Chaby G, Martin L, Perrussel M, Sassolas B, Sigal ML, Kaassis C, Lespessailles E, Nseir A, Estève E. Alopecia areata during anti-TNF alpha therapy: nine cases. Ann Dermatol Venereol. 2011; **138**: 285–93. DOI: 10.1016/j.annder.2011.01.047

[83] Pan Y, Rao NA. Alopecia areata during etanercept therapy. Ocul Immunol Inflamm. 2009; **17**: 127–9. DOI: 10.1080/09273940802596559

[84] Pelivani N, Hassan AS, Braathen LR, Hunger RE. Alopecia areata universalis elicited during treatment with adalimumab. Dermatology. 2008; **216**: 320–3. DOI: 10.1159/000113945

[85] Tauber M, Buche S, Reygagne P, Berthelot JM, Aubin F, Ghislain PD, Cohen JD, Coquerelle P, Goujon E, Jullien D, Brixi H, Jeudy G, Guennoc X, Martin A, Brénaut E, Hoppé E, Bertolotti A, Bardin T, Delaporte E, Allez M, Bachelez H, Seneschal J, Viguier M, Groupe de Recherche sur Psoriasis de Société Française de, Dermatologie, Club Rhumatismes et Inflammation (CRI), Groupe d'étudesthérapeutiques des affections inflammatoires du tube digestif (GETAID). Alopecia areata occurring during anti-TNF therapy: a national multicenter prospective study. J Am Acad Dermatol. 2014; **70**: 1146–9. DOI: 10.1016/j.jaad.2014.03.005

[86] Ferran M, Calvet J, Almirall M, Pujol RM, Maymó J. Alopecia areata as another immune-mediated disease developed in patients treated with tumour necrosis factor-α blocker agents: report of five cases and review of the literature. J Eur Acad Dermatol Venereol. 2011; **25**: 479–84. DOI: 10.1111/j.1468-3083.2010.03770.x

[87] Gorcey L, Gordon Spratt EA, Leger MC. Alopecia universalis successfully treated with adalimumab. JAMA Dermatol. 2014; **150**: 1341–4. DOI: 10.1001/jamadermatol.2014.1544

[88] Meng Y, Dongmei L, Yanbin P, Jinju F, Meile T, Binzhu L, Xiao H, Ping T, Jianmin L. Systematic review and meta-analysis of ustekinumab for moderate to severe psoriasis. Clin Exp Dermatol. 2014; **39**: 696–707. DOI: 10.1111/ced.12390

[89] Mease PJ. Inhibition of interleukin-17, interleukin-23 and the TH17 cell pathway in the treatment of psoriatic arthritis and psoriasis. Curr Opin Rheumatol. 2015; **27**: 127–33. DOI: 10.1097/BOR.0000000000000147

[90] Johnsson HJ, McInnes IB. Interleukin-12 and interleukin-23 inhibition in psoriatic arthritis. Clin Exp Rheumatol. 2015; **33**: S115-8.

[91] Barahmani N, Lopez A, Babu D, Hernandez M, Donley SE, Duvic M. Serum T helper 1 cytokine levels are greater in patients with alopecia areata regardless of severity or atopy. Clin Exp Dermatol. 2010; **35**: 409–16. DOI: 10.1111/j.1365-2230.2009.03523.x

[92] Guttman-Yassky E, Ungar B, Noda S, Suprun M, Shroff A, Dutt R, Khattri S, Min M, Mansouri Y, Zheng X, Estrada YD, Singer GK, Suarez-Farinas M, Krueger JG, Lebwohl MG. Extensive alopecia areata is reversed by IL-12/IL-23p40 cytokine antagonism. J Allergy Clin Immunol. 2016; **137**: 301–4. DOI: 10.1016/j.jaci.2015.11.001

[93] Verros C, Rallis E, Crowe M. Letter: alopecia areata during ustekinumab administration: co-existence or an adverse reaction?. Dermatol Online J. 2012; **18**: 14.

[94] Słowińska M, Kardynal A, Warszawik O, Czuwara J, Rudnicka L. Alopecia areata developing parallel to improvement of psoriasis during ustekinumab therapy. J Dermatol Case Rep. 2010; **4**: 15–7. DOI: 10.3315/jdcr.2010.1041

[95] Tauber M, Beneton N, Reygagne P, Bachelez H, Viguier M. Alopecia areata developing during ustekinumab therapy: report of two cases. Eur J Dermatol. 2013; **23**: 912–3. DOI: 10.1684/ejd.2013.2221

[96] Garnock-Jones KP. Secukinumab: a review in moderate to severe plaque psoriasis. Am J Clin Dermatol. 2015;**16**: 323–30. DOI: 10.1007/s40257-015-0143-7

[97] Gaspari AA, Tyring S. New and emerging biologic therapies for moderate-to-severe plaque psoriasis: mechanistic rationales and recent clinical data for IL-17 and IL-23 inhibitors. Dermatol Ther. 2015; **28**: 179–93. DOI: 10.1111/dth.12251

[98] Tanemura A, Oiso N, Nakano M, Itoi S, Kawada A, Katayama I. Alopecia areata: infiltration of Th17 cells in the dermis, particularly around hair follicles. Dermatology. 2013; **226**: 333–6. DOI: 10.1159/000350933

[99] Atwa MA, Youssef N, Bayoumy NM. T-helper 17 cytokines (interleukins 17, 21, 22, and 6, and tumor necrosis factor-α) in patients with alopecia areata: association with clinical type and severity. Int J Dermatol. 2016; **55**: 666–72. DOI: 10.1111/ijd.12808

[100] Lew BL, Cho HR, Haw S, Kim HJ, Chung JH, Sim WY. Association between IL17A/IL17RA gene polymorphisms and susceptibility to alopecia areata in the Korean population. Ann Dermatol. 2012; **24**: 61–5. DOI: 10.5021/ad.2012.24.1.61

[101] Forchhammer S, Ghoreschi K. Update on the treatment of psoriasis and psoriatic arthritis-role of apremilast. Psoriasis: Targets and Therapy. 2015; **15**: 125–8.

[102] Poole RM, Ballantyne AD. Apremilast: first global approval. Drugs. 2014;**74**:825–37. DOI: 10.1007/s40265-014-0218-4

[103] Schafer PH, Day RM. Novel systemic drugs for psoriasis: mechanism of action for apremilast, a specific inhibitor of PDE4. J Am Acad Dermatol. 2013; **68**: 1041–2. DOI: 10.1016/j.jaad.2012.10.064

[104] Schafer PH, Parton A, Gandhi AK, Capone L, Adams M, Wu L, Bartlett JB, Loveland MA, Gilhar A, Cheung YF, Baillie GS, Houslay MD, Man HW, Muller GW, Stirling DI. Apremilast, a cAMP phosphodiesterase-4 inhibitor, demonstrates anti inflammatory activity in vitro and in a model of psoriasis. Br J Pharmacol. 2010; **159**: 842–55. DOI: 10.1111/j.1476-5381.2009.00559.x

[105] Keren A, Shemer A, Ullmann Y, Paus R, Gilhar A. The PDE4 inhibitor, apremilast, suppresses experimentally induced alopecia areata in human skin in vivo. J Dermatol Sci. 2015; **77**: 74–6. DOI: 10.1016/j.jdermsci.2014.11.009

[106] Ghoreschi K, Gadina M. Jakpot! New small molecules in autoimmune and inflammatory diseases. Exp Dermatol. 2014; **23**: 7–11. DOI: 10.1111/exd.12265

[107] Seavey MM, Dobrzanski P. The many faces of Janus kinase. Biochem Pharmacol. 2012; **83**: 1136–45. DOI: 10.1016/j.bcp.2011.12.024

[108] Roskoski R Jr. Janus kinase (JAK) inhibitors in the treatment of inflammatory and neoplastic diseases. Pharmacol Res. 2016; **111**: 784–803. DOI: 10.1016/j.phrs.2016.07.038

[109] Jabbari A, Nguyen N, Cerise JE, et al. Treatment of an alopecia areata patient with tofacitinib results in regrowth of hair and changes in serum and skin biomarkers. Exp Dermatol. 2016; **25**: 642–3. DOI: 10.1111/exd.13060

[110] Jabbari A, Dai Z, Xing L, et al. Reversal of alopecia areata following treatment with the JAK1/2 inhibitor baricitinib. EBioMedicine. 2015; **2**: 351–5. DOI: 10.1016/j.ebiom.2015.02.015

[111] Craiglow BG, King BA. Killing two birds with one stone: oral tofacitinib reverses alopecia universalis in a patient with plaque psoriasis. J Invest Dermatol. 2014; **134**: 2988–9. DOI: 10.1038/jid.2014.260

[112] Gupta AK, Carviel JL, Abramovits W. Efficacy of tofacitinib in treatment of alopecia universalis in two patients. J Eur Acad Dermatol Venereol. 2016; **30**: 1373–8. DOI:10.1111/jdv.13598

[113] Anzengruber F, Maul JT, Kamarachev J, et al. Transient efficacy of tofacitinib in alopecia areata universalis. Case Rep Dermatol. 2016; **8**: 102–6. DOI: 10.1159/000445182

[114] Bissonnette R, Papp KA, Poulin Y, Gooderham M, Raman M, Mallbris L, Wang C, Purohit V, Mamolo C, Papacharalambous J, Ports WC. Topical tofacitinib for atopic dermatitis: a phase 2a randomised trial. Br J Dermatol. 2016. Doi: 10.1111/bjd.14871. [Epub ahead of print]

[115] Ports WC, Khan S, Lan S, Lamba M, Bolduc C, Bissonnette R, Papp K. A randomized phase 2a efficacy and safety trial of the topical Janus kinase inhibitor tofacitinib in the treatment of chronic plaque psoriasis. Br J Dermatol. 2013; **169**: 137–45. DOI: 10.1111/bjd.12266

[116] Liew SH, Nichols KK, Klamerus KJ, Li JZ, Zhang M, Foulks GN. Tofacitinib (CP-690,550), a Janus kinase inhibitor for dry eye disease: results from a phase 1/2 trial. Ophthalmology. 2012; **119**: 1328–35. DOI: 10.1016/j.ophtha.2012.01.028

[117] Fukuyama T, Ehling S, Cook E, Bäumer W. Topically administered Janus-Kinase inhibitors tofacitinib and oclacitinib display impressive antipruritic and anti-inflammatory responses in a model of allergic dermatitis. J Pharmacol Exp Ther. 2015; **354**: 394–405. DOI: 10.1124/jpet.115.223784

[118] Herrero-Beaumont G, Martínez Calatrava MJ, Castañeda S. Abatacept mechanism of action: concordance with its clinical profile. Reumatol Clin. 2012; **8**: 78–83. DOI: 10.1016/j.reuma.2011.08.002

[119] Furst DE, Breedveld FC, Kalden JR, Smolen JS, Burmester GR, Emery P, Keystone EC, Schiff MH, van Riel PL, Weinblatt ME, Weisman MH. Updated consensus statement on biological agents for the treatment of rheumatic diseases, 2006. Ann Rheum Dis. 2006;**65**:iii2-15. DOI: 10.1136/ard.2006.061937

[120] Bonelli M, Göschl L, Blüml S, Karonitsch T, Hirahara K, Ferner E, Steiner CW, Steiner G, Smolen JS, Scheinecker C. Abatacept (CTLA-4Ig) treatment reduces T cell apoptosis and regulatory T cell suppression in patients with rheumatoid arthritis. Rheumatology (Oxford). 2016; **55**: 710–20. DOI: 10.1093/rheumatology/kev403

[121] Noble S, Goa KL. Aldesleukin (recombinant interleukin-2). BioDrugs. 1997; **7**: 394–422.

[122] Schmidinger M, Hejna M, Zielinski CC. Aldesleukin in advanced renal cell carcinoma. Expert Rev Anticancer Ther. 2004; **4**: 957–80. DOI: 10.1586/14737140.4.6.957

[123] Atkins MB, Lotze MT, Dutcher JP, Fisher RI, Weiss G, Margolin K, Abrams J, Sznol M, Parkinson D, Hawkins M, Paradise C, Kunkel L, Rosenberg SA. High-dose recombinant interleukin 2 therapy for patients with metastatic melanoma: analysis of 270 patients treated between 1985 and 1993. J Clin Oncol. 1999; **17**: 2105–6.

[124] Klatzmann D, Abbas AK. The promise of low-dose interleukin-2 therapy for autoimmune and inflammatory diseases. Nat Rev Immunol. 2015; **15**: 283–94. DOI: 10.1038/nri3823

[125] Tembhre MK, Sharma VK. T-helper and regulatory T-cell cytokines in the peripheral blood of patients with active alopecia areata. Br J Dermatol. 2013; **169**: 543–8. DOI: 10.1111/bjd.12396

[126] Han YM, Sheng YY, Xu F, Qi SS, Liu XJ, Hu RM, Miao Y, Huang GQ, Yang QP. Imbalance of T-helper 17 and regulatory T cells in patients with alopecia areata. J Dermatol. 2015; **42**: 981–8. DOI: 10.1111/1346-8138.12978

[127] Shin BS, Furuhashi T, Nakamura M, Torii K, Morita A. Impaired inhibitory function of circulating CD4+CD25+ regulatory T cells in alopecia areata. J Dermatol Sci. 2013; 70: 141–3. DOI: 10.1016/j.jdermsci.2013.01.006

[128] Castela E, Le Duff F, Butori C, Ticchioni M, Hofman P, Bahadoran P, Lacour JP, Passeron T. Effects of low-dose recombinant interleukin 2 to promote T-regulatory cells in alopecia areata. JAMA Dermatol. 2014; **150**: 748–51. DOI: 10.1001/jamadermatol.2014.504

[129] Beck LA, Thaçi D, Hamilton JD, Graham NM, Bieber T, Rocklin R, Ming JE, Ren H, Kao R, Simpson E, Ardeleanu M, Weinstein SP, Pirozzi G, Guttman-Yassky E, Suárez-Fariñas M, Hager MD, Stahl N, Yancopoulos GD, Radin AR. Dupilumab treatment in adults with moderate-to-severe atopic dermatitis. N Engl J Med. 2014;**371**: 130–9. DOI: 10.1056/NEJMoa1314768

[130] Simpson EL, Bieber T, Eckert L, Wu R, Ardeleanu M, Graham NM, Pirozzi G,Mastey V. Patient burden of moderate to severe atopic dermatitis (AD): insights from a phase 2b clinical trial of dupilumab in adults. J Am Acad Dermatol. 2016; **74**: 491–8. DOI: 10.1016/j.jaad.2015.10.043

[131] Thaçi D, Simpson EL, Beck LA, Bieber T, Blauvelt A, Papp K, Soong W, Worm M, Szepietowski JC, Sofen H, Kawashima M, Wu R, Weinstein SP, Graham NM, Pirozzi G, Teper A, Sutherland ER, Mastey V, Stahl N, Yancopoulos GD, Ardeleanu M. Efficacy and safety of dupilumab in adults with moderate-to-severe atopic dermatitis inade-

quately controlled by topical treatments: a randomised, placebo-controlled, dose-ranging phase 2b trial. Lancet. 2016; **387**: 40–52. DOI: 10.1016/S0140-6736(15)00388-8

[132] Chung KF. Dupilumab: a potential new treatment for severe asthma. Lancet. 2016; **388**: 3–4. DOI: 10.1016/S0140-6736(16)30311-7

[133] Wenzel S, Castro M, Corren J, Maspero J, Wang L, Zhang B, Pirozzi G,Sutherland ER, Evans RR, Joish VN, Eckert L, Graham NM, Stahl N, Yancopoulos GD, Louis-Tisserand M, Teper A. Dupilumab efficacy and safety in adults with uncontrolled persistent asthma despite use of medium-to-high-dose inhaled corticosteroids plus a long-acting β2 agonist: a randomised double-blind placebo-controlled pivotal phase 2b dose-ranging trial. Lancet. 2016; **388**: 31–44. DOI: 10.1016/S0140-6736(16)30307-5

[134] Chu SY, Chen YJ, Tseng WC, Lin MW, Chen TJ, Hwang CY, Chen CC, Lee DD, Chang YT, Wang WJ, Liu HN. Comorbidity profiles among patients with alopecia areata: the importance of onset age, a nationwide population-based study. J Am Acad Dermatol. 2011; **65**: 949–56. DOI: 10.1016/j.jaad.2010.08.032

[135] Gilhar A, Etzioni A, Paus R. Alopecia areata. N Engl J Med. 2012;**366**:1515–25. DOI: 10.1056/NEJMra1103442

[136] Barahmani N, Schabath MB, Duvic M, National Alopecia Areata Registry. History of atopy or autoimmunity increases risk of alopecia areata. J Am Acad Dermatol. 2009; **61**: 581–91. DOI: 10.1016/j.jaad.2009.04.031

[137] Hussein YM, Ahmad AS, Ibrahem MM, Elsherbeny HM, Shalaby SM, El-Shal AS, Sabbah NA. Interleukin 13 receptors as biochemical markers in atopic patients. J Investig Allergol Clin Immunol. 2011; **21**: 101–7.

Chapter 18

Cosmetic Procedures in the Treatment of Alopecia

Selda Pelin Kartal, Cemile Altunel and
Bilgen Gencler

Additional information is available at the end of the chapter

http://dx.doi.org/10.5772/66747

Abstract

Alopecia has a significant negative impact on the quality of life. Unfortunately, there is no satisfactory cure for most types of alopecia. Alopecia is divided into cicatricial and noncicatricial types. Androgenetic alopecia, alopecia areata, and telogen effluvium are common forms of noncicatricial alopecias. In order to treat or improve the appearance, various procedures that are being applied for different types of alopecia including mesotherapy, microneedling, platelet-rich plasma, low-level light therapy, and stem-cell therapy with variable outcomes are reviewed in this chapter.

Keywords: alopecia, hair loss, mesotherapy, microneedling, platelet-rich plasma, low-level light therapy, stem-cell therapy

1. Introduction

Alopecia (hair loss) is a common problem in dermatology setting and it has a significant negative impact on the quality of life. Therefore, most patients seek for treatment in order to improve their appearance although there is no satisfactory cure for most types of alopecia. Alopecia is divided into cicatricial and noncicatricial types. Androgenetic alopecia (AGA), alopecia areata (AA), and telogen effluvium are common forms of noncicatricial alopecias. Telogen effluvium is the diffuse hair shedding caused by physiological, hormonal metabolic stress, or by drugs. AGA is caused by the effect of dihydrotestosterone (DHT) on hair follicles leading to their miniaturization. It is seen in different appearances in males and females. In males, AGA presents as hairline recession and vertex balding. Unlike in men, female pattern hair loss (FPHL) is characterized by diffuse hair thinning over the crown with retention of the frontal hairline. AA is caused by autoimmune destruction of hair follicles involving cell-based and humoral immunity [1].

Various cosmetic procedures are being applied for different types of alopecia including mesotherapy, microneedling, platelet-rich plasma (PRP), low-level light therapy, and stem-cell therapy with variable outcomes [2, 3].

In this chapter, the above-mentioned cosmetic treatments for alopecia are briefly described.

2. Mesotherapy in alopecia treatment

2.1. Introduction

Mesotherapy is a noninvasive technique in which active substances are delivered just below the epidermis via superficial microinjections. Various substances including vitamins, medications, plant extracts, and other bioactive compounds including vasodilators, finasteride, and minoxidil can be injected intradermally or subcutaneously to reach the target tissues in mesotherapy [4].

There is evidence regarding the clinical efficacy of mesotherapy in the treatment of thermal burns, local pain, local fat contouring, and skin aging [5–8].

Although evidence-based studies regarding the efficacy of mesotherapy in different types of alopecia are lacking, in recent years, mesotherapy is increasingly being used in the treatment of telogen effluvium, androgenetic alopecia, and alopecia areata [9–11].

2.2. Method

Before starting hair mesotherapy, informed consent should be taken from the patient. After cleaning the scalp with antiseptic solution, the substances can be given by intraepidermal, papular, nappage, or point-by-point technique. In hair mesotherapy usually 4–6 mm, 27–32 G special mesotherapy needles are applied a depth of 4–6 mm about 1–2 cm apart. Although superficial intradermal technique is most commonly used, nappage technique can also be used manually or by mesotherapy gun. Hair mesotherapy can also be applied by using mesoroller device [9–11]. Each session lasts for 10–30 min [9]. There is no standardized protocol for the frequency of sessions and it depends on the decision of the applier and the indication it is done for. Hair mesotherapy is commonly applied at intervals of 1–4 weeks [10, 11]. Frequently accepted schedule is once a week for the initial weeks then with longer intervals and maintenance treatment in every 2–3 months [12]. Some clinics prefer to apply mesotherapy once in two weeks for at least 10 sessions and then once a month for 5 months [10].

2.3. Mechanism of action

Although the exact mechanism how the mesotherapy works is not known, several theories have been speculated. According to Pistor, skin may be a point for stimulation which is triggered by mesotherapy that sends inhibitory signals reaching to the lateral medullary center of the spinal cord. These inhibitory signals have been suggested to be either produced by the needling itself or the pharmacologic substances given during mesotherapy. The negative signals are suggested to restore the pathologic mechanisms causing alopecia [13]. The target tissue of hair mesotherapy is mostly the dermis including the circulatory, neuronal, and immune component. Also, epidermis and subcutaneous tissue are affected by the procedure of diffusion of substances. According to mesodermic theory, mesotherapy acts on the tissues derived from mesoderm including capillary and venous spaces, neuronal components, and immune cells of the skin [13, 14]. Another explanation is the third circulation theory that, after blood (first) and the lymphatic (second) circulation, interstitial compartment between skin cells are considered as the third space of circulation. Mesotherapy is suggested to target the interstitial compartment that the substances administered via mesotherapy diffuse through interstitial compartment to the deep target tissues without being rapidly washed out by vessels [13].

The aim of hair mesotherapy is to restore the abnormal physiology causing alopecia by stimulating various biological responses via injecting the active substances into scalp. Additionally, mechanical stimulation by needling itself creates a biologic response that is expected to stimulate mesodermal changes [10, 15]. Hair mesotherapy offers the prevention of hair loss, activation of new hair growth, and the improvement in the quality of existing hair. By hair mesotherapy, local microcirculation is increased, which improves the environment of hair follicle for better growth. Additionally, nutritional supply is provided to the hair follicle and the excess of dihydrotestosterone (DHT) is suggested to be neutralized [16].

2.4. Solutions and substances

There is no standardized formulation used in hair mesotherapy and the various ingredients can be given depending on the indication. Generally, cocktails containing mixture of different ingredients used in hair mesotherapy and they can be applied in alternation depending on the clinical response. It is important to remember that there may be interactions between the injected substances that interfere with the efficacy. However, there is no definite protocol for the compounds and the concentrations [9–11, 15]. Commonly used substances in hair mesotherapy include minoxidil, finasteride, dutasteride, biotin, tretinoin, pantothenic acid, pyridoxine, procaine, dexpanthenol, azelaic acid, T3/T4, and other vitamins and minerals [9–12]. These compounds have different biologic effects. Especially, buflomedil, minoxidil, finasteride, dutasteride, biotin, vitamins, and organic silicium are proposed to stimulate new hair growth [10]. Many of these substances have vasodilator effect. The main effects of the commonly used substances in hair mesotherapy are as follows:

Buflomedil is an α-2 receptor antagonist and a weak calcium channel blocker. It has vasodilatory effect [10, 17]. Minoxidil also has vasodilatory effect. It is the only drug that is proven to increase hair growth by prolonging the anagen phase [10, 11]. Some authors do not use minoxidil more than 1/2 cc in the cocktail since it may be painful for the patient [10]. Procaine is a well known anesthetic that provides patient comfort. It has vasodilator activity and enhances the absorption of other drugs [10, 11]. Ginkgo biloba increases perifollicular blood flow. It also has antiedema and antioxidant effect. It contains diterpene which inhibits platelet activating factor and decreases platelet aggregation [10, 11]. Conjoctyl (organic silicium, salicylate of monometilsilanotriol) has an antioxidant and vasodilatory effect [10]. Dexpanthenol (Vitamin B5) is involved in the hair development. It is converted into pantothenic acid which is a precursor for the synthesis of coenzyme A, important in the carbohydrate metabolism [10, 11]. Biotin acts as a coenzyme and growth factor. It has a role in the carboxylation and fatty acid metabolism [10, 11]. Vitamin C acts as an antioxidant and helps in collagen production [18]. Vitamin A (retinoic acid) has a regulatory role in the growth of epidermal cells and keratinization process. It induces dermal fibroblastic activity and collagen production [18]. Pyridoxine (Vitamin B6) stimulates hair growth and augments the effects of zinc [11]. Cobalt, copper, lithium, magnesium, manganese, phosphorus, selenium, sulphur, and zinc can be used as trace elements [10]. Zinc acts as a 5-α reductase inhibitor [11]. Recently intradermal injection of copper has been suggested to be beneficial in AGA most likely by balancing the steroid-converting enzyme activity, enhancing the anagen phase of hair cycle, simultaneous transition to the telogen phase, and stimulation of the proliferation of dermal papilla cells [19]. Finasteride is an inhibitor of 5-α reductase enzyme and selectively interfere with the androgen activity on skin [18]. Dutasteride is a second generation 5-α reductase inhibitor. While finasteride inhibits type II enzyme, dutasteride inhibits both type I and type II [18]. Heparin and heparin-like mesoglycan acts as vasodilator [11]. X adene contains vitamin B complex and increases blood flow [11]. Azelaic acid inhibits 5-α reductase activity [11]. Calcitonin and cyproterone acetate can also be used in hair mesotherapy [10].

A test trichogram should be performed one year after to evaluate the clinical efficacy of hair mesotherapy. Additionally, mesotherapy injection technique has been suggested to decrease the pain and provide the distribution of drug more evenly during intralesional corticosteroid therapy for AA [20]. Shulaia et al. have reported successful results in AA patients treated with mesotherapy using nicotinic acid, vitamin C, pentoxifylline, and trace elements (Zn, Se, and placentex) over a period of 28 weeks [21].

2.5. Contraindications and side effects

The contraindications of hair mesotherapy are as follows: allergy to the substances used in mesotherapy, diabetes, liver, renal and cardiac failure, pregnancy, lactation, use of medication for anticoagulation, infection, or lesion on the area [11, 22]. Side effects of hair mesotherapy are edema, bruising, itching, pain, and headache [10, 23]. Also, side effects related to the systemic absorption of substances may be observed [11]. Contrarily, alopecia has been reported as a side effect following hair mesotherapy. In one case report, one patient developed cicatricial alopecia after heparinoid vasodilator mesoglycan and reversible alopecia has occurred in the second patient due to homoeopathic agents [24]. Additionally, cutaneous infections caused by nontuberculous mycobacteria have been observed after mesotherapy. Although these infections are mostly reported after mesotherapy for lipolysis, physicians should keep in mind that they can be seen after hair mesotherapy [11, 25–27]. Moreover, multifocal scalp abscesses with subcutaneous fat necrosis and scarring alopecia have been reported as a complication of hair mesotherapy. This complication has been attributed to the improper application technique [28]. Recently, frontal edema due to %5 minoxidil solution after hair mesotherapy has been reported [29].

http://dx.doi.org/10.5772/66747

2.6. Evidence for efficacy

Unfortunately, there is scanty scientific data on the role of mesotherapy in the treatment of alopecia. Abdallah et al. have found hair mesotherapy more effective than placebo in 28 male AGA patients by using a dutasteride containing solution (dutasteride 5 mg, D-panthenol 500 mg, biotin 20 mg, and pyridoxine 200 mg) after 11 weeks of treatment. They also observed a negative correlation between the duration of AGA and response to treatment which is suggested to be associated with the replacement of terminal hair follicles with epithelial remnants of telogen follicles [30]. In another study, 90 male AGA patients were divided into three groups as group A (30 patients) receiving pure dutasteride, group B (30 patients) receiving dutasteride containing solution (dutasteride 5 mg, dexpanthenol 500 mg, biotin 20 mg, and pyridoxine 200 mg), and group C (30 patients) receiving saline. According to the results, there was no statistically significant difference between groups, however, dutasteride containing solution was found to be superior according to trichogram results [31]. Ozdoğan et al. have treated 15 male and 8 female AGA patients with mesotherapy using 2% minoxidil, biotin, dexpanthenol, herbal complex, and procaine once a week. Hair mesotherapy was found to be significantly effective in the improvement of hair quantity and hair thickness after 10 weeks [32]. A mesotherapy solution containing dutasteride 0.5 mg, biotin 20 mg, pyridoxin 200 mg, and D-panthenol 500 mg was used in 86 female AGA patients and the results were compared with control group receiving saline solution. A decrease in hair loss and improvement in both photographic assessment and hair density after 12 sessions were observed [23]. Topical application of minoxidil 2% (30 patients) was compared with the intraepidermal injection of the drug (30 patients) on 60 females with FPHL and it was concluded that the mesotherapeutic application of minoxidil revealed significantly better results compared to topical application of the drug in both self assessment and trichogram tests [33]. Freund et al. have treated 40 male AGA patients with mesotherapy using botulinum toxin. They have applied two injections at 24-week intervals after a 12 weeks period without treatment. After 48 weeks of first injection, statistically significant increase in mean hair counts was observed. They suggested that botulinum toxin relaxes the scalp muscles and reduces the pressure on the perforating vessels resulting in the increase of blood flow and oxygen concentration. Furthermore, they reported that there is an increased oxygenation of the scalp so the hair follicles may be associated with enhanced conversion of testosterone to estradiol which favors high oxygen concentrations [34].

Recently, in a systematic review, two unpublished trials (NCT01655108, EUCTR2013-002740-85-ES) have been reported on the efficacy of mesotherapy for the treatment of FPHL. First trial (54 patients) has compared the application of minoxidil 0.5% (27 patients) with saline 0.9% (27 patients) using mesotherapy technique. Although the study is ongoing, the results regarding the increase in hair volume and decrease in the extent of hair loss were better in minoxidil group. The second was a randomized, double-blind, and placebo-controlled clinical trial evaluating the efficacy of plasma rich in growth factors (PRGF-Endoret) on 24 male and female AGA patients by comparing with saline solution. The results of the study are awaiting publication [35].

3. Microneedling in the treatment of alopecia

3.1. Introduction

Microneedling is a medical procedure done by a drum-shaped roller device with hundreds of micron-sized microneedles (0.5–1.5 mm in length) projecting on it. Before the treatment, local anesthetics should be applied to the area.

3.2. Method

Roller device is applied in vertical, horizontal, and diagonal directions. By rolling the device across the skin, these microneedles pierce the stratum corneum and create numerous transient microchannels over the applied surface without damaging the epidermis [36, 37]. Microneedling provides direct entry to viable epidermis where it acts on, and does not contact with the dermal nerves and capillaries [37].

Generally, microneedling is applied at 4–6 week intervals in order to wait for new collagen synthesis. For acne scars, 3–4 treatment sessions may be required [36]. However, there is no standard protocol for the application of microneedling in alopecia treatment.

3.3. Mechanism of action

Microtrauma caused by puncturing of the skin induces the collagen synthesis and neo-angiogenesis through the wound healing response [36, 37]. Microneedling leads the stimulation of stem cells and activation of growth factors [38–40]. It increases the blood flow to the hair follicles [40]. Also, it was reported that the expression of hair growth related genes are induced after microneedling [41]. Additionally, transient micropores formed through the procedure allow the delivery of molecules into the epidermis. Therefore, after microneedling many cosmeceutical agents have been suggested to be delivered deep to the skin [37, 42, 43]. Accordingly, in mesotherapy, substances can be given with mesoroller device, as mentioned above [11].

3.4. Side effects

Erythema is rapidly recovered in 24–48 hours of treatment. No serious side effects have been associated with microneedling [37, 43]. Patients can complaint from mild pain [42]. As the microchannels close immediately after the application, infection is not expected after the procedure [36]. In order to avoid potential side effects, appropriate sterilization of the device and the use of only fully licensed and tested agents together with microneedling are important [37].

3.5. Evidence for efficacy

The effect of microneedling has been investigated on 100 men with AGA. Authors randomized the patients into two groups. First group (50 men) treated with weekly microneedling and 5% minoxidil twice daily (except the day of microneedling) and second group only treated with 5% minoxidil twice daily. After 12 weeks of treatment, the results regarding mean change in hair count were statistically better in the microneedling plus minoxidil group [38]. Additionally, the authors evaluated the supplementary effect of microneedling on four men with AGA who were on oral finasteride and topical 5% minoxidil therapy. New hair growth was seen after 8–10 sessions. Patients treated weekly for the first four weeks, then 11 sessions were applied at 2-week intervals. After 6 months of treatment grade +2 to +3 response was seen in all patients on photographic assessment. Regarding the patient's subjective assessment scale three patients showed more than 75% satisfaction and one patient showed more than 50% satisfaction. After 18 months of follow up, the results of microneedling were reported to be sustained [44].

Lee et al. applied microneedling in conjunction with topical growth factors on eleven FPHL patients. In their scalp-split, single-blinded, and placebo-controlled trial, they treated patients weekly for five sessions. One half of the scalp was treated with a solution containing growth factors (basic fibroblast growth factor, insulin-like growth factor-1, vascular endothelial growth factor, stem cell factor, keratinocyte growth factor-2, superoxide dismutase-1, and Noggin) plus microneedling, whereas the other half was treated with saline plus microneedling. The increase in hair shaft density and hair count was significant in growth factor plus microneedling group. Also patients' satisfaction was reported to be higher in the same group compared to saline group [42].

Other than AGA, the effect of microneedling was also assessed in resistant AA. Deepak et al. reported three cases of AA (one patchy AA, two alopecia universalis) that were previously unsuccessfully treated with contact sensitizers, topical tacrolimus, minoxidil, and corticosteroids and oral mini pulse betamethasone. Authors applied microneedling with a solution containing triamcinolone acetonide, mesotherapy cocktail (growth factors, copper tripeptide-1, multivitamins, amino acids, and minerals), and minoxidil 2–5%. Marked clinical response was seen in all the three of cases after 4–6 sessions. The authors suggested that scalp roller therapy might be an effective and safe complementary intervention for the treatment of resistant AA [43].

In another study, two cases of patchy AA were successfully treated with microneedling plus topical triamcinolone. After three sessions which were applied at 3-week intervals, both patients showed marked response and no recurrence was seen after 3 months follow up [40].

The role of photodynamic therapy (PDT) with methyl 5-aminolevulinic acid (MAL) has been studied for the treatment of AA with variable results. The lack of response has been attributed to the inadequate transepidermal penetration of the drug. With regard to facilitator effect of microneedling in drug delivery, the efficacy of roller therapy in the penetration of MAL in PDT of AA has been evaluated in two studies. Patients are treated with PDT with MAL with only half scalp application of microneedling. In both study, as none of the patients showed hair growth, authors concluded that PDT with MAL may not be an effective strategy for AA, regardless of adjunctive microneedling to enhance the drug passage deep into the skin [45, 46].

Recently, an animal study has demonstrated that micro injury caused by microneedling induced hair regrowth in two pomeranian dogs with alopecia X (hair cycle arrest) [47]. In another animal study assessing the hair growth effect of mycophenolic acid (MP), microneedling was found to accelerate the stimulatory growth of topical MP on anagen follicles [48].

4. Platelet-rich plasma in the treatment of alopecia

4.1. Platelets

Platelets are one of the shapely structured elements of the peripheral blood and do not have cell nuclei. The number of platelets ranges from 150,000 to 350,000/mm^3 in peripheral blood and they are functioning primarily in hemostasis [49]. They take active role in wound healing, angiogenesis, and inflammation owing to the numerous proteins, cytokines, and bioactive factors they contain [49, 50]. In addition, they induce the migration and adherence of bone marrow-origin cells into angiogenesis territory and the differentiation of endothelial cell progenitors to the mature endothelial cells [51].

The platelets have three main storage sites; α granules, dense granules, and lysosomes [52]. The major growth factors (GF) and cytokines already stored in α granules are; transforming growth factor-β (TGF-β), platelet-derived growth factor (PDGF), insulin-like growth factor (IGF-I, IGF-II), fibroblast growth factor (FGF), epidermal growth factor (EGF), vascular endothelial growth factor (VEGF), and endothelial cell growth factor (ECGF) [49, 53, 54]. The activation of platelets induces degranulation of GFs which are already restored. The secreted GFs bind to the transmembrane receptors on mesenchymal stem cells, osteoblasts, fibroblasts, endothelial cells, and epidermal cells and then induce the internal signal transduction pathway. They initiate the healing process such as cell proliferation, differentiation, chemotaxis, angiogenesis, matrix formation, osteoid production, and collagen synthesis [49, 53].

The dense granules of the platelets have bioactive factors such as serotonin, histamine, dopamine, calcium, adenosine triphosphate (ATP), adenosine diphosphate (ADP), and catecholamine. These substances have significant effects in wound healing. They have effects such as boosting the capillary permeability, vasoconstriction, hauling and activating the macrophages, tissue modulation, and regeneration [49, 54].

4.2. Platelet-rich plasma

PRP is an autologous, biologically active concentration, composed of many growth factors (GF), cytokines, and plasma proteins [55]. It came into use since 1970s owing to its effects to promote the wound healing to a cellular level [54]. Platelet concentration in PRP is at least 1,000,000/μg/L in 5 mL and the growth factor concentration is 3–5 times higher than peripheral blood [49]. Platelet gel concentration which is higher or lower than 1,500,000 was associated with decreased angiogenic features of endothelial cells [56].

There are four different PRP subgroups available; pure PRP, leukocyte and PRP (L-PRP), platelet-rich fibrin matrix (PRFM), and leukocyte- and platelet-rich fibrin matrix. Clinically, pure PRP and L-PRP are widely used. The one widely used in cosmetic dermatology is the pure PRP [57].

In vitro studies indicate a dose-dependent positive correlation between the platelet concentration and human mesenchymal stem cells and fibroblast proliferation and type 1 collagen production [58]. It is reported that PRP increased the proliferation of fibroblasts and their transformation into myofibroblasts as well as the synthesis of collagen and matrix remodeling proteins [59, 60].

4.3. Preparation of platelet-rich plasma

PRP is prepared with 20–60 mL of plasma [61] by means of automatic devices under aseptic conditions at 20–22°C. It must be prepared using anticoagulants containing citrate dextrose solution formula A (ACD-A) or sodium citrate in order to inhibit PRP aggregation [53]. The blood elements are separated according to their molecular weights by means of centrifugal method in manual double spin method. Respectively, red blood cells (RBC) are the heaviest, white blood cells (WBC) are moderate, and the platelets are the lightest ones. The platelets are first separated from RBC and WBC by means of light-spin centrifuge that they become available in concentrated form in the top part of buffy coat layer. Subsequently, heavy-spin centrifuge separates the supernatant plasma and more concentrated platelets are obtained. Bottom part of the tube holds the platelets and the upper part retains the platelet-poor plasma (PPP). Thrombin is used as an activator to obtain coagulation and thus "activated PRP" is extracted by means of GF degranulation [49, 53]. Approximately, 70% of GFs is released in 10 min and almost 100% is released in an hour and a small amount of GF continues to be produced for up to 8–10 days during the life of platelets [62]. For this reason, PRP should be administered soon after it is prepared.

The platelet-rich fibrin matrix (PRFM) is developed to retard GF secretion from the platelets, which is a dense fibrin matrix generated by adding $CaCl_2$ during the secondary centrifuge that induces the conversion of autogenous thrombin from prothrombin. Platelet activation decreases as the thrombin amount reduces, so the platelets secrete their GFs slowly in a period of 7 days. Therefore, it is used in fat grafting and soft tissue augmentation. At the same time, fibrin matrix serves as a building block in wound healing [49, 57].

L-PRP is a subtype of PRP consisting of the platelet, leucocyte, and red blood cells. It is produced by the collection of PPP and all buffy coats following the centrifuge of anticoagulant blood. Whereas Leukocyte-PRFM is a subform made up of platelet and leucocyte-rich fibrin polymerized clot. It is produced without using anticoagulant and activator [57].

Another platelet activation type is the method which stimulates PDGF and VEGF secretion and enables collagen-PRP gel formation, performed by using type I collagen [63].

A great number of commercial kits came into use in addition to manual PRP preparation. However, different technologies introduce products with different biology and unclear effect profile. There are various PRP preparation methods in the literature, which contain different protocols, different centrifugal techniques, and different cellular components [61].

4.4. Indications

Various indications of PRP in dermatology are outlined in **Table 1** [53, 57, 64].

4.5. Method

The patients should be informed and a signed consent form should always be obtained prior to the application. The patient is required stop taking anticoagulants such as aspirin and

Alopecia; androgenetic alopecia, and alopecia areata
Skin rejuvenation
Dermal volume augmentation
Scar revision; acne, and traumatic scars
Striae distensae
Chronic wounds
Fat grafting
Laser resurfacing
Lichen sclerosus

Table 1. Dermatological indications of PRP.

other nonsteroidal antiinflammatory medications at least 2 weeks before the application. Local anaesthesia should be given, if required, under aseptic circumstances. Different application methods are available, which may be preferred by the clinicians and for the comfort of the patient. First method is the retrograde injection of PRP deep-to-surface at a rate of 0.05–0.1 mL/cm^2 per each centimeter. The second one is the administration of PRP either by puncturing holes over the scalp by means of 1 mm microneedle roller or by means of mesotherapy gun. The third method is the application of PRP before or after the implantation in order to assist the hair transplantation, keeping the follicular grafts in PRP for 15 minutes prior to implantation or the application in order to speed up the wound healing in donor's excision line [53].

There is no consensus on the parameters such as the frequency, depth (interfollicular, intradermal, or subcutaneous), and the dose of the application.

4.6. Contraindications

Contraindications of PRP are listed on **Table 2** [63–65].

Pregnancy and breastfeeding period
Acute and chronic infections
Autoimmune disorders
Sensitivity to blood and blood products
Hepatopathy (liver disease)
Malignancies
Thrombocytopenia and hypofibrinogenemia

Table 2. Contraindications of PRP.

4.7. Side effects

The incidence of adverse effects is quite low since PRP application is an autologous one. Local side effects due to injection such as rash, ecchymosis, pain, and infection are mild and temporal. It does not have any risk of transmitting infections such as hepatitis B (HBV), hepatitis C (HCV), and human immunodeficiency virus (HIV). Risk of allergy is low as the patient's own blood is used [53, 65].

4.8. Evidence for efficacy of platelet-rich plasma in various conditions

4.8.1. Androgenetic alopecia

AGA is characterized by progressive hair follicle miniaturization and its treatment is quite challenging [66, 67]. The two medications approved by Food and Drug Administration (FDA) are minoxidil and finasteride. Dermatologists and plastic surgeons tend to prefer new treatment methods due to limited effects and adverse effect profile of these agents. In recent years, a good number of studies have been carried out on the effectivity of PRP in an AGA treatment.

4.8.1.1. The mechanism of platelet-rich plasma in androgenetic alopecia

PRP enhances the proliferation of dermal papilla (DP) cells and protect the cells against apoptosis by increasing Bcl-2 protein level. Moreover, it stimulates the Akt signalization which has antiapoptotic effects on cell survival and also stimulates extracellular signal-regulated kinase (ERK) that regulates the cell growth. In this way, it promotes cell growth and extends the survival of hair follicles. B-catenin is expressed in the external root sheath in the bulge area of human anagen hair follicle and ensures the differentiation of stem cells into the hair follicle cells and other adult cells. B-catenin activity in DP cells of the patients treated with PRP is upregulated, inducing the differentiation of stem cells into hair follicle cells and stimulating the hair growth. In addition, FGF-7 expression in DP cells increases, ensuring that the anagen phase of hair growth cycle is extended. Enhanced VEGF and PDGF boosts the perifollicular vascular plexus with proangiogenic effect. Active PRP injected to the mice *in vivo* is indicated to induce the acceleration of telogen-to-anagen transition [68].

The first study performed on PRP indicated that both the survival of follicular units are increased and follicular density is augmented in the patients of hair plantation since the follicular grafts were soaked in PRP for 15 minutes prior to implantation [69]. Various studies in the literature indicated that PRP stimulates a number of active features such as growth rate, hair count, hair density, hair shaft diameter, hair root strength, anagen hair, telogen hair, terminal hair density, epidermal keratinocytes, hair follicular bulge cells, and lead to increase in small blood vessels in hair follicle, prevents dermal papilla apoptosis, extent anagen phase, and enhances hair regrowth [70–74]. The carrier which contains dalteparin/protamine micro particles (DP MP) (low-molecular-weight heparin) was used to enhance the efficiency of PRP. DP MP ensures adsorption, stabilization, and slow secretion of GFs. PRP containing DP MP is observed to increase the hair thickness significantly compared to PRP alone [75]. In another study, PRP containing CD34$^+$ cell has been tried on patients with AGA and a significant increase has been observed in hair thickness [76].

4.8.2. Alopecia areata

AA targets the anagen hair follicles in which spontaneous remission may be observed [77–79]. Although immunosuppressive agents can generally be used in the treatment of AA and regarded as an organ specific autoimmune disease, there is not any curative or preventive treatment of the disease [80]. Therefore, PRP has been introduced in recent years as an alternative treatment.

4.8.2.1. The mechanism of platelet-rich plasma on alopecia alopecia

PRP has also an antiinflammatory effect in addition to its effect on the induction of proliferation. Endogen lipid molecules called "lipoxin" derived from cellular arachidonic acid serve in the resolution of the inflammation. Lipoxins retard the arrival of new neutrophils into the inflammation area and support the neutrophil apoptosis to organize the resolution. PRP promotes lipoxin A4 (LXA4) secretion and suppresses the cytokine secretions to limit the inflammation [81]. The fact that inflammatory cytokines play a part in the etiopathogenesis of AA led to an argument that PRP could be effective in AA treatment with antiinflammatory effect.

There is limited number of studies in the literature on the use of PRP in the treatment of AA. A recent study indicated a significant increase in hair growth, an increase in Ki-67 which is the cellular proliferation marker and a degradation in the rate of relapse, in AA patients treated with intralesional PRP, compared with the patients treated with both placebo and intralesional triamcinolone acetonide (TrA). Furthermore, it has been observed that both groups taking PRP and TrA had less rash and irritancy as well as reduced dystrophic hair in dermoscopy. A complete remission rate of 60% has been achieved in the group treated with PRP at the end of the treatment [79].

In another study carried out with 20 AA patients, PRP was well tolerated, no adverse effect was observed and improvement in hair growth was seen. Minimal response to treatment and relapse was observed in only one patient [82].

PRP treatment applied on an ophiasis-type alopecia areata patient, resistive to corticosteroid treatment, yielded a successful result and hair regrowth was observed. PRP is suggested to be an alternative treatment in AA patients resistive to corticosteroid treatment and in the patients with side effects of steroid injection [83].

5. Laser and light sources in the treatment of alopecia

Laser (light amplification by stimulated emission of radiation)/light sources have become popular in dermatology practice on various disorders. Recently, these devices have been tried for the treatment of male and female pattern hair loss and alopecia areata with variable success rates. The laser beam having the coherent, monochromatic, and polarized characteristics that differs it from the ordinary light. The low-energy laser light penetrates the surface in a defined position and does not damage the skin [84]. There is a consensus among many authors that current laser/light sources are safe methods if they can be used properly and also these treatment modalities can be used alone or in combination with other treatments. The literature reveals that the texture and quality of hair improves even if there is no hair regrowth by the use of laser/light sources [85].

5.1. Androgenetic alopecia

AGA is the most common form of hair loss that may affect up to 70% of men and 40% of women in their lifetime [86, 87]. The aim of the treatment is to stop miniaturization and induce hair thickening and regrowth [88]. Finasteride and minoxidil are the most common therapeutic drugs used for AGA [87]. But new treatment modalities are under investigation. Laser/light sources for AGA have become popular in the last few years.

Photobiomodulation is a term that is used to describe the effects of lower level light energy (650–900 nm) on the cellular level. The exact mechanism of photobiomodulation that stops or reduces hair loss in patients is not well known [85, 89]. Low-level visible light treatment (LLLT) modulates the gen expression of 5α-reductase and vascular endothelial growth factor (VEGF) and consequently stimulates hair growth through androgen metabolism and angiogenesis [90]. It was previously reported that helium-neon (He-Ne) laser (632.8 nm) irradiation stimulates cellular activities like deoxyribonucleic acid (DNA) and protein synthesis, mitochondrial electron transport, and adenosine triphosphate (ATP) generation [91]. Low-level laser irradiation prolonged the duration of anagen phase and caused the catagen and telogen follicles to reenter into the anagen phase in a study in mice treated with He-Ne laser. It was revealed that He-Ne laser with a dose of 1 J/cm^2 shows stimulatory effects on hair growth with a significant increase in percentage of anagen, but a suppression of hair growth was observed at a dose of 5 J/cm^2. Cells with low growth rate or under stress conditions, give better response to low-level laser irradiation [90]. Low level of reactive oxygen species (ROS) occurred due to low doses of irradiation show stimulatory effects on cell metabolism, while high level of ROS due to high doses of irradiation show inhibitory effects [92–94].

Subsequently, paradoxical hypertrichosis was reported for many times after using laser and intense pulsed light (IPL) photoepilation therapy for hair removal [95–99]. It is not exactly known, how these light sources can induce hair growth. One possible mechanism is the activation of silent hair follicles or the synchronization of hair growth cycles by direct light stimulation [89]. Radmanesh et al. identified different mechanisms for developing hypertrichosis after the IPL. First, certain wavelengths of IPL show photostimulator effects on hair follicle germinative and stem cells, directly or indirectly and facilitate hair regeneration and growth. The stem cells in the bulge area of the hair follicle are usually inactive. The second mechanism is the stimulation of the secretion of the mediators and cytokines that stimulate hair growth by IPL. Keratinocyte growth factor and fibroblast growth factor are two well known trichostimulatory cytokines and they have stimulatory effects on hair follicles and epidermal cells. They maintain epidermal proliferation and hair growth. The individual differences and the properties of the devices may also affect the paradoxical hypertrichosis [98].

There are various studies showing the positive effects of laser/light treatments in AGA. In a previous study, the effects of laser on cancer were investigated in mice. The dorsal hair of mice was shaved and the low-powered ruby laser (694 nm) therapy was given toward this area. They did not find any evidence of cancer but observed accelerated hair growth in laser-treated sides [100]. In a clinical study, seven patients with a diagnosis of AGA were exposed to LLLT twice weekly for 20 min for 3–6 months. An increase in the number of terminal hair, a decrease in the number of vellus hair, and an increase in shaft diameter were observed in this study but these changes were not statistically significant [89].

To assess the effect of a 1550 nm fractional erbium-glass laser in a female pattern hair loss, 28 patients received 10 treatments at 2-week interval. At the end of the study, a marked increase in hair density and hair shaft thickness and significant improvement at the frontal hair recess were seen in patients. It was revealed that 1550 nm fractional erbium-glass laser may be a safe and effective treatment option for female pattern hair loss (FPHL) [101]. In a clinical study, the effects of a 1550 nm fractional erbium-glass laser on the hair cycle in an alopecia mouse model and on the treatment of male pattern hair loss were investigated. In the human pilot study, an increase in hair density and an improvement of growth rate were observed. In the animal study, the effect on hair stimulation was dependent upon the energy levels, densities, and irradiation intervals. Fractional laser irradiation can promote anagen hair growth and induce transition from the telogen phase to the anagen phase. It was shown that Wnt 5-α and β-catenin expressions play a role in hair growth were induced by laser irradiation [102].

In a study of 32 patients with male and female androgenetic alopecia, the efficacy and safety of LLLT were evaluated. A Laser comb (655 nm) was used as monotherapy or as a concomitant therapy with minoxidil and finasteride. Eight patients showed significant improvement, 20 patients showed moderate improvement while no improvement was observed in four patients. Improvement was observed in both monotherapy and the dual therapy group [103]. Previously, a Laser comb has been tested in 110 patients with AGA in a double-blind, sham device-controlled, multicenter, and 26-week trial. Significant increase in mean terminal hair density was observed in patients in the LLLT group when compared to patients in the sham device group [104]. Jimenez et al. reported a statistically significant increase in terminal hair density after 26 weeks of low-level laser comb device treatment compared with sham treatment in patients with FPHL and male pattern hair loss (MPHL) [105].

5.2. Alopecia areata

As there is no cure for alopecia areata which is an autoimmune disease and may improve spontaneously in 34–50% of patients, clinicians search for new treatment modalities such as laser/light sources [86, 106, 107].

There are limited studies about laser irradiation for alopecia areata. In a study, clinicians used 308 nm xenon chloride excimer laser (XeCl) for two patients with alopecia areata for 11–12 sessions within a 9–11 weeks period. They observed homogeneous and thick hair growth. The exact mechanism was not clear, but immunosuppressive effects of laser irradiation by inducing T-cell apoptosis and interrupting autoaggressive immune cascade were held responsible [108]. In a study with nine patients with AA, 308-nm excimer laser was used for lesions twice a week for 12–24 sessions. They observed hair regrowth in patients with AA partialis [109].

In a previous study, researchers chose a single representative lesion that was unresponsive to the other treatments. One half of the lesion was exposed to the 308-nm laser while the other part was not treated. After 27 sessions, only the treated area showed hair regrowth, suggesting it was not a spontaneous recovery [110].

The 308-nm excimer laser was used for patients with AA twice a week for 24 sessions. And it is reported as an effective treatment for patchy AA of the scalp and in some cases with AA of the beard area, but patchy lesions of the extremities and alopecia totalis were unresponsive [111]. It was also used for children with patchy AA successfully. Atopic diathesis was considered as a poor prognostic factor in this study [112].

Waiz et al. used pulsed infrared diode (904 nm) laser on 16 patients with 34 resistant alopecia areata patches. They observed hair regrowth with a rate of 94%. They suggest that laser may alter the cellular membrane or change the exposed antigen which was previously hidden to become hidden again [84].

Yoo et al. treated a patient with recalcitrant AA with fractional laser therapy weekly for 24 weeks. Hair regrowth was observed after 1 month treatment. After 3 months 30–40% of lesions were covered with terminal hair. Complete recovery occurred after 6 months of fractional laser therapy. One of the possible mechanisms of fractional laser induced hair regrowth is inducing T-cell apoptosis or decreasing inflammation. Another mechanism is about microscopic thermal columns in the dermis that were made by laser therapy. A healing process starts including lymphocyte infiltrations. It may scatter perifollicular lymphocyte infiltration and cause a decrease in perifollicular lymphocytic infiltration. Fractional laser may stop disease progression by increasing anagen phase. Furthermore, minor trauma and wound healing induced by fractional laser therapy may facilitate hair growth [113].

Three patients with ophiasis, a special pattern of AA, were enrolled in a study. Two of the patients were treated with nonablative 1550 nm erbium glass fractional laser (NAFL) and one of the patients treated with both NAFL and ablative 10,600 nm carbon dioxide fractional laser (AFL). The clinicians observed that patients who have AA for 1 year or less respond to treatment better than patients with long-term disease. They considered NAFL treatment may have beneficial effects on early ophiasis lesions [114].

6. Stem-cell therapy in alopecia

6.1. Hair follicle, stem cells, and dermal papilla

Hair follicle (HF) is a complex structure that contains important units in the development of hair shaft including dermal papilla, matrix, and bulge region [3].

The HF undergoes cycles of growth and degeneration that a new hair shaft is formed in each cycle [115]. The signaling in this cycling is not completely understood. Fundamentally, there is a bidirectional communication between the mesenchymal and stem cells within the hair follicle that controls the formation, growth, and cycling of hair follicle [3, 116, 117].

Dermal papilla (DP) is located at the bottom of hair follicle (hair bulb) and consists of specialized mesenchymal cells which produce signals regulating the hair cycling of follicular epithelium and also driving the formation of hair follicle [116, 117]. Bulge region of hair follicle houses epithelial stem cells that become progenitor cells forming the hair follicle. Upon the stimulatory signals from DP cells, progenitor cells move down to the deep dermis where they turn into matrix cells which differentiate to form different parts of hair follicle [3, 117, 118]. It can be understood from these information that although the immediate formation of hair shaft and follicle is achieved by the matrix cells in the DP, reservoir stem cells reside in the upward bulge region that maintain the follicle regeneration [115].

Stem cells are characterized by the capacity of self-renewal and ability to differentiate into various cell lineages. Hair follicle stem cells (HFSCs) which are found in hair bulge are quiescence cells that divide infrequently [3]. HFSCs are multipotent that they can give rise to all cells of a hair follicle, sebaceous gland, and interfollicular epidermis [3, 115, 118]. In addition, hair follicle bears other types of stem cells including interfollicular epidermal stem cells, sebaceous gland stem cells, follicle nestin + pluripotent stem cells, etc. [3, 115].

The induction of hair cycling and hair follicle regeneration from the HFSCs is a complex process which starts with the signals from DP cells. This interaction involves several signaling pathways, growth factors, specific protein ligand-receptor binding, upregulation of various hair-related genes and activation of different transcription factors [3, 116, 118].

6.2. The rationale behind the stem-cell therapy in the treatment of alopecia

As the current treatment options for most types of alopecia including AGA and AA are not satisfactory, new therapies are still being under investigation for various types of alopecia. Development of bioengineering technologies has provided the use of HFSCs as a promising treatment in the management of alopecia. Since the conventional drugs for alopecia are unable to target all the pathophysiologic factors, stem-cell therapy is considered as a potential solution to correct the main pathology in various types of alopecias [3, 115, 117, 118].

It has been suggested that the distinct pathophysiologic pathways may be targeted by stem cell therapies in different diseases. An important point is that in order to specifically manage the alopecia, it is important to clarify the exact etiologic mechanism underlying various types of alopecias [3, 118]. For example, in AGA, the main etiology is that the HF is miniaturized by the effect of 5-DHT and the signaling that drives the HF regeneration is impaired. Although the stem cells in bulge region are undamaged, the production of new hair formation is interrupted in AGA [3, 116]. Another example for the impaired induction of hair formation by the destruction of DP region is the chemotherapy induced alopecia. Induction of hair generation by DP cells has been suggested to be achieved by stem-cell therapy in this type of alopecia [116]. In AA, DP (bulbar region of HF) is attacked by the immune cells [3, 115]. Stem-cell therapy has been suggested to be effective in the suppression of autoimmune destruction and recovery of immune balance in AA patients [119]. In cicatricial alopecia, inflammation leads to the destruction of the bulge region where the normal immune privilege has been lost by pathologic triggers and stem cells are destroyed [115]. Producing a new hair follicle unit via transplantation of stem cells has been suggested as a major innovation for the treatment of most forms of alopecias including scarring alopecia [3, 115, 117, 118].

6.3. Preliminary hair follicle generation studies and obstacles in stem cell therapies

As the epithelial-mesenchymal interaction is crucial in the development of HF, it is essential to coculture DP cells with stem cells in order to generate a complete HF in laboratory condition. However, it has to be in mind that it is not easy to obtain and grow stem cells in laboratory experiments and their turnover is low [115, 117].

Marazzi et al. have isolated human follicle DP and bulge cells and cultured them in human skin sample (organotypical culture). After injection of the cultured bulge and DP cells into deep dermis, epidermis forming ability of the cells was assessed. The authors suggested their methodology as a relevant source of bioengineered hair follicles for hair transplantation therapies in alopecia [120].

In a previous report, mouse embryonic skin-derived stem cells were used to form a hair germ and the resultant bioengineered follicle germ was intracutaneously transplanted to create a structurally correct hair follicle. On the back skin of a nude mouse, the transplanted follicle germ was able to form hair shaft, construct appropriate connection with surrounding tissue, and undergo cycling [121]. As the transplantation of a mature bioengineered hair follicle rather than follicle germ is considered to be more favorable in hair regeneration, Asakawa et al. in their animal study, have shown that ectopic transplantation of bioengineered hair follicles (created by follicle germ cells from embryonic pelage skin and regenerated *in vitro* culture) could develop a fully functional hair follicle in host. Authors reported that the results of the study have indicated transplantation of the bioengineered hair follicles could replace the conventional FUT therapy in alopecia treatment [122].

An important problem in the hair follicle regeneration studies is that cultured DP cells lose their inductive capacity after a few passages. Attempts including co-culturing with keratinocytes and adding growth factors to the medium have been done to effectively expand DP cells *in vitro* culture [117]. As the laboratory conditions and *in vitro* assays are far from the *in vivo* ambience of DP cells, to better simulate the real hair follicle, three-dimensional (3D) dermal spheric cultures have been generated [123]. To further increase the inductive capacity of DP cells and to enhance the reproducibility of assays, novel membranes for spheric culturing have been used [124]. One of the most important obstacles in hair regeneration studies is the results of animal or *in vitro* studies differ from those on human. Despite an intact HF can be formed in murine and embryonic cell experiments, incomplete HF are formed with human DPCs. Subcutaneous implantation of isolated human HFSCs and human scalp DPCs resulted in the formation of hair follicle-like structures in nude mice [125]. To overcome this problem strategies such as culturing DPCs with keratinocytes have been formulated [126]. Recently an acellular dermal matrix has been used to grow human epithelial and dermal cells from scalp tissue with promising results [127]. Recently, human DP cells from scalp tissue have been embedded into dermal–epidermal composites (DECs) and formation of complete HF has been observed [128].

By ongoing studies, it was realized that not only the close environment of HF but also the macro environment of HF is important in the growth induction of HF. As the adipocyte stem cells (ASCs) secrete growth factors and stimulate hair growth pathways and the activation of hair follicle stem cell by adipocyte lineage cells has been shown, ASCs and ASC-conditioned medium (ASC-CM) have been investigated in hair regeneration studies. DPCs which are cultured in ASC-CM showed increased proliferation. These studies suggested a role for ASCs in alopecia treatment [117, 129].

Bone marrow mesenchymal stem cells (BM-MSCs) have also been used to induce hair induction *in vitro* assays and tested for HF formation capacity in mouse models [116].

6.4. Studies on the stem-cell therapy in alopecia

In a randomized placebo-controlled trial, topical application of a commercially available solution containing HFSCs in male patients with AGA was found to be effective in the induction of hair growth and reduction of hair loss [130]. Supernatant of BM-MSC culture overexpressing Wnt1a has been shown to increase hair producing ability of DP cells. Additionally, intradermal injection of concentrated solution of the above mentioned supernatant enhanced the transition from telogen to anagen in mouse. Also, negative effect of a 5-DHT on hair related genes was restored with the addition of Wnt-CM. Study indicated a role for Wnt1a from MSCs in hair regeneration therapies for alopecia [116].

The effect of intradermal injection of commercially available ASC-CM product (containing hepatocyte growth factor, fibroblast growth factor-1, granulocyte colony-stimulating factor, granulocyte macrophage-colony-stimulating factor, interleukin-6, vascular endothelial growth factor, and transforming growth factor β-3) to 22 AGA patients (11 males, 11 females) has been studied. Patients were treated in six sessions at 3–5- week interval. Six male patients were also on finasteride treatment. Half-side comparison study has been undertaken in 10 patients. Hair counts were increased in all patients according to trichogram assays. In comparison study, hair count was increased in both side of the scalp, however, the increase was higher in the treatment side compared to the placebo side. The response in the placebo side is suggested to be related to the effect of injection itself or the diffusion of the solution to the other side [131].

In another study with the same product, 27 patients with FPHL were treated with the solution (ASC-CM) weekly with concurrent use of microneedling roller. Retrospective assessment of the results revealed significant increment in the hair density and thickness after 12 sessions [129].

An evidence to the alternative mechanisms of stem-cell therapy is the "stem cell educator therapy" which has been used for its immune modulation effect in nine AA patients. Cord blood stem cells (CB-SCs) have been used to be introduced to patient's blood in a closed loop system. Patient's lymphocytes are separated and cocultured with CB-SCs *in vitro* and returned to patient's circulation after "education." A significant suppression of CD8Tcell attacking and upregulation of the co inhibitory molecules resulted in the diminishment of autoimmune destruction and reversal of immune balance by shifting the immune response toward Th2. As only a small portion of lymphocytes encounter with CB-SCs, the educated immune response has been suggested to be expanded systemically leading a generalized outcome [119].

In a recent review, an unpublished study (NCT01286649) has been reported investigating the efficacy of injecting human autologous HF dermal sheath cup cells which have been taken by punch biopsy from the scalp of patients with AGA. The results of the study await publication [118].

6.5. Contraindications and side effects of stem-cell therapy in alopecia treatment

The presence of skin disease, inflammation or infection, having an allergic, autoimmune disease or cancer, pregnancy, and the usage of anticoagulant therapy are reported as contraindications of stem-cell therapy [131]. Most of the studies on stem-cell therapy in alopecia treatment reported no severe adverse effects [119, 129, 132]. Patients can feel pain when injection technique is used which can be overcome by nerve blockages, local anesthesia, cooling, or prescription of nonsteroidal antiinflammatory drugs [131].

7. Conclusions

Although the scientific data to support the validity of mesotherapy as a treatment option in alopecia is still lacking, there is an increasing interest in its use. Hair mesotherapy is not yet approved in the treatment of alopecia and the existing studies give variable results. Therefore, long-term studies on a large cohort of patients are necessary to document its efficacy and safety in alopecia treatment and to standardize the treatment protocols. Hair mesotherapy can be used as an alternative intervention in the treatment of AA, AGA, and telogen effluvium in patients without systemic diseases.

Despite the increasing interest in microneedling in the treatment of different types of alopecia, further randomized controlled trials are required to assess the efficacy of microneedling on alopecia.

Literature suggests PRP as an effective tool in AGA patients. PRP can be considered as an alternative treatment in AA patients not responsive to corticosteroid treatment or in the patients developing side effects due to steroid injections.

LLLT seems to be a safe and effective treatment option for patients with AGA, but more long-term placebo-controlled studies are needed to define the beneficial effects of laser/light sources for the management of this disease. The effects of laser/light sources are shown in many studies as mentioned above in AA. However, larger placebo-controlled studies should be performed to evaluate the beneficial and adverse effects of these devices.

There is no conclusive data regarding the efficacy, applicability, and method of stem-cell therapy in the treatment of alopecia, however, it still remains as a potential intervention. Further studies are required with improved techniques to overcome challenges in regenerating intact HFs before clinical use. Also the cost and availability of such bioengineering therapies must be taken into consideration. Similar to the current follicular unit transplantation (FUT) therapy, in future, it is expected to transplant a complete HF created by stem cell technology and be able to treat various types of alopecia.

Author details

Selda Pelin Kartal[1]*, Cemile Altunel[2] and Bilgen Gencler[1]

*Address all correspondence to: pelin@dr.com

1 Ministry of Health Ankara Diskapi Yildirim Beyazit Education and Research Hospital Dermatology Clinic, Ankara, Turkey

2 Ankara Nato Hospital, Dermatology Clinic, Ankara, Turkey

References

[1] Qi J, Garza LA. An overview of alopecias. Cold Spring Harb Perspect Med. 2014;4(3). pii:a013615. DOI: 10.1101/cshperspect.a013615.

[2] Levy LL, Emer JJ. Female pattern alopecia: current perspectives. Int J Womens Health. 2013;5:541–56. DOI: 10.2147/IJWH.S49337.

[3] Santos Z, Avci P, Hamblin MR. Drug discovery for alopecia: gone today, hair tomorrow. Expert Opin Drug Discov. 2015;10:269–92. DOI: 10.1517/17460441.2015.1009892.

[4] Mysore V. Mesotherapy in management of hairloss - is it of any use? Int J Trichology. 2010;2:45–6. DOI: 10.4103/0974-7753.66914.

[5] Buz A, Görgülü T, Olgun A, Kargi E. Efficacy of glutathione mesotherapy inburns: an experimental study. Eur J Trauma Emerg Surg. 2015;42:775. DOI: 10.1007/s00068-015-0607-8.

[6] Mammucari M, Maggiori E, Lazzari M, Natoli S. Should the general practitioner consider mesotherapy (intradermal therapy) to manage localized pain? Pain Ther. 2016;5:123–6. DOI: 10.1007/s40122-016-0052-3.

[7] Chen DL, Cohen JL, Green JB. Injectable agents affecting subcutaneous fats. Semin Cutan Med Surg. 2015;34:134–7. DOI: 10.12788/j.sder.2015.0166.

[8] Prikhnenko S. Polycomponent mesotherapy formulations for the treatment of skin aging and improvement of skin quality. Clin Cosmet Investig Dermatol. 2015;8:151–7. DOI: 10.2147/CCID.S76721.

[9] Konda D, Thappa DM. Mesotherapy: what is new? Indian J Dermatol Venereol Leprol. 2013;79:127–34. DOI: 10.4103/0378-6323.104689.

[10] Kutlubay Z, Karakus Ö. Hair mesotherapy. Hair Ther Transplant. 2012;2:1–3.

[11] Inanır I, Gençoğlan G. Hair mesotherapy. Turkiye Klinikleri J Cosm Dermatol-Special Topics. 2014;7:22–5.

[12] Nusbaum AG, Rose PT, Nusbaum BP. Nonsurgical therapy for hair loss. Facial Plast Surg Clin North Am. 2013;21:335–42. DOI: 10.1016/j.fsc.2013.04.003.

[13] Handog EB, Gabriel TG. Mesotherapy. In: Baran R, Maibach H, editors. Textbook of Cosmetic Dermatology. 4th ed. London: Informa Healthcare; 2010. pp. 411–12.

[14] Herreros FO, Moraes AM, Velho PE. Mesotherapy: a bibliographical review. An Bras Dermatol. 2011;86:96–101.

[15] Petit P. Mesotherapy and aging skin. Acta Dermatovenerol Croat. 2010;18:209–14.

[16] Dolar N. The mesotherapy of scalp. Turkiye Klinikleri J Cosm Dermatol-Special Topics. 2008;1:26–32.

[17] Gokdemir G. Has the effect of mesotherapy been proved? Turkderm. 2009;43:12–6.

[18] Gokdemir G. Mesotherapy and platelet-rich plasma for the treatment of hair loss. Turkderm. 2014;48:74–9.

[19] Skalnaya MG, Tkachev VP. Trace elements content and hormonal profiles in women with androgenetic alopecia. J Trace Elem Med Biol. 2011;25:50–3. DOI: 10.1016/j.jtemb.2010.10.006.

[20] Ferrando J, Moreno-Arias GA. Multi-injection plate for intralesional corticosteroid treatment of patchy alopecia areata. Dermatol Surg. 2000;26:690–1.

[21] Shulaia T, Kiladze N, Babilashvili I. Mesotherapy in treatment of alopecia areata. J Exp Clin Med. 2007;1:19–22.

[22] Bulam H, Ayhan S, Sezgin B, Özmen S, Çenetoğlu S. Mesotherapy: Is it the miracle at the edge of the needle or not? Turk Plast Surg. 2013;21:16–9.

[23] Moftah N, Moftah N, Abd-Elaziz G, Ahmed N, Hamed Y, Ghannam B, Ibrahim M. Mesotherapy using dutasteride-containing preparation in treatment of female pattern hair loss: photographic, morphometric and ultrustructural evaluation. J Eur Acad Dermatol Venereol. 2013;27:686–93. DOI: 10.1111/j.1468-3083.2012.04535.

[24] Duque-Estrada B, Vincenzi C, Misciali C, Tosti A. Alopecia secondary to mesotherapy. J Am Acad Dermatol. 2009;61:707–9. DOI: 10.1016/j.jaad.2008.11.896.

[25] Galmés-Truyols A, Giménez-Duran J, Bosch-Isabel C, Nicolau-Riutort A, Vanrell-Berga J, Portell-Arbona M, Seguí-Prat B, Gumá-Torá M, Martí-Alomar I, Rojo-Arias MÁ, Ruiz-Veramendi M. An outbreak of cutaneous infection due to *Mycobacterium abscessus* associated to mesotherapy. Enferm Infecc Microbiol Clin. 2011;29:510–4. DOI: 10.1016/j.eimc.2011.03.006.

[26] Regnier S, Cambau E, Meningaud JP, Guihot A, Deforges L, Carbonne A, Bricaire F, Caumes E. Clinical management of rapidly growing mycobacterial cutaneous infections in patients after mesotherapy. Clin Infect Dis. 2009;49:1358–64. DOI: 10.1086/606050.

[27] Rivera-Olivero IA, Guevara A, Escalona A, Oliver M, Pérez-Alfonzo R, Piquero J, Zerpa O, de Waard JH. Soft-tissue infections due to non-tuberculous mycobacteria following mesotherapy. What is the price of beauty. Enferm Infecc Microbiol Clin. 2006;24:302–6.

[28] Kadry R, Hamadah I, Al-Issa A, Field L, Alrabiah F. Multifocal scalp abscess with subcutaneous fat necrosis and scarring alopecia as a complication of scalp mesotherapy. J Drugs Dermatol. 2008;7:72–3.

[29] Gungor S, Kocaturk E, Topal IO. Frontal edema due to topical application of %5 minoxidil solution following mesotherapy injections. Int J Trichology. 2015;7:86–7. DOI: 10.4103/0974-7753.160124.

[30] Abdallah M, El-Zawahry K, Besar H. Mesotherapy using dutasteride-containing solution in male pattern hair loss: a controlled pilot study. PALD. 2009;20:137–45.

[31] Sobhy N, Aly H, Shafee AE, Deeb MA. Evaluation of the effect of injection of dutasteride as mesotherapeutic tool in treatment of androgenetic alopecia in males. Our Dermatol Online. 2013;4:40–5.

[32] Ozdogan S, Erdal M, Oktar FD, Tan S. Hair mesotherapy in treatment of alopecia. J Clin Analytic Med. 2011;2:5–8.

[33] Azam MH, Morsi HM. Comparative study between 2% minoxidil topical spray vs. intradermal injection (mesotherapy) for treatment of androgenetic alopecia in female patients: a controlled, 4-month randomized trial. EDOJ. 2010;6:1–12.

[34] Freund BJ, Schwartz M. Treatment of male pattern baldness with botulinum toxin: a pilot study. Plast Reconstr Surg. 2010;126:246–8.

[35] van Zuuren EJ, Fedorowicz Z, Schoones J. Interventions for female pattern hair loss. Cochrane Database Syst Rev. 2016;5:CD007628. DOI: 10.1002/14651858.

[36] Doddaballapur S. Microneedling with dermaroller. J Cutan Aesthet Surg. 2009;2:110–1. DOI: 10.4103/0974-2077.58529.

[37] McCrudden MT, McAlister E, Courtenay AJ, González-Vázquez P, Singh TR, Donnelly RF. Microneedle applications in improving skin appearance. Exp Dermatol. 2015;24:561–6. DOI: 10.1111/exd.12723.

[38] Dhurat R, Sukesh M, Avhad G, Dandale A, Pal A, Pund P. A randomized evaluator blinded study of effect of microneedling in androgenetic alopecia: a pilot study. Int J Trichology. 2013;5:6–11. DOI: 10.4103/0974-7753.114700.

[39] Kim BJ, Lim YY, Kim HM, Lee YW, Won CH, Huh CH, Kang H. Hair follicle regeneration in mice after wounding by microneedle roller. Int J Trichology. 2012;4:117–30.

[40] Chandrashekar B, Yepuri V, Mysore V. Alopecia areata-successful outcome with microneedling and triamcinolone acetonide. J Cutan Aesthet Surg. 2014;7:63–4. DOI: 10.4103/0974-2077.129989.

[41] Jeong K, Lee YJ, Kim JE, Park YM, Kim BJ, Kang H. Repeated microneedle stimulation induce the enhanced expression of hair-growth-related genes. Int J Trichology. 2012;4:117–30.

[42] Lee YB, Eun YS, Lee JH, Cheon MS, Park YG, Cho BK, Park HJ. Effects of topical application of growth factors followed by microneedle therapy in women with female pattern hair loss: a pilot study. J Dermatol. 2013;40:81–3. DOI: 10.1111/j.1346-8138.2012.01680.

[43] Deepak SH, Shwetha S. Scalp roller therapy in resistant alopecia areata. J Cutan Aesthet Surg. 2014;7:61–2. DOI: 10.4103/0974-2077.129988.

[44] Dhurat R, Mathapati S. Response to microneedling treatment in men with androgenetic alopecia who failed to respond to conventional therapy. Indian J Dermatol. 2015;60:260–3. DOI: 10.4103/0019-5154.156361.

[45] Yoo KH, Lee JW, Li K, Kim BJ, Kim MN. Photodynamic therapy with methyl 5-aminolevulinate acid might be ineffective in recalcitrant alopecia totalis regardless of using a microneedle roller to increase skin penetration. Dermatol Surg. 2010;36:618–22. DOI: 10.1111/j.1524-4725.2010.01515.

[46] Lee JW, Yoo KH, Kim BJ, Kim MN. Photodynamic therapy with methyl 5-aminolevulinate acid combined with microneedle treatment in patients with extensive alopecia areata. Clin Exp Dermatol. 2010;35:548–9. DOI: 10.1111/j.1365-2230.2009.03695.x.

[47] Stoll S, Dietlin C, Nett-Mettler CS. Microneedling as a successful treatment for alopecia X in two Pomeranian siblings. Vet Dermatol. 2015;26:387–90, e88. DOI: 10.1111/vde.12236.

[48] Jeong KH, Joo HJ, Kim JE, Park YM, Kang H. Effect of mycophenolic acid on proliferation of dermal papilla cells and induction of anagen hair follicles. Clin Exp Dermatol. 2015;40:894–902. DOI: 10.1111/ced.12650.

[49] Foster TE, Puskas BL, Mandelbaum BR, Gerhardt MB, Rodeo SA. Platelet-rich plasma: from basic science to clinical applications. Am J Sports Med. 2009;37:2259–72. DOI: 10.1177/0363546509349921.

[50] Nachman RL, Rafii S. Platelets, petechiae, and preservation of the vascular wall. N Engl J Med. 2008;359:1261–70. DOI: 10.1056/NEJMra0800887.

[51] Jurk K, Kehrel BE. Platelets: physiology and biochemistry. Semin Thromb Hemost. 2005;31:381–92.

[52] Rendu F, Brohard-Bohn B. The platelet release reaction: granules' constituents, secretion and functions. Platelets. 2001;12:261–73.

[53] Arshdeep, Kumaran MS. Platelet-rich plasma in dermatology: boon or a bane? Indian J Dermatol Venereol Leprol. 2014;80:5–14. DOI: 10.4103/0378-6323.125467.

[54] Sánchez-González DJ, Méndez-Bolaina E, Trejo-Bahena NI. Platelet-rich plasma peptides: key for regeneration. Int J Pept. 2012;2012:532519. DOI: 10.1155/2012/532519.

[55] Dohan Ehrenfest DM, Rasmusson L, Albrektsson T. Classification of platelet concentrates: from pure platelet-rich plasma (P-PRP) to leucocyte- and platelet-rich fibrin (L-PRF). Trends Biotechnol. 2009;27:158–67.

[56] Giusti I, Rughetti A, D'Ascenzo S, Millimaggi D, Pavan A, Dell'Orso L, Dolo V. Identification of an optimal concentration of platelet gel for promoting angiogenesis in human endothelial cells. Transfusion. 2009;49:771–78. DOI: 10.1111/j.1537-2995.2008.02033.x.

[57] Leo MS, Kumar AS, Kirit R, Konathan R, Sivamani RK. Systematic review of the use of platelet-rich plasma in aesthetic dermatology. J Cosmet Dermatol. 2015;14:315–23. DOI: 10.1111/jocd.12167.

[58] Liu Y, Kalén A, Risto O, Wahlström O. Fibroblast proliferation due to exposure to a platelet concentrate in vitro is pH dependent. Wound Repair Regen. 2002;10:336–40.

[59] Cho JW, Kim SA, Lee KS. Platelet-rich plasma induces increased expression of G1 cell cycle regulators, type I collagen, and matrix metalloproteinase-1 in human skin fibroblasts. Int J Mol Med. 2012;29:32–6. DOI: 10.3892/ijmm.2011.803.

[60] Kushida S, Kakudo N, Suzuki K, Kusumoto K. Effects of platelet-rich plasma on proliferation and myofibroblastic differentiation in human dermal fibroblasts. Ann Plast Surg. 2013;71:219–24. DOI: 10.1097/SAP.0b013e31823cd7a4.

[61] Dhurat R, Sukesh M. Principles and methods of preparation of platelet-rich plasma: a review and author's perspective. J Cutan Aesthet Surg. 2014;7:189–97. DOI: 10.4103/0974-2077.150734.

[62] Marx RE. Platelet-rich plasma (PRP): what is PRP and what is not PRP? Implant Dent. 2001;10:225–8.

[63] Fufa D, Shealy B, Jacobson M, Kevy S, Murray MM. Activation of platelet-rich plasma using soluble type I collagen. J Oral Maxillofac Surg. 2008;66:684–90. DOI: 10.1016/j.joms.2007.06.635.

[64] Lynch MD, Bashir S. Applications of platelet-rich plasma in dermatology: a critical appraisal of the literature. J Dermatolog Treat. 2016;27:285–9. DOI: 10.3109/09546634.2015.1094178.

[65] Sarıcaoglu H, Gunay IT. Platelet rich plasma applications. Turkiye Klinikleri J Cosm Dermatol-Special Topics. 2012;5:34–7.

[66] Kaliyadan F, Nambiar A, Vijayaraghavan S. Androgenetic alopecia: an update. Indian J Dermatol Venereol Leprol. 2013;79:613–25. DOI: 10.4103/0378-6323.116730.

[67] Gupta AK, Carviel JL. Meta-analysis of efficacy of platelet-rich plasma therapy for androgenetic alopecia. J Dermatolog Treat. 2016;6:1–4.

[68] Li ZJ, Choi HI, Choi DK, Sohn KC, Im M, Seo YJ, Lee YH, Lee JH, Lee Y. Autologous platelet-rich plasma: a potential therapeutic tool for promoting hair growth. Dermatol Surg. 2012;38:1040–6. DOI: 10.1111/j.1524-4725.2012.02394.

[69] Uebel CO, da Silva JB, Cantarelli D, Martins P. The role of platelet plasma growth factors in male pattern baldness surgery. Plast Reconstr Surg. 2006;118:1458–67.

[70] Alves R, Grimalt R. Randomized placebo-controlled, double-blind, half-head study to assess the efficacy of platelet-rich plasma on the treatment of androgenetic alopecia. Dermatol Surg. 2016;42:491–7. DOI: 10.1097/DSS.0000000000000665.

[71] Gentile P, Garcovich S, Bielli A, Scioli MG, Orlandi A, Cervelli V. The effect of platelet-rich plasma in hair regrowth: a randomized placebo-controlled trial. Stem Cells Transl Med. 2015;4:1317–23. DOI: 10.5966/sctm.2015-0107.

[72] Singhal P, Agarwal S, Dhot PS, Sayal SK. Efficacy of platelet-rich plasma in treatment of androgenic alopecia. Asian J Transfus Sci. 2015;9:159–62. DOI: 10.4103/0973-6247.162713.

[73] Park KY, Kim HK, Kim BJ, Kim MN. Letter: Platelet-rich plasma for treating male pattern baldness. Dermatol Surg. 2012;38:2042–4. DOI: 10.1111/dsu.12037.

[74] Gkini MA, Kouskoukis AE, Tripsianis G, Rigopoulos D, Kouskoukis K. Study of platelet-rich plasma injections in the treatment of androgenetic alopecia through an one-year period. J Cutan Aesthet Surg. 2014;7:213–9. DOI: 10.4103/0974-2077.150743.

[75] Takikawa M, Nakamura S, Nakamura S, Ishirara M, Kishimoto S, Sasaki K, Yanagibayashi S, Azuma R, Yamamoto N, Kiyosawa T. Enhanced effect of platelet-rich plasma containing a new carrier on hair growth. Dermatol Surg. 2011;37:1721–9. DOI: 10.1111/j.1524-4725.2011.02123.

[76] Kang JS, Zheng Z, Choi MJ, Lee SH, Kim DY, Cho SB. The effect of CD34+ cell-containing autologous platelet-rich plasma injection on pattern hair loss: a preliminary study. J Eur Acad Dermatol Venereol. 2014;28:72–9. DOI: 10.1111/jdv.12062.

[77] Hordinsky MK. Overview of alopecia areata. J Investig Dermatol Symp Proc. 2013;16:13–5. DOI: 10.1038/jidsymp.2013.4

[78] Gilhar A, Etzioni A, Paus R. Alopecia areata. N Engl J Med. 2012;366:1515–25. DOI: 10.1056/NEJMra1103442.

[79] Trink A, Sorbellini E, Bezzola P, Rodella L, Rezzani R, Ramot Y, Rinaldi F. A randomized, double-blind, placebo- and active-controlled, half-head study to evaluate the effects of platelet-rich plasma on alopecia areata. Br J Dermatol. 2013;169:690–4. DOI: 10.1111/bjd.12397.

[80] Alkhalifah A. Topical and intralesional therapies for alopecia areata. Dermatol Ther. 2011;24:355–63. DOI: 10.1111/j.1529-8019.2011.01419.

[81] El-Sharkawy H, Kantarci A, Deady J, Hasturk H, Liu H, Alshahat M, Van Dyke TE. Platelet-rich plasma: growth factors and pro- and anti-inflammatory properties. J Periodontol. 2007;78:661–9.

[82] Singh S. Role of platelet-rich plasma in chronic alopecia areata: our centre experience. Indian J Plast Surg. 2015;48:57–9. DOI: 10.4103/0970-0358.155271.

[83] Donovan J. Successful treatment of corticosteroid-resistant ophiasis-type alopecia areata (AA) with platelet-rich plasma (PRP). JAAD Case Rep. 2015;1:305–7. DOI: 10.1016/j.jdcr.2015.07.004.

[84] Waiz M, Saleh AZ, Hayani R, Jubory SO. Use of the pulsed infrared diode laser (904 nm) in the treatment of alopecia areata. J Cosmet Laser Ther. 2006;8:27–30.

[85] Avram MR, Leonard RT Jr, Epstein ES, Williams JL, Bauman AJ. The current role of laser/light sources in the treatment of male and female pattern hair loss. J Cosmet Laser Ther. 2007;9:27–8.

[86] Iorizzo M, Tosti A. Treatments options for alopecia. Expert Opin Pharmacother. 2015;16: 2343–54. DOI: 10.1517/14656566.2015.1084501.

[87] McElwee KJ, Shapiro JS. Promising therapies for treating and/or preventing androgenic alopecia. Skin Therapy Lett. 2012;17:1–4.

[88] Tsuboi R, Itami S, Inui S, Ueki R, Katsuoka K, Kurata S, Kono T, Saito N, Manabe M, Yamazaki M, Guidelines Planning Committee for the management of androgenetic alopecia. Guidelines for the management of androgenetic alopecia (2010). J Dermatol. 2012;39:113–20. DOI: 10.1111/j.1346-8138.2011.01361.x.

[89] Avram MR, Rogers NE. The use of low-level light for hair growth: part I. J Cosmet Laser Ther. 2009;11:110–7. DOI: 10.1080/14764170902842531.

[90] Shukla S, Sahu K, Verma Y, Rao KD, Dube A, Gupta PK. Effect of helium-neon laser irradiation on hair follicle growth cycle of Swiss albino mice. Skin Pharmacol Physiol. 2010;23:79–85. DOI: 10.1159/000265678.

[91] Karu T. Primary and secondary mechanisms of action of visible to near-IR radiation on cells. J Photochem Photobiol B. 1999;49:1–17.

[92] Grossman N, Schneid N, Reuveni H, Halevy S, Lubart R. 780 nm low power diode laser irradiation stimulates proliferation of keratinocyte cultures: involvement of reactive oxygen species. Lasers Surg Med. 1998;22:212–8.

[93] Pal G, Dutta A, Mitra K, Grace MS, Romanczyk TB, Wu X, Chakrabarti K, Anders J, Gorman E, Waynant RW, Tata DB. Effect of low intensity laser interaction with human skin fibroblast cells using fiber-optic nano-probes. J Photochem Photobiol B. 2007;86:252–61.

[94] Kim YG, Pak SC, Lee SR. Hairless mouse epidermal antioxidants and lipid peroxidation assessed by He-Ne laser. Lasers Surg Med. 2000;27(5):420–6.

[95] Bouzari N, Firooz AR. Lasers may induce terminal hair growth. Dermatol Surg. 2006;32:460.

[96] Alajlan A, Shapiro J, Rivers JK, MacDonald N, Wiggin J, Lui H. Paradoxical hypertrichosis after laser epilation. J Am Acad Dermatol. 2005;53:85–8.

[97] Moreno-Arias GA, Castelo-Branco C, Ferrando J. Side-effects after IPL photodepilation. Dermatol Surg. 2002;28:1131–4.

[98] Radmanesh M. Paradoxical hypertrichosis and terminal hair change after intense pulsed light hair removal therapy. J Dermatolog Treat. 2009;20:52–4. DOI: 10.1080/09546630802178224.

[99] Bernstein EF. Hair growth induced by diode laser treatment. Dermatol Surg. 2005; 31:584–6.

[100] Mester E, Szende B, Gärtner P. The effect of laser beams on the growth of hair in mice. Radiobiol Radiother. 1968;9:621–6.

[101] Lee GY, Lee SJ, Kim WS. The effect of a 1550 nm fractional erbium-glass laser in female pattern hair loss. J Eur Acad Dermatol Venereol. 2011;25:1450–4. DOI: 10.1111/j.1468-3083.2011.04183.

[102] Kim WS, Lee HI, Lee JW, Lim YY, Lee SJ, Kim BJ, Kim MN, Song KY, Park WS. Fractional photothermolysis laser treatment of male pattern hair loss. Dermatol Surg. 2011;37:41–51. DOI: 10.1111/j.1524-4725.2010.01833.

[103] Munck A, Gavazzoni MF, Trüeb RM. Use of low-level laser therapy as monotherapy or concomitant therapy for male and female androgenetic alopecia. Int J Trichology. 2014;6:45–9. DOI: 10.4103/0974-7753.138584.

[104] Leavitt M, Charles G, Heyman E, Michaels D. HairMax Laser Comb laser phototherapy device in the treatment of male androgenetic alopecia: a randomized, double-blind, sham device-controlled, multicentre trial. Clin Drug Investig. 2009;29:283–92. DOI: 10.2165/00044011-200929050-00001.

[105] Jimenez JJ, Wikramanayake TC, Bergfeld W, Hordinsky M, Hickman JG, Hamblin MR, Schachner LA. Efficacy and safety of a low-level laser device in the treatment of male and female pattern hair loss: a multicenter, randomized, sham device-controlled, double-blind study. Am J Clin Dermatol. 2014;15:115–27. DOI: 10.1007/s40257-013-0060-6.

[106] Brzezińska-Wcisło L, Bergler-Czop B, Wcisło-Dziadecka D, Lis-Święty A. New aspects of the treatment of alopecia areata. Postepy Dermatol Alergol. 2014;31:262–5. DOI: 10.5114/pdia.2014.40923.

[107] Tosti A, Duque-Estrada B. Treatment strategies for alopecia. Expert Opin Pharmacother. 2009;10:1017–26. DOI: 10.1517/14656560902876368.

[108] Gundogan C, Greve B, Raulin C. Treatment of alopecia areata with the 308-nm xenon chloride excimer laser: case report of two successful treatments with the excimer laser. Lasers Surg Med. 2004;34:86–90.

[109] Zakaria W, Passeron T, Ostovari N, Lacour JP, Ortonne JP. 308-nm excimer laser therapy in alopecia areata. J Am Acad Dermatol. 2004;51:837–8.

[110] Raulin C, Gundogan C, Greve B, Gebert S. Excimer laser therapy of alopecia areata--side-by-side evaluation of a representative area. J Dtsch Dermatol Ges. 2005;3:524–6.

[111] Al-Mutairi N. 308-nm excimer laser for the treatment of alopecia areata. Dermatol Surg. 2007;33:1483–7.

[112] Al-Mutairi N. 308-nm excimer laser for the treatment of alopecia areata in children. Pediatr Dermatol. 2009;26:547–50. DOI: 10.1111/j.1525-1470.2009.00980.x.

[113] Yoo KH, Kim MN, Kim BJ, Kim CW. Treatment of alopecia areata with fractional photothermolysis laser. Int J Dermatol. 2010;49:845–7. DOI: 10.1111/j.1365-4632.2009.04230.x.

[114] Cho S, Choi MJ, Zheng Z, Goo B, Kim DY, Cho SB. Clinical effects of non-ablative and ablative fractional lasers on various hair disorders: a case series of 17 patients. J Cosmet Laser Ther. 2013;15:74–9. DOI: 10.3109/14764172.2013.764436.

[115] Mokos ZB, Mosler EL. Advances in a rapidly emerging field of hair follicle stem cell research. Coll Antropol. 2014;38(1):373–8.

[116] Dong L, Hao H, Xia L, Liu J, Ti D, Tong C, Hou Q, Han Q, Zhao Y, Liu H, Fu X, Han W. Treatment of MSCs with Wnt1a-conditioned medium activates DP cells and promotes hair follicle regrowth. Sci Rep. 2014; 25;4:5432. DOI: 10.1038/srep05432.

[117] Zhang P, Kling RE, Ravuri SK, Kokai LE, Rubin JP, Chai JK, Marra KG. A review of adipocyte lineage cells and dermal papilla cells in hair follicle regeneration. J Tissue Eng. 2014; 27;5:2041731414556850. DOI: 10.1177/2041731414556850.

[118] Falto-Aizpurua L, Choudhary S, Tosti A. Emerging treatments in alopecia. Expert Opin Emerg Drugs. 2014;19(4):545–56. DOI: 10.1517/14728214.2014.974550. Epub 2014 Oct.

[119] Review. Erratum in: Expert Opin Emerg Drugs. 2015;20(2):347.

[120] Li Y, Yan B, Wang H, Li H, Li Q, Zhao D, Chen Y, Zhang Y, Li W, Zhang J, Wang S, Shen J, Li Y, Guindi E, Zhao Y. Hair regrowth in alopecia areata patients following Stem Cell Educator therapy. BMC Med. 2015; 20;13:87. DOI: 10.1186/s12916-015-0331-6.

[121] Marazzi M, Crovato F, Bucco M, Sironi MC, Tosca MC, Antonioli B, Chlapanidas T, Lucconi G, Rapisarda V, Scalise A, Vigo D, Faustini M, Torre ML. GMP-compliant culture of human hair follicle cells for encapsulation and transplantation. Cell Transplant. 2012;21(1):373–8. DOI: 10.3727/096368911X565010. Epub 2011 Mar 25.

[122] Toyoshima KE, Asakawa K, Ishibashi N, Toki H, Ogawa M, Hasegawa T, Irié T, Tachikawa T, Sato A, Takeda A, Tsuji T. Fully functional hair follicle regeneration through the rearrangement of stem cells and their niches. Nat Commun. 2012; 17;3:784. DOI: 10.1038/ncomms1784.

[123] Asakawa K, Toyoshima KE, Ishibashi N, Tobe H, Iwadate A, Kanayama T, Hasegawa T, Nakao K, Toki H, Noguchi S, Ogawa M, Sato A, Tsuji T. Hair organ regeneration via the bioengineered hair follicular unit transplantation. Sci Rep. 2012;2:424. DOI: 10.1038/srep00424. Epub 2012 May 28.

[124] Higgins CA, Richardson GD, Ferdinando D, Westgate GE, Jahoda CA. Modelling the hair follicle dermal papilla using spheroid cell cultures. Exp Dermatol. 2010;19(6):546–8. DOI: 10.1111/j.1600-0625.2009.01007.x.

[125] Balana ME, Charreau HE, Leirós GJ. Epidermal stem cells and skin tissue engineering in hair follicle regeneration. World J Stem Cells. 2015; 26;7(4):711–27. DOI: 10.4252/wjsc.v7.i4.711. Review.

[126] Tan T, Hu ZQ. Follicular cell implantation for induce hair follicle growth in nude mice. Nan Fang Yi Ke Da Xue Xue Bao. 2009;29(10):1987–9. Chinese.

[127] Qiao J, Zawadzka A, Philips E, Turetsky A, Batchelor S, Peacock J, Durrant S, Garlick D, Kemp P, Teumer J. Hair follicle neogenesis induced by cultured human scalp dermal papilla cells. Regen Med. 2009;4(5):667–76. DOI: 10.2217/rme.09.50.

[128] Leiros GJ, Kusinsky AG, Drago H, Bossi S, Sturla F, Castellanos ML, Stella IY, Balañá ME. Dermal papilla cells improve the wound healing process and generate hair bud-like structures in grafted skin substitutes using hair follicle stem cells. Stem Cells Transl Med. 2014;3:1209–19 [PMID: 25161315 DOI: 10.5966/sctm.2013-0217]

[129] Thangapazham RL, Klover P, Wang JA, et al. Dissociated human dermal papilla cells induce hair follicle neogenesis in grafted dermal-epidermal composites. J Invest Dermatol. 2014;134:538–40.

[130] Shin H, Ryu HH, Kwon O, Park BS, Jo SJ. Clinical use of conditioned media of adipose tissue-derived stem cells in female pattern hair loss: a retrospective case series study. Int J Dermatol. 2015;54(6):730–5. DOI: 10.1111/ijd.12650.

[131] Buonocore D, Nobile V, Michelotti A, Marzatico F. Clinical efficacy of a cosmetic treatment by Crescina(®) human follicle stem cell on healthy males with androgenetic alopecia. Dermatol Ther (Heidelb). 2013; 20;3(1):53–62. DOI: 10.1007/s13555-013-0021-2. Print 2013 Jun. Erratum in: Dermatol Ther (Heidelb). 2013;3(1):113.

[132] Fukuoka H, Suga H. Hair regeneration treatment using adipose-derived stem cell conditioned medium: follow-up with trichograms. Eplasty. 2015; 26;15:e10. eCollection 2015.

Chapter 19

Alternative Medicine for Hair Loss

Gurkan Yardimci

Additional information is available at the end of the chapter

http://dx.doi.org/10.5772/66593

Abstract

In recent years, people have begun to give further emphasis to the external beauty, especially for their hair. Except drugs with proven effectiveness, complementary and alternative treatment options that have not yet been clarified of their effectiveness and side effect profiles have been used for centuries. Many plants or their extracts are widely used to prevent hair loss and treat alopecia (e.g., androgenetic alopecia, alopecia areata, or traction alopecia) worldwide, especially in Far Eastern countries. The mechanisms of action of these plants are still unknown. Although there are little randomized-controlled studies investigating the effectiveness in the treatment of hair loss, reported results have demonstrated that complementary and alternative medicine will become much more popular in the near future.

Keywords: hair loss, complementary, alternative, medicine, herbal, acupuncture, hypnosis

1. Introduction

The social and sexual communication roles of hair as well as its protective function have absolutely undeniable for both sexes for many years [1, 2]. Although the loss of hair is not a life-threatening condition, the loss of hair at an early age or sudden onset hair loss may cause serious psychological distress, thus it may directly affect the quality of life negatively [1, 3]. For this reason, patients with suffering from hair loss should be considered finically in order to distinguish ordinary hair shedding from pathologic hair loss. A loss of 100 or less hair falling per day should not be considered as pathological hair loss. But in case of hair loss more than 100 per day, a pathological condition should be mentioned [3].

Hair loss is a common dermatological problem that has been estimated to affect between 0.2 and 2% of the world's population. There are several factors leading to hair loss including major physical-emotional stress, chemotherapy, genetic predisposition, dihydrotestosterone (DHT), excessive sebum, cardiovascular diseases, smoking, and endogenous substances [3]. The common hair diseases that dermatologists are often faced in daily practice are androgenetic alopecia (AGA), alopecia areata (AA), telogen effluvium, anagen effluvium, and traumatic alopecia such as trichotillomania and traction alopecia [1]. AGA, known as male pattern hair loss in men and as female pattern hair loss in women, is the most common form of hair loss in adults [1, 4, 5]. Approximately 60% of males between the ages 30 and 50 years and 17% of women under 50 years of age suffer from AGA [4]. The role of DHT which is reduced from testosterone by enzyme 5α-reductase is clearly known in the mechanism of AGA [6]. In early stage, the process begins with shortening of the anagen phase and continuous miniaturization of sensitive follicles [1]. During this process, terminal hairs are replaced by vellus hairs which are shorter, finer and nonpigmented in the frontal and vertex regions of the scalp [3, 4]. Year after year, permanent baldness occurs at the site of miniaturized hair [1]. AA is a common, chronic inflammatory disease that is characterized by non-scarring alopecic patches on the scalp. It affects approximately 2% of the United States (US) population [7, 8]. Although the mechanism of AA is exactly unknown, it is thought that a necessary secondary event or cofactor such as febrile illness, pregnancy, or a major life crisis in addition to genetic predisposition [8, 9]. Even though AA may regress spontaneously, the disease may remain stable or even may spread to the entire scalp (known as alopecia totalis) or body (known as alopecia universalis). Telogen effluvium is a disease that occurs as a result of passing of a portion of hair from anagen phase to telogen phase. It is characterized by diffuse hair shedding. While trichotillomania is an impulse control disorder, traction alopecia is association with patients' hairstyle. These two diseases that occur after recurrent and chronic trauma are frequently seen in females than males. Both of them can result with permanent scarring [9].

In recent years, complementary and alternative medicine (CAM) is becoming increasingly popular all over the world. In fact, CAM is still the only option to cure and treat some diseases in some regions of Africa, Asia, and South America [10]. Alternative medicine refers to the use of CAM in place of conventional medicine, while complementary medicine refers to the use of CAM along with conventional medicine [11]. According to The National Center for Complementary and Alternative Medicine (NCCAM) in the United States, CAM is defined as 'a group of diverse medical and health-care system, practices, and products that are not presently considered to be a part of conventional medicine' [12]. In some countries like Korea, oriental medicine has been officially approved and has gained support from legal system using the licensing system [13]. The number of visits to alternative care practitioners increased by about 1.5 times in 7 years (from 427 billion in 1990 to 629 billion in 1997) in the United States [14]. The National Health Interview Survey estimated that in 2007 alone, 38% of adults in the United States used CAM [15].

CAM is separated by NNCAM into four categories: alternative medical systems, biologically based therapies, manipulative and body-based therapies, and mind-body therapies. The details of these therapies are shown in **Table 1** [16]. In a survey study conducted in the United Kingdom (UK) in 2010, the most popular CAM therapies were reported as acupuncture, hypnotherapy, and chiropractic, while the least preferred CAM were noted as aromatherapy, reflexology, and medical herbalism [17]. The annual expenditure on CAM is about \$30 billion in the United States and £1.6 billion in the UK [18, 19].

Alternative medical system	Acupuncture
	Ayurveda
	Homeopathy
	Naturopathy
Biologically based therapies	Chelation
	Folk medicine
	Nonvitamin nonmineral natural products
	Diet-based therapies
	Megavitamin therapy
Manipulative and body-based therapies	Chiropractic care
	Massage
Mind-body therapies	Biofeedback
	Relaxation techniques
	Hypnosis
	Yoga
	Tai Chi
	Qi Gong
	Healing rituals
	Energy healing
	Reiki

Table 1. Various treatments used in complementary and alternative medicine.

Similarly, using of CAM is quite often among patients suffering from dermatologic disorders such as acne, atopic dermatitis, psoriasis, dermatophytes, actinic keratosis, vitiligo, hair loss, cosmetic indications, melanoma, and lupus erythematosus [20–27]. A survey data from UK indicated that 35–69% of patients who have various skin diseases have used CAM in their lifetime [27]. The prevalence of CAM use by dermatology patients were 25.7 and 41% in Singapore [28] and Taiwan [29], respectively, while it ranges from 33.5 [30] to 43.7% in Turkey [31]. As the most frequently complementary medicines used by patients to treat their dermatological diseases have been reported as homeopathy, herbalism, diets, and food supplements in the UK [19, 27], the most used types of CAM have been recorded as herbal remedies, special diet, and megavitamin in Taiwan [29]. In one study, positive feedbacks from patients using CAM, especially herbal therapies, were noteworthy for both skin-related and non-skin-related conditions. Approximately 85% of patients with skin-related conditions, many of those with chronic diseases such as acne and eczema, noted improvement with CAM use [32]. To treat hair loss, the first two groups shown in **Table 1** are more preferred than the others.

Ideal treatment of hair loss should include the drugs that have both 5α-reductase inhibition effect and hair growth promoter substances, together. The most used conventional treatments are topical minoxidil, finasteride, dutasteride, combination of cyproterone acetate and estrogen, spironolactone, flutamide, topical progesterone, cimetidine, zinc sulfate, topical niacin, topical aminexil, topical ketoconazole, and cyclosporine-A [2]. In particular, minoxidil and finasteride are widely used for treating hair loss. But adverse effects of all of these agents have limited to their usage [1, 2]. Hence, patients suffer from hair loss have begun to turn to alternative therapies, even though there is little scientific evidence to prove their effectiveness.

2. Complementary and alternative medicines for hair loss

2.1. Herbal drugs

Herbal medicine is extremely popular since ancient times in Ayurveda, Siddha, Chinese, and Unani systems of medicine [3, 33]. Many plants and/or their extracts have been used to prevent hair loss and treat alopecia. These plants and their properties are summarized in **Table 2.**

2.1.1. *Thuja orientalis*

Thuja orientalis (T. orientalis, family *Cupressaceae)*, also known as *T. occidentalis* in Eastern or Arbor vitae or white cedar, is a plant that is widely distributed in East Asia [34, 35]. In addition to grown as an ornamental tree in Europe, it has been used to treat various diseases concerning respiratory system, skin disorders, and urinary system. Nowadays, it is often used in homeopathy and evidence-based phytotherapy [35]. It has also been traditionally used to promote hair growth in the oriental medicine. Although *T. orientalis* has a strong 5α-reductase inhibitor effect, the exact mechanism of hair-promoting effect of *T. orientalis* is still unknown. In the literature, there are few studies investigating the association between *T. orientalis* and hair growth. In animal studies, it was demonstrated that topically application of *T. orientalis* extract induced an earlier anagen phase and prolonged the mature anagen phase. In immunohistochemistry analysis, it was also shown that the expression levels of β-catenin and sonic hedgehog (Shh) were upregulated in *T. orientalis* extract-treated group at 14 days, compared to those in the control or 1% minoxidil-treated group. In mice treated with *T. orientalis*, authors observed an increase in both the number and size of hair follicles [34, 36]. Even, cubosomal suspension of *T. orientalis* extract was found to be more effective due to increased skin penetration of the *T. orientalis* [37].

2.1.2. *Citrullus colocynthis*

Citrullus colocynthis (C. colocynthis) Shrad (family *Cucurbitaceae)*, known as *Indrayan*, is one of the numerous herbal drugs recommended by the traditional system of medicine for hair growth promotion in India [38, 39]. It contains β-sitosterol, campesterol, stigmasterol, α-spinasterol, and cucurbitacin glycosides. It has several pharmacological effects such as immunostimulating, antiandrogenic, antibacterial, and hypoglycaemic in addition to hair-promoting effect [39]. There are few animal studies evaluating hair growth-promoting activities of the *C. colocynthis*. Roy et al. reported that topical application of *C. colocynthis* plant, especially petroleum ether extracts, had an astonishing effect on hair growth initiation time, complete hair growth,

http://dx.doi.org/10.5772/66593

Botanical name	Family	Possible mechanisms of action
Thuja orientalis	*Cupressaceae*	Inhibition of 5α-reductase enzyme
Citrullus colocynthis	*Cucurbitaceae*	Antiandrogenic effect
Rosmarinus officinalis	*Lamiaceae*	Increasing the circulation of the scalp
Camellia sinensis	*Theaceae*	Inhibition of 5α-reductase enzyme
Asiasari radix	*Aristolochiaceae*	Inducing early telogen-to-anagen conversion
Allium cepa L.	*Liliaceae*	Unknown
Polygonum multiflorum	*Polygonaceae*	Proliferation of dermal papilla cells, expression of FGF-7, up-regulating Shh and β-catenin expression
Allium tuberosum Rottler ex Spreng	*Liliaceae*	Stimulating expression of IGF-1
Cucurbita pepo	*Cucurbitaceae*	Inhibition of 5α-reductase enzyme
Serenoa repens	*Arecaceae*	Inhibition of 5α-reductase enzyme, decreasing DHT uptake by hair follicle, decreasing the binding of DHT to androgenetic receptors
Panax ginseng C.A. Meyer	*Araliaceae*	Expression of VEGF, antiapoptotic activity
Eclipta alba	*Asteraceae*	Anagen phase induction, reducing level of TGF-β1
Zizyphus jujuba	*Rhamnaceae*	Unknown
Allium sativum	*Liliaceae*	Unknown
Avicennia marina	*Acanthaceae*	Inhibition of 5α-reductase enzyme
Phyllanthus niruri	*Euphorbiaceae*	Inhibition of 5α-reductase enzyme
Oryza sativa		Inhibition of 5α-reductase enzyme
Sophora flavescens Aiton	*Leguminosae*	Inhibition of 5α-reductase enzyme, vasodilator and antiandrogen effects
Chrysanthemum zawadskii var. latilobum	*Asteraceae*	Anti-inflammatory effect
Scutellaria baicalensis	*Lamiaceae*	Inhibiting nuclear translocation of the androgen receptor, enhance proliferation of human dermal papilla cells
Cuscuta reflexa Roxb	*Convulvulaceae*	Inhibition of 5α-reductase enzyme
Pueraria thomsonii	*Leguminosae*	Inhibition of 5α-reductase enzyme
Curcuma aeruginosa	*Zingiberaceae*	Inhibition of 5α-reductase enzyme
Hura crepitans	*Euphorbiaceae*	Inhibition the neurotrophin (NT)-4 activation
Tobacco leaves	*Solanaceae*	Inhibition of 5α-reductase enzyme
Tectona grandis Linn	*Verbinaceae*	Unknown
Boehmeria nipononivea	*Urticaceae*	Inhibition of 5α-reductase enzyme

Table 2. Some plants used for hair loss and their properties.

and the length of hair follicle in albino rats. In qualitative studies, hair growth was initiated in the denuded area on the 4th day and 5th day with 5 and 2% ointment of petroleum ether extract of *C. colocynthis*, respectively. But, hair growth initiation was noted on the 6th day and the second week in minoxidil-treated standard group and in control group, respectively. Complete hair growth was recorded on the 16th, 18th, 19th, and 24th days in the 5% petroleum ether extract group, 2% petroleum ether extract group, minoxidil group, and control group, respectively. In quantitative studies, at 30 days after treatments with extracts of *C. colocynthis*, anagenic population were recorded as 67 and 47% in the minoxidil group and control group, whereas it was noted as 75 and 72% in the 5 and 2% petroleum ether extract groups, respectively. In both 2 and 5% petroleum ether extract groups, approximately 50% of hair population had length of 0.5 mm and above at 30 days after treatment [38]. In another study, Dhanotia et al. evaluated the hair growth-promoting activities of the petroleum ether extract from the fruit of *C. colocynthis* on albino mice using a testosterone-induced alopecia model. As a result of both qualitative and quantitative studies on hair growth, they suggested to present the inhibition of androgenic activity and altered anagen/telogen ratio and follicular density [39]. Polyherbal formulation including *C. colocynthis* was also shown to present hair growth-promoting activity on rats. Hair growth initiation time was markedly reduced to one-third on treatment with the prepared formulation compared to control group. The time required for complete hair growth was also reduced by 32%. Quantitative analysis of hair growth cycle after treatment with formulations and 2% minoxidil solution (positive control group) exhibited greater number of hair follicles in anagenic phase compared with control [40].

2.1.3. *Rosmarinus officinalis*

Rosmarinus officinalis (R. officinalis), commonly known as Rosemary, is a plant that belongs to family *Lamiaceae* and naturally grows in all Mediterranean countries [41, 42]. It has antiandrogenic effect and hair growth-promoting activity apart from antioxidative, anti-inflammatory, antibacterial, and antitumor effects [43]. In CAM, *R. officinalis* is often used in aromatherapy to treat anxiety-related conditions and increase alertness, although it has occasionally been used to stimulate hair growth [41]. The exact mechanism of hair growth is still unclear, but it is believed to act by increasing the circulation of the scalp. Murata et al. showed that topical administration of *R. officinalis* extracts solution (2 mg/day/mouse) improved hair regrowth in the testosterone-treated C57BL/6NCrSIc mice. They also showed significant promotion of hair growth after 16 days of topical administration. Among the some constituents of *R. officinalis* [i.e., rosmarinic acid, ursolic acid, 12-methoxycarnosic acid (12-MCA)], it was demonstrated that inhibitory activity of 12-MCA on 5α-reductase was higher than rosmarinic acid and ursalic acid (82.4, 14.2, and 2.5% inhibition at 200 μg/ml, respectively) [43].

2.1.4. Green tea

Green tea (*Camellia sinensis*, family *Theaceae*) is a well-known plant since ancient times, especially in China. It has been regarded to possess numerous pharmacological effects such as antimetastatic, anticancer, hepatoprotective, antidiabetic, antiobesity, anti-atherosclerotic, antibacterial, antiviral, anti-inflammatory, and antioxidant effects. It has been preferred in various dermatological diseases due to its mentioned beneficial effects worldwide. Human papilloma virus (HPV)-induced cervical cancer, genital warts, acne, rosacea, wound healing, atopic dermatitis, and keloids are diseases that green tea is commonly used. Apart from these diseases, it can be used to prevent or treat AGA by selectively inhibiting 5α-reductase activity. Catechins, a group of very active flavonoids, are a major component of green tea representing 60–80% of all polyphenols [44, 45]. There are four major catechins in green tea: epigallocatechin-3-gallate (ECGC), epigallocatechin (EGC), epicatechin gallate, and epicatechin [46, 47]. ECGC is the most highly bioactive catechin among these constituents [45]. In a study, EGCG was found to cause significant human hair follicle elongation ex vivo. Indeed, it was also shown proliferative and antiapoptotic effects of ECGC on dermal papilla cells through the upregulations of phosphorylated *Erk* and *Akt* and by an increase in the ratio of Bcl-2/Bax ratio [48]. Esfandiari et al. also reported that 33% of the mice that received 50% fraction of polyphenol extract from dehydrated green tea in their drinking water had significant hair regrowth within a period of 6 months compared with control group received regular drinking water [49].

2.1.5. *Asiasari radix*

Asiasari radix (A. radix, family *Aristolochiaceae)* or the radix of *Asiasarum heterotropoides var. mandshuricum* F. Maekawa usually grows in Korea, Japan, and China. *A. radix* is also called as *'seshin'* in Korea, as *'saishin'* in Japan, or Chinese wild ginger in English [50, 51]. It is used to treat various oral mucosal diseases such as aphthous stomatitis, gingivitis, local pain, and toothache apart from hair loss. A study from Korea showed its potent hair growth effect in mice. Though *A. radix* had not inhibitory effect on 5α-reductase enzyme, authors suggested that the extract of the plants induced early telogen-to-anagen conversion. They also demonstrated expression of vascular endothelial growth factor (VEGF) in human dermal papilla cells cultured in vitro [52].

2.1.6. *Allium cepa L*

Onion juice (*Allium cepa* L., family *Liliaceae)* may be used in patients with AA because of garlic-like activity. Both herbal medicines have similar chemical constituents, especially *Allicin*. The exact mechanism of onion juice in the treatment of AA is still unknown [53, 54]. In the study by *Sharquie and Al-Obaidi*, at 4 and 6 weeks after topical application of onion juice twice a day, hair regrowth was observed as 73.9 and 86.9% of patients with AA, respectively. Patients should be informed about skin irritation on the skin surface in contact with the onion juice [53].

2.1.7. *Polygonum multiflorum*

Polygonum multiflorum (*P. multiflorum,* family *Polygonaceae*) is a very popular plant that has been widely used to treat various diseases in traditional Chinese medicine due to its different pharmacological effects such as antiaging, immunomodulating, antihyperlipidemia, hepatoprotective, anticancer, and anti-inflammatory. Besides these pharmacological effects, some studies have been reported related to hair growth promotion activity and hair-blacking effect [55, 56]. An active component of *P. multiflorum,* known as 2,3,5,4′-tetrahydroxystilbene-2-O-β-D-glucoside (THSG), has melanogenesis-stimulating effect in melanocytes [55]. A new compound isolated from *P. multiflorum*, known as torachrysone-8-O-β-D-glucoside, induces a strong increase in the proliferation of dermal papilla cells and significantly increases the hair-fiber length of rat vibrissa follicles [57]. Li et al. investigated hair growth promotion activities and their possible mechanism of *P. multiflorum* Radix (PMR) and *P. multiflorum* Radix Preparata (PMRP), both of them originated from *P. multiflorum*, in C57BL/6J mice. While hair covered skin ratio was higher in oral PMR groups than in PMRP groups, hair covered skin ratio was lower in topical PMR groups compared with topical PMRP groups. It was also demonstrated that the most possible cytokines regarding hair growth-promoting activity were fibroblast growth factor-7 (FGF-7) and Shh [58]. Another animal study suggested that anagen phase was induced in resting hair follicles through upregulating Shh and β-catenin expression after topical application of *P. multiflorum* [55].

2.1.8. Allium tuberosum Rottler ex Spreng

Allium tuberosum Rottler ex Spreng (*ATRES*, family *Liliaceae*) is one of the Allium species like *Allium tuberosum* and *Allium cepa* L. It is widely distributed in East Asia and has been used for treating abdominal pain, diarrhea, hematemesis, and asthma in traditional medicine. Choline acetyltransferase activity of *ATRES* was also reported [54, 59]. In the first study, evaluating the hair growth-promoting activity and its mechanism of action, *ATRES* has strong hair-promoting activity through stimulating expression of insulin-like growth factor-1 (IGF-1). Especially, the n-butanol extract of *ATRES* was found to have most hair growth-promoting activity among the other compared groups including minoxidil, ethanol, n-hexane, distilled water groups on telogenic C57BL6/N mice [59].

2.1.9. Pumpkin seed oil

Pumpkin seed oil (PSO, family *Cucurbitaceae*) has been used for treating symptomatic benign prostatic hyperplasia through its inhibitory effect on 5α-reductase and antiandrogenic effect [60, 61]. In a randomized, double-blind, placebo-controlled study, self-rated improvement score, and self-rated satisfaction scores in the PSO-treated group were higher compared with the placebo group after oral administration of PSO at dosage of 400 mg/day for 24 weeks. At 24 weeks, mean hair count was recorded as increase of 40 and 10% in the PSO-treated group and placebo group, respectively. But, there was no significant difference in hair thickness between groups [60].

2.1.10. Serenoa repens

Serenoa repens (*S. repens*, family *Arecaceae*) is a native plant in West India and is grown in large quantities on the Atlantic southeast coast of North America. Saw palmetto is extracted from the berries of this plant. It is one of the herbal medicines that have inhibitory effect on both types 1 and 2 of 5α-reductase enzyme. In addition to inhibitory effect on 5α-reductase, *S. repens* may also decrease DHT uptake by hair follicle and decrease the binding of DHT to androgenetic receptors [62, 63]. Anti-inflammatory effect has been demonstrated with a composition containing saw palmetto, carnitine, and thioctic acid in hair follicle keratinocytes [64]. Both oral and topical use of *S. repens* could be effective for treating androgen-induced alopecia in both sexes [63]. In an open label study, 50 male patients with mild to moderate AGA were treated with *S. repens* 320 mg/day for 24 months. After this period, only 38% of patients had an increase in hair growth. But, this improvement was lower than the group treated with finasteride (68% of patients) [62]. Satisfactory results were also observed after application of topical products containing *S. repens* extract for 24 weeks in male patients with AGA [65]. Recommended dose is 320 mg/day orally [63]. Side effects of *S. repens* are minimal. The most known side effects are related to gastric symptoms, although contact dermatitis, feeling of coldness, mild burning sensation, undesirable smell, itching, and acne are the reported adverse events after topical application [63, 65, 66].

2.1.11. Ginseng

Ginseng (family *Araliaceae*) is traditionally used as an important herbal medicine in East Asian countries such as China, Korea, and Japan. It is divided into three categories: fresh ginseng, red ginseng, and white ginseng [67, 68]. Red ginseng is extracted from the steamed root of *Panax ginseng C.A.* Meyer, or known as Korean ginseng, and has various effects such as anti-aging, antidiabetic, immunoregulatory, anticancer, neuroregulation, lipid-regulating and antithrombotic activities, and wound- and ulcer-healing activity [68, 69]. In addition to these properties, it has also been used for treating numerous hair diseases such as AGA and AA due to its promoting hair growth activity [70, 71]. There are very important chemical constitutes such as polysaccharides, ginsenosides (or known as saphonins), alkaloids, glucosides, and phenolic acid in ginseng [68]. Ginsenosides are the major pharmacologically active ingredients of ginseng. To date, approximately 70 ginsenosides have been isolated from ginseng. In a study, it has been demonstrated that ginsenoside Rg3 had upregulated the expression of VEGF in human dermal papilla cells and mouse hair follicles [72]. Antiapoptotic activity of *fructus panax ginseng* was also shown in human dermal papilla cells [73].

2.1.12. Eclipta alba (L.) Hassk

Eclipta alba (L.) *Hassk.* (*E. alba*, family *Asteraceae*) is a medicinal plant commonly used for treating gastrointestinal disorders, respiratory tract disorders, fever, liver disorders, skin disorders, spleen enlargement, and cuts and wounds as well as hair loss and graying of hair. Numerous pharmacological activities including hepatoprotective, hair growth-promoting activity, antidiabetic, analgesic, anti-inflammatory, neuropharmacological activities, antioxidant, antimicrobial, antimalarial, cardiovascular effects, immunomodulatory, antiepilepsy, anticancer, antiulcer, and antihelmintic activities have been demonstrated. *E. alba* phytoconstituents including wedelolactone, eclalbasaponins, α-amyrin, oleanolic acid, ursolic acid, luteolin, and apigenin are responsible from main medicinal effects [74]. Hair growth-promoting activity has been investigated on animals. The methanol extract of *E. alba* has been tested for its efficacy for hair growth in pigmented C57/BL6 mice. While the transition of telogen phase to anagen phase of hair growth was observed in approximately 87.5% animals treated with 3.2 mg/15 cm^2 of methanol extract of *E. alba*, 50% of the animals treated with 1.6 mg/15 cm^2 of methanol extract of *E. alba* was observed transition from telogen phase to anagen phase of hair growth. The rate of anagen induction was dependent on concentration of methanol extract of *E. alba* [75]. The petroleum ether extract of *E. alba* was also investigated for its hair growth stimulatory effects in nude mice. This fraction of *E. alba* significantly reduced the levels of transforming growth factor-β1 (TGF-β1) expression during early anagen and anagen-catagen transition, so that authors suggested that the duration of terminal differentiation was extended [76]. Roy et al. also reported that the petroleum ether and ethanol extracts of *E. alba* (incorporated into ointment base in concentration of 2 and 5%, respectively) significantly reduced the time taken for hair growth initiation and completion in albino rats treated with the extracts [77].

2.1.13. *Zizyphus jujuba*

The plant, *Zizyphus jujuba* (*Z. jujuba*, family *Rhamnaceae*), is a widely distributed both in the Mediterranean regions and in the tropical and subtropical region of Asia and America. It can be used for several diseases such as diabetes, diarrhea, skin infections, liver complaints, urinary disorders, obesity, fever, pharyngitis, bronchitis, anemia, insomnia, and cancer [78]. There is no sufficient data related to its hair growth-promoting effect. In a study by Yoon et al., a greater effect on length of hair was reported in mice treated with 1 and 10% of *Z. jujuba* essential oil after 21 days of treatment as compared to control group. Although the length of hair was measured as 9.96 mm with 1% of oil and 10.02 mm with 10% of oil, respectively, the length of hair was measured as 8.94 mm in the control group [79].

2.1.14. *Allium sativum*

Allium sativum (family *Liliaceae*), known as garlic, is one of the most popular herbal medicine and can be used in the treatment of various dermatologic conditions such as psoriasis, AA, keloid scar, wound healing, cutaneous corn, viral and fungal infection, leishmaniasis, and skin-aging and rejuvenation. Constituents of garlic include enzymes (e.g., alliinase), sulfur-containing compounds (e.g., alliin), compounds produced enzymatically from alliin (e.g., allicin), arginine, oligosaccharides, flavanoids, and selenium [80]. In a double-blind randomized-controlled study, Hajheydari et al. reported that combination of topical garlic gel and betamethasone valerate cream was more effective than betamethasone valerate cream alone in patients with localized AA at the 3rd month. The number of total and terminal hairs in the group treated with garlic gel was significantly higher than those of the control group at the third months [81].

2.1.15. *Avicennia marina*

Avicennia marina (*A. marina*), also known as grey or white mangrove, is a traditional herbal plant belonging to family of *Acanthaceae*. However, it is traditionally used to treat various skin diseases in Egypt, antiandrogenic activity of *A. marina* and a compound, avicequinone C, isolated from the hearthwood of *A. marina* was firstly reported by Jain et al. [82. The results revealed that *A. marina* was a potent 5α-reductase type 1 inhibitor, reducing the 5α-DHT production by 52% at the final concentration of 10 μg/mL [82]. Moreover, among the thirty different extracts, the highest inhibitory activity was observed from the crude extract of *A. marina* at a final concentration of 10 g/ml through the reduction in 5α-DHT formation by more than 50% [83].

http://dx.doi.org/10.5772/66593

2.1.16. *Phyllanthus niruri*

Phyllanthus ninuri (*P. niruri*, family *Euphorbiaceae*) is a widely used plant of genus *Phyllanthus* in traditional medicine. It is also known as *'chanka piedra,' 'bhuiamlki,' 'zhuzicao,' 'dukung anak,' 'quebra-pedra,'* and *'chanca piedra.' P. niruri* usually grows in tropical and subtropical regions in Central and South American countries, India and East Asia and has several biologic activities such as antidiabetic, analgesic, wound healing, and immunomodulatory effects. It is traditionally used to cure of jaundice, fever, malaria, stomachache, urolithiasis, vaginal candidiasis, varicella, and tuberculosis by people living in these countries [84, 85]. Newly, inhibitory activity of petroleum ether extract of *P. niruri* on 5α-reductase type 2 enzyme was shown, and it has been suggested to be useful in the treatment testosterone-induced alopecia [85].

2.1.17. Rice bran

It has been believed that rice bran extract, which is produced by milled rice (*Oryza sativa*), has antioxidant, anticancer, and antihyperlipidemic effects as well as 5α-reductase inhibitory activity [86]. The compounds having antioxidant activity are phenolic acids, flavonoids, anthocyanins, proanthocyanidins, tocopherols, tocotrienols, γ-oryzanol, and phytic acid [87]. Very few studies exist to support the claims of the efficacy of rice bran. The hair growth-promoting activity of rice bran supercritical CO_2 extract (RB-SCE) and its two components (linoleic acid and γ-oryzanol) were shown using real-time reverse transcriptase-polymerase chain reaction in C57BL/6 mice by Choi et al. [86]. In a double-blinded randomized-controlled study, dermal application of 0.5% of RB-SCE (8 ml/day) to the head skin significantly increased hair density and hair diameter in male patients with alopecia for 16 weeks [88].

2.1.18. *Sophora flavescens Aiton*

Sophora flavescens Aiton (*S. flavescens*, family *Leguminosae*) is one of the important plants used in traditional Chinese medicine [89, 90]. It has been used for treating viral hepatitis, cancer, viral myocarditis, heat dysentery, hemafecia, jaundice, anuresis, leucorrhoea with reddish discharge, vulval swelling, pruritus vulvae, eczema, and trichomonas vaginalis [90, 91]. It is a strong inhibitor of 5α-reductase enzyme in addition to its vasodilatory and antiandrogen effects. Despite lack of proper clinical trials to support its efficacy for hair loss, the mechanism of affect on hair loss treatment is thought to be through these activities. It was demonstrated that the isolated two pterocarpans, L-maackiain and medicarpin, promoted the proliferation of human hair keratinocytes [89].

2.1.19. *Laminaria japonica*

Laminaria japonica (*L. japonica*) is a kind of brown algae and called as *'kombu'* in Japanese, *'dashima'* in Korean, and *'haidai'* in Chinese. The most consumed countries of *L. japonica* are Far Eastern countries such as Korea, Japan, and China. *L. japonica* is believed to have beneficial effects for health; however, the mechanism of beneficial effects is not fully understood [92, 93]. The combination of *L. japonica* extract and *Cistanche tubulusa* extract has the potential to promote hair growth. Oral administration of both *L. japonica* extract at dosage of 54 mg/kg and *Cistanche tubulusa* extract at dosage of 162 mg/kg exhibited an excellent hair regrowth activity on mice. It has been thought that anti-inflammatory activities of the both plant extracts could play an important role to prevent hair loss and improve alopecia [94].

2.1.20. Chrysanthemum zawadskii var. latilobum

Chrysanthemum zawadskii var. latilobum (*C. zawadskii*, family *Asteraceae*) has been used for the treatment of pneumonia, bronchitis, cough, common cold, pharyngitis, bladder-related disorders, gastrointestinal disorders, and hypertension in traditional medicine for ages. Essential oil of the plant contains 27 hydrocarbons, 12 alcohols, 7 ketones, 4 esters, 1 aldehyde, 1 amine, and 3 miscellaneous components [95, 96]. Although recent studies have expressed anti-inflammatory effect and protective effects from liver damage of *C. zawadskii*, there is little experimental evidence suggesting that the extract stimulates hair growth in humans and animals. In mice study, topical methanol extract of *C. zawadskii* was more effective compared to minoxidil-treated group. In the *C. zawadskii*-treated and minoxidil-treated groups, while the maximum hair scores in the first hair-growth generation were recorded as 2.5 ± 0.29 and 2.5 ± 0.28, hair coverage scores in the second hair-growth generation were noted as 2 ± 0.41 and 1.5 ± 0.29, respectively. Rapid hair loss seen in minoxidil-treated mice was not observed in *C. zawadskii*-treated group after the first hair growth generation [95].

2.1.21. Scutellaria baicalensis

Scutellaria baicalensis (*S. baicalensis*, family *Lamiaceae*), also known as *Huang Qin*, mostly grows in China, Japan, Korea, Mongolia, and Russia [97, 98]. *S. baicalensis* is likely to have hair growth-promoting effect by means of its active substances. It has been reported that the compound possessing this activity is an active flavonoid isolated from *S. baicalensis* named *'Baicalin'*. In recent years, it has also suggested that both the extract of *S. baicalensis* and baicalin inhibit nuclear translocation of the androgen receptor stimulated by DHT in human dermal papilla cells and enhance proliferation of human dermal papilla cells in vitro [98].

2.1.22. Cuscuta reflexa Roxb

Cuscuta reflexa Roxb. (*C. reflexa*, family *Convulvulaceae*) is a parasitic plant that is used as herbal medicine. It is also known as *'Tukhm-e-Kasoos (dodder),' 'Aftimoon,'* or *'Kasoos'* in Unani Tibbi, *'Akashabela,'* or *'Amarabela'* in Hindi, *'Swarnalata'* in Bengali, and *'Akakhilata'* in Assamese, in vernacular [99, 100]. It commonly grows on different host plants, mostly thorny herbs in all geographical regions of India [99, 101]. Many pharmacological activities such as relaxant and spasmolytic action, positive inotropic and cardiotonic activities, cholinergic action, anti-HIV, antioxidant, anti-steroidogenic, antibacterial, hepatoprotective, hypoglyceamic, diuretic, anti-convulsant, anti-inflammatory and anticancer activities as well as hair growth activity have been previously reported [100]. A number of experimental observations have indicated that *C. reflexa* has hair growth-promoting and 5α-reductase inhibitory activities. Hair growth was shown after treatment of the petroleum ether extract solution (250 mg/kg, orally) of *C. reflexa* and the ethanolic extract solution (250 mg/kg, orally) of *C. reflexa* in male albino rats with cyclophosphamide-induced alopecia at 19 days [99]. In another animal study by Pandit et al. suggested that petroleum ether extract of *C. reflexa* reversed androgen-induced alopecia by inhibiting conversion of testosterone to DHT [101]. Polyherbal formulation including *C. reflexa* was also shown to present hair growth-promoting activity on rats. Hair growth initiation time was markedly reduced to one-third on treatment with the prepared formulation compared to control group. The time required for complete hair growth was also reduced by 32%. Quantitative analysis of hair growth cycle after treatment with formulations and 2% minoxidil solution (positive control group) exhibited greater number of hair follicles in anagenic phase compared with control [40].

2.1.23. *Ishige sinicola*

Ishige sinicola (*I. sinicola*) is a brown alga that has antibacterial and anti-inflammatory effects against acne. In 2013, a study firstly demonstrated that *I. sinicola* extract and its component, octaphlorethol A, have the potential to promote hair growth via the proliferation of dermal papilla cells followed by the activation of β-catenin pathway, and the 5α-reductase inhibition [102].

2.1.24. *Grateloupia elliptica*

G. elliptica is the edible seaweed in some Asian countries. Although it is thought that potential anticancer activity, there is no enough evidence investigating the protective effect against hair loss and hair growth-stimulating effect of *G. elliptica* [103, 104]. Possible mechanisms including the proliferation of dermal papilla cells, inhibition of 5α-reductase enzyme, increase in prostaglandin E2 (PGE2) production, decrease in pro-inflammatory cytokine production, and inhibitory activity against *Pityrosporum ovale* (P. ovale) have been shown in the prevention of hair loss. A study showed that *G. elliptica* extract promoted the proliferation of dermal papilla cells by 169.5% at the concentration of 100 μg/ml compared with the vehicle-treated control group. The study also indicated that *G. elliptica* extract inhibited 5α-reductase enzyme and this activity increased with dosage [104].

2.1.25. *Puerariae flos*

Puerariae flos (the flowers of *Pueraria thomsonii*, family *Leguminosae*) extract (PF-ext) has inhibitory activity on testosterone 5α-reductase. The two major compounds, soyasaponin I and kaikasaponin III, are responsible for this inhibitory activity. In addition to inhibitory activity on testosterone 5α-reductase of both compounds, soyasaponin I possesses hepatoprotective, sialyltransferase inhibitory, and renin inhibitory activities, while kaikasaponin III possesses anti-hepatotoxic, hypoglycemic, hypolipidemic, and anti-herpes virus activities [105, 106]. Inhibitory activity of PF-ext on 5α-reductase is stronger than *Puerariae Radix* extract (PR-ext). In testosterone-sensitive male mice, hair regrowth was improved after the application of PF-ext solution in a dose-dependent manner via antiandrogenic activity. PF-ext can stimulate the induction of the hair cycle to anagen phase, but this mechanism has not been proven definitely [105].

2.1.26. *Curcuma aeruginosa*

Curcuma aeruginosa (*C. aeruginosa*, family *Zingiberaceae*) is a native plant of India and Southeast Asia. The rootstock of *C. aeruginosa* has long been used in traditional medicine for various indications such as dysmenorrhea, exanthemas and fungal infections. The oils derived from this plant consist of 1,8-cineole, curserenone, furanogermenone, camphor, (Z)-3-hexenol, zedoarol, furanodienone, curcumenol, isocurcumenol, β-alemene, curzerene, and germacrone, among others. *C. aeruginosa* hexane extract effects by inhibiting 5α-reductase activity, consecutively impairing the conversion of testosterone to DHT [107, 108]. Pumthong et al. investigated the effect of *C. aeruginosa* hexane extract on male-pattern baldness with a randomized, double-blind, placebo-controlled study. The study has shown that 5% hexane extract of *C. aeruginosa* especially combined with 5% minoxidil increased hair growth and decreased hair shedding [107].

2.1.27. *Hura crepitans*

Hura crepitans (*H. crepitans*, family *Euphorbiaceae*) has been used as a traditional medicine to treat some diseases such as Hansen's disease and syphilis in the Amazon region. A compound in *H. crepitans*, daphne factor F3, can play an effective role the mechanism of the hair growth. But, interestingly, the amount of daphne factor F3 is very important for hair growth. While *H. crepitans* from Peru possesses hair regrowth activity, *H. crepitans* from Brazil is not affect hair growth. Because, the daphne factor F3 content of *H. crepitans* from Peru is about 30 times more than *H. crepitans* from Brazil [109, 110]. It has been suggested that *H. crepitans* inhibits the retardation of hair regrowth by DHT through inhibition the neurotrophin (NT)-4 activation induced by DHT [109].

2.1.28. *Tobacco leaves*

Tobacco leaves (family *Solanaceae*) are used in traditional medicine for promoting of hair growth. The leaves also used to treat bronchitis, asthma, skin diseases, headache, etc. Alkaloid nicotine is the main constituent of tobacco leaves. Alkaloids such as nicotine, nicotianin, nicotinine, nicoteine, and nicoteline, which are the constituent parts of tobacco leaves, selectively inhibit 5α-reductase activity. The microbial bio transformed extract of tobacco leaves in cow urine has been investigated to treat AGA, and it has been found that it promotes hair growth at concentration dependent manner. The study confirms that 30% concentrated lotion treatment is at par with 2% minoxidil treatment in potentiating hair growth promotion in male albino Wister rats [111, 112].

2.1.29. *Tectona grandis Linn*

Tectona grandis Linn. (*T. grandis*, family *Verbinaceae*) (teak tree) has been used to cure many diseases in traditional Indian medicine. *T. grandis* is called as '*saka*' in Sanskrit, '*sagun*' in Hindi, '*sagwan*' in Marathi, and teak tree in English. It has also been used as a hypoglycaemic agent. According to the traditional Indian medicine, *T. grandis* roots are useful in anuria and urinary retention. The flowers have used to treat bronchitis, biliousness, and urinary discharge. The oil from the seeds is useful in scabies. The wood is used to relax and sedate the gravid uterus, heal headache and burning pains, cure liver problems, and even dysentery. *T. grandis* has been investigated in some studies for its anti-inflammatory and wound healing effects and is used as a topical treatment for burn wounds [113, 114]. Jaybhaye et al. investigated the effect of petroleum ether extract of *T. grandis Linn.* seeds on hair growth activity of albino mice. According to this study, topical application of the petroleum ether extract of *T. grandis* induced hair growth initiation and was superior to standard therapy with minoxidil 2% solution. The combination of the petroleum ether extract (5%) with 2% minoxidil has the strongest effect on hair growth initiation [113].

2.1.30. *Boehmeria nipononivea*

Boehmeria nipononivea (*B. nipononivea*, family *Urticaceae*) is a Japanese plant and the use of acetone extract derived from this plant has been investigated for treatment of androgen-dependent alopecia. One study indicates that the acetone extract of *B. nipononivea* has 5α-reductase inhibitory activity. The acetone extract derived from *B. nipononivea* was investigated on mice for its hair growth effect, and it resulted with a significant hair regrowth starting on 15th day and continues until 22th day. The 5α-reductase inhibitory activity of the acetone extract of *B. nipononivea* is attributed to fatty acids contains such as α-linolenic acid, palmitic acid, oleic acid, elaidic acid, and stearic acid. The study reveals that both the acetone extract of *B. nipononive* and three fatty acids (α-linolenic, elaidic, and stearic acids) have 5α-reductase activity and stimulates hair regrowth [115].

2.2. Acupuncture

Acupuncture is an ancient holistic system of Chinese medicine and has been practiced there so many years. China had the cultural and traditional exchange with its neighbors, and therefore, it spread to all over the world in time. Today, it is one of the most frequently used forms of complementary medicine [116].

Acupuncture aims to bring a complete cure, not only managing the outstanding symptom but to heal the whole body. Even though various acupuncture techniques are available, the fundamental techniques are needling, moxibustion, cupping, suction, and acupressure. Over the centuries, acupuncture has been used to treat a wide variety of diseases including skin disorders such as acne, alopecia, eczema and dermatitis, pruritus, pityriasis, psoriasis, rosacea, systemic lupus, urticaria, herpes zoster, chicken pox, impetigo, leprosy, and vitiligo. The exact mechanism of action of acupuncture treatment in skin disorders is not clear but investigations revealed that acupuncture stimulation effects on three key points: the hypothalamus-pituitary-adrenal axis, the autonomic nervous system, and brain-derived neurotrophic factor. There may be an increase on serum levels of cortisol by the effect of acupuncture. It has also been demonstrated by functional MRI that manual needle acupuncture distinctively activates the hypothalamus-limbic system [116].

Degranulation of mast cells significantly increases in autoimmune diseases such as AA and chronic inflammation. A mouse model for AA study has shown that severe mast cell degranulation and accumulation around the anagen hair follicle cause a self-attack of the hair follicle cells by migration of the inflammatory cells. This attack induces the hair matrix cell phase to the telogen phase that results with hair loss. Acupuncture treatment reduces T_1-cell attacks on hair bulb and activates blood circulation by warming the local collaterals; therefore, it may help to reduce hair loss. The same mouse study indicated that electro-acupuncture reduces mast cell degranulation in the dermis. It is reported that may be the cause of the pathological changes causing AA but reliable evidence is not yet available [117, 118].

Even though acupuncture treatment in dermatological diseases is safe and inexpensive, improperly performed acupuncture can cause potentially serious adverse effects such as vasovagal events, local infections, damage to internal organs, pneumothorax, spinal cord injury, and hepatitis B infection [116].

2.3. Hypnotherapy

The hypnotic phenomenon has been used over thousands of years, and it is a form of trance induction. Recently, the use of hypnotic therapy in somatic medicine has been supported by the British Medical Association in 1955 and the American Medical Association in 1958. A hypnotic trance can be described as an altered state of consciousness with "inward focus." It can be differed from other states of consciousness by electroencephalography (EEG) and imaging modalities. A hypnotic state can be induced by a therapist or an individual can induce hypnotic trace in himself or herself (self-hypnosis) [119, 120].

Hypnosis has been used for several indications such as induction of anesthesia or to heal irritable bowel syndrome and psychosomatic diseases as well as a variety of skin disorders including AA and trichotillomania. Nowadays, medical hypnosis is performed by physicians whom have received appropriate training in many countries all over the world. For some selected skin disorders, with proper training and selection of appropriate patients, medical hypnosis can relieve symptoms and in some cases can cure the illness [119, 120].

Hypnosis is a cost-effective and nontoxic therapy and can be used in dermatological treatment especially in patients with psychosomatic component [119, 120]. In a preliminary study, hypnotic sessions including relaxing suggestions and symptoms-oriented suggestions were held as a complementary or the only treatment once every 3 weeks in patients with severe AA, alopecia totalis, or alopecia universalis. Twelve of 21 patients showed significant improvement after 4–13 (mean 5.5) sessions of hypnosis, while treatment success could not be achieved in 9 patients. But also, minimal relapses were observed in all patients responded well [121]. In another prospective cohort study, it has been suggested that hypnosis had no significant contribution on hair regrowth in patients with refractory AA [122].

Despite confusing conclusions have been reported about the efficacy in the treatment of AA, hypnosis seems to be salubrious in the treatment of both children and adolescents with trichotillomania. Cohen et al. reported that complete resolution of their complaints was seen in two children after 7–8 weeks and in one child after 16 weeks. Even if just a recurrence was observed in one patient during follow-up, the patient completely recovered again with hypnotic retreatment [123]. *Iglesias A* observed that three pediatric cases completely disappeared to their trichotillomania behavior after 7 or less hypnotic sessions [124]. In addition to children, hair pulling was significantly reduced with imaginative techniques in adolescents with trichotillomania [125]. According to these results, hypnotherapeutic approach

http://dx.doi.org/10.5772/66593

can be considered as a quite effective and preferred option in both children and adolescents with trichotillomania.

3. Side effects

The side effects reported after CAM is often minimal. Contact dermatitis was reported with onion juice in patients with AA, thus patients should be informed about skin irritation on the skin surface in contact with the onion juice (**Figure 1**) [53]. *S. repens* that can be used as both orally and topically may cause undesirable adverse effects such as mild stomach discomfort, contact dermatitis, feeling of coldness, mild burning sensation, undesirable smell, itching, and acne [63, 65, 66]. Vasovagal events, local infections, damage to internal organs, pneumothorax, spinal cord injury, and hepatitis B infection are some of the side effects that can be encountered after acupuncture therapy [116]. Prurigo nodularis also reported on extremities of a patient shortly after acupuncture [126].

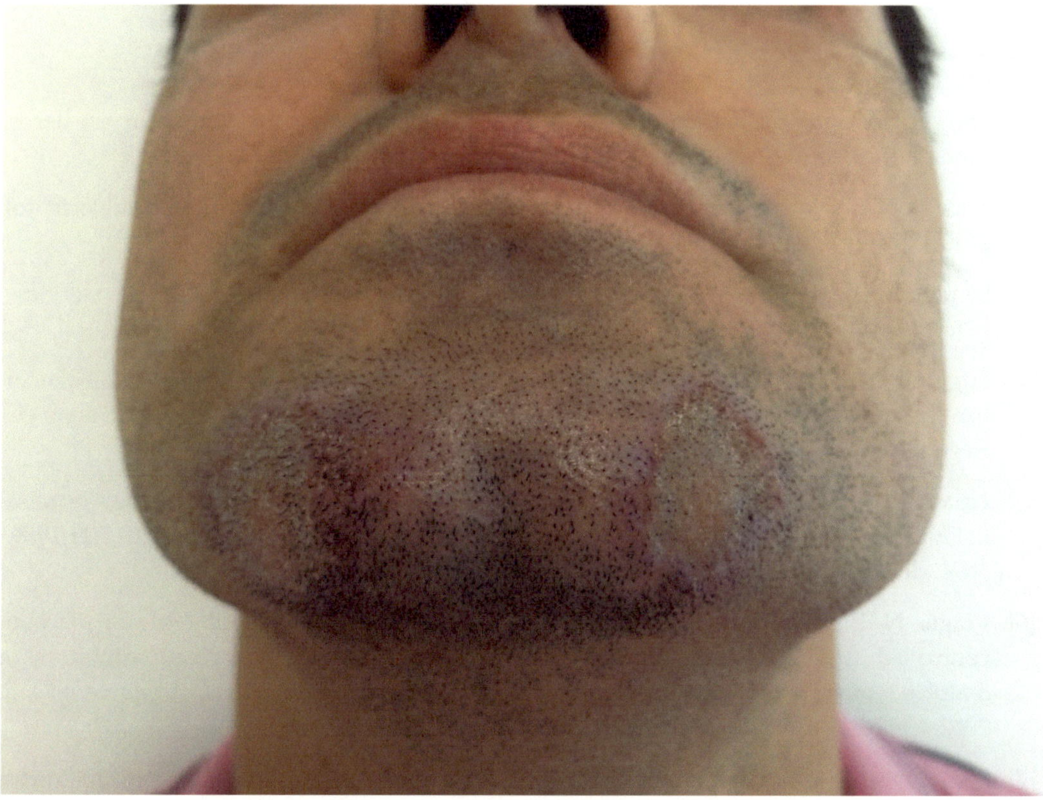

Figure 1. Contact dermatitis developed after topical application of onion and garlic on face of a patient with AA.

4. Conclusion

In recent years, although the increasingly widespread use of CAM, scientific data are still not enough. The observed results with herbal medicine are promising in the treatment of hair loss, especially AGA and AA. According to acceptable results, hypnosis may be an effective and safe alternative option in patients with hair loss, especially AA and trichotillomania. Even so, there is need for more scientific data proving its effectiveness and reliability.

Author details

Gurkan Yardimci

Address all correspondence to: dr.gurkanyardimci@gmail.com

Istanbul Medipol University Health Care Practice & Research Center Esenler Hospital, Istanbul, Turkey

References

[1] Patel S, Sharma V, Chauhan NS, Thakur M, Dixit VK. Hair growth: focus on herbal therapeutic agent. Curr Drug Discov Technol. 2015;**12**:21–42.

[2] Lourith N, Kanlayavattanakul M. Hair loss and herbs for treatment. J Cosmet Dermatol. 2013;**12**:210–222. doi:10.1111/jocd.12051

[3] Semalty M, Semalty A, Joshi GP, Rawat MS. Hair growth and rejuvenation: an overview. J Dermatolog Treat. 2011;**22**:123–132. doi:10.3109/09546630903578574

[4] Higgins CA, Christiano AM. Regenerative medicine and hair loss: how hair follicle culture has advanced our understanding of treatment options for androgenetic alopecia. Regen Med. 2014;**9**:101–111. doi:10.2217/rme.13.87

[5] Huang M, Zhou X. Appraisal of guidelines for androgenetic alopecia using the Appraisal of Guidelines for Research and Evaluation II instrument. J Eval Clin Pract. 2015;**21**:1089–1094. doi:10.1111/jep.12474

[6] Prager N, Bickett K, French N, Marcovici G. A randomized, double-blind, placebo-controlled trial to determine the effectiveness of botanically derived inhibitors of 5-alpha-reductase in the treatment of androgenetic alopecia. J Altern Complement Med. 2002;**8**:143–152. doi:10.1089/acm.2002.8.143

[7] Papadopoulos AJ, Schwartz RA, Janniger CK. Alopecia areata. Pathogenesis, diagnosis, and therapy. Am J Clin Dermatol. 2000;**1**:101–105.

[8] Meidan VM, Touitou E. Treatments for androgenetic alopecia and alopecia areata: current options and future prospects. Drugs. 2001;**61**:53–69.

[9] Harrison S, Sinclair R. Optimal management of hair loss (alopecia) in children. Am J Clin Dermatol. 2003;**4**:757–770.

[10] Barikani A, Beheshti A, Javadi M, Yasi M. Knowledge, attitude and practice of general practitioners toward complementary and alternative medicine: a cross-sectional study. Acta Med Iran. 2015;**53**:501–506.

[11] Kalaaji AN, Wahner-Roedler DL, Sood A, Chon TY, Loehrer LL, Cha SS et al. Use of complementary and alternative medicine by patients seen at the dermatology department of a tertiary care center. Complement Ther Clin Pract. 2012;**18**:49–53. doi:10.1016/j.ctcp.2011.05.003

[12] National Institutes of Health, National Center for Complementary and Alternative Medicine (NCCAM). Complementary, alternative, or integrative health: what's in a name? Available from: https://nccih.nih.gov/health/integrative-health. [Accessed November 14, 2014.]

[13] Kim GW, Park JM, Chin HW, Ko HC, Kim MB, Kim JY et al. Comparative analysis of the use of complementary and alternative medicine by Korean patients with androgenetic alopecia, atopic dermatitis and psoriasis. J Eur Acad Dermatol Venereol. 2013;**27**:827–835. doi:10.1111/j.1468-3083.2012.04583.x

[14] Neldner KH. Complementary and alternative medicine. Dermatol Clin. 2000;**18**:189–193.

[15] Landis ET, Davis SA, Feldman SR, Taylor S. Complementary and alternative medicine use in dermatology in the United States. J Altern Complement Med. 2014;**20**:392–398. doi:10.1089/acm.2013.0327

[16] Fuhrmann T, Smith N, Tausk F. Use of complementary and alternative medicine among adults with skin disease: updated results from a national survey. J Am Acad Dermatol. 2010;**63**:1000–1005. doi:10.1016/j.jaad.2009.12.009

[17] Perry R, Dowrick C, Ernst E. Complementary medicine and general practice in an urban setting: a decade on. Prim Health Care Res Dev. 2014;**15**:262–267. doi:10.1017/S1463423613000182

[18] Mainardi T, Kapoor S, Bielory L. Complementary and alternative medicine: herbs, phytochemicals and vitamins and their immunologic effects. J Allergy Clin Immunol. 2009;**123**:283–924. doi:10.1016/j.jaci.2008.12.023

[19] Baron SE, Goodwin RG, Nicolau N, Blackford S, Goulden V. Use of complementary medicine among outpatients with dermatologic conditions within Yorkshire and South Wales, United Kingdom. J Am Acad Dermatol. 2005;**52**:589–954. doi:10.1016/j.jaad.2004.11.058

[20] Malhi HK, Tu J, Riley TV, Kumarasinghe SP, Hammer KA. Tea tree oil gel for mild to moderate acne; a 12 week uncontrolled, open-label phase II pilot study. Australas J Dermatol. 2016 Mar 21. doi:10.1111/ajd.12465

[21] Goddard AL, Lio PA. Alternative, complementary, and forgotten remedies for atopic dermatitis. Evid Based Complement Alternat Med. 2015;**2015**:676897. doi:10.1155/2015/676897

[22] Bartosińska JP, Pietrzak A, Szepietowski J, Dreiher J, Maciejewski R, Chodorowska G. Traditional Chinese medicine herbs-are they safe for psoriatic patients? Folia Histochem Cytobiol. 2011;**49**:201–205.

[23] Chen YJ, Chen YY, Wu CY, Chi CC. Oral Chinese herbal medicine in combination with phototherapy for vitiligo: a systematic review and meta-analysis of randomized controlled trials. Complement Ther Med. 2016;**26**:21–27. doi:10.1016/j.ctim.2016.02.009

[24] Reuter J, Wölfle U, Korting HC, Schempp C. Which plant for which skin disease? Part 2: Dermatophytes, chronic venous insufficiency, photoprotection, actinic keratoses, vitiligo, hair loss, cosmetic indications. J Dtsch Dermatol Ges. 2010;**8**:866–873. doi:10.1111/j.1610-0387.2010.07472.x

[25] Huebner J, Mohr P, Simon JC, Fluck M, Berking C, Zimmer L et al. Use of complementary medicine in metastatic melanoma patients treated with ipilimumab within a clinical trial. J Dtsch Dermatol Ges. 2016;**14**:508–513. doi:10.1111/ddg.12750

[26] Loquai C, Dechent D, Garzarolli M, Kaatz M, Kaehler KC, Kurschat P et al. Risk of interactions between complementary and alternative medicine and medication for comorbidities in patients with melanoma. Med Oncol. 2016;**33**:52. doi:10.1007/s12032-016-0764-6

[27] Ernst E. The usage of complementary therapies by dermatological patients: a systematic review. Br J Dermatol. 2000;**142**:857–861.

[28] See A, Teo B, Kwan R, Lim R, Lee J, Tang MB et al. Use of complementary and alternative medicine among dermatology outpatients in Singapore. Australas J Dermatol. 2011;**52**:7–13. doi:10.1111/j.1440-0960.2010.00709.x

[29] Chen YF, Chang JS. Complementary and alternative medicine use among patients attending a hospital dermatology clinic in Taiwan. Int J Dermatol. 2003;**42**:616–621.

[30] Gönül M, Gül U, Cakmak SK, Kiliç S. Unconventional medicine in dermatology outpatients in Turkey. Int J Dermatol. 2009;**48**:639–644. doi:10.1111/j.1365-4632.2009.04043.x

[31] Bilgili SG, Ozkol HU, Karadag AS, Calka O. The use of complementary and alternative medicine among dermatology outpatients in Eastern Turkey. Hum Exp Toxicol. 2014;**33**:214–221. doi:10.1177/0960327113494904

[32] Sivamani RK, Morley JE, Rehal B, Armstrong AW. Comparative prevalence of complementary and alternative medicine use among outpatients in dermatology and primary care clinics. JAMA Dermatol. 2014;**150**:1363–1365. doi:10.1001/jamadermatol.2014.2274

[33] Thas JJ. Siddha medicine—background and principles and the application for skin diseases. Clin Dermatol. 2008;**26**:62–78. doi:10.1016/j.clindermatol.2007.11.010

[34] Zhang NN, Park DK, Park HJ. Hair growth-promoting activity of hot water extract of *Thuja orientalis*. BMC Complement Altern Med. 2013;**13**:9. doi:10.1186/1472-6882-13-9

[35] Naser B, Bodinet C, Tegtmeier M, Lindequist U. *Thuja occidentalis* (*Arbor vitae*): a review of its pharmaceutical, pharmacological and clinical properties. Evid Based Complement Alternat Med. 2005;**2**:69–78. doi:10.1093/ecam/neh065

[36] Park WS, Lee CH, Lee BG, Chang IS. The extract of *Thujae occidentalis* semen inhibited 5alpha-reductase and androchronogenetic alopecia of B6CBAF1/j hybrid mouse. J Dermatol Sci. 2003;**31**:91–98.

[37] Seo SR, Kang G, Ha JW, Kim JC. In vivo hair growth-promoting efficacies of herbal extracts and their cubosomal suspensions. J Ind Eng Chem. 2013;19:1331–1339. doi:10.1016/j.jiec.2012.12.037

[38] Roy RK, Thakur M, Dixit VK. Effect of *Citrullus colocynthis* on hair growth in albino rats. Pharm Biol. 2007;**45**:739–744. doi:10.1080/13880200701585709

[39] Dhanotia R, Chauhan NS, Saraf DK, Dixit VK. Effect of Citrullus colocynthis Schrad fruits on testosterone-induced alopecia. Nat Prod Res. 2011;**25**:1432–1443. doi:10.1080/14786410802632820

[40] Roy RK, Thakur M, Dixit VK. Development and evaluation of polyherbal formulation for hair growth-promoting activity. J Cosmet Dermatol. 2007;**6**:108–112. doi:10.1111/j.1473-2165.2007.00305.x

[41] Ulbricht C, Abrams TR, Brigham A, Ceurvels J, Clubb J, Curtiss W et al. An evidence-based systematic review of rosemary (Rosmarinus officinalis) by the Natural Standard Research Collaboration. J Diet Suppl. 2010;**7**:351–413. doi:10.3109/19390211.2010.525049

[42] Angioni A, Barra A, Cereti E, Barile D, Coïsson JD, Arlorio M et al. Chemical composition, plant genetic differences, antimicrobial and antifungal activity investigation of the essential oil of Rosmarinus officinalis L. J Agric Food Chem. 2004;**52**:3530–3535. doi:10.1021/jf049913t

[43] Murata K, Noguchi K, Kondo M, Onishi M, Watanabe N, Okamura K et al. Promotion of hair growth by Rosmarinus officinalis leaf extract. Phytother Res. 2013;**27**:212–217. doi:10.1002/ptr.4712

[44] Suzuki Y, Miyoshi N, Isemura M. Health-promoting effects of green tea. Proc Jpn Acad Ser B Phys Biol Sci. 2012;**88**:88–101.

[45] Zink A, Traidl-Hoffmann C. Green tea in dermatology—myths and facts. J Dtsch Dermatol Ges. 2015;**13**:768–775. doi:10.1111/ddg.12737

[46] Barbosa NS, Kalaaji AN. CAM use in dermatology. Is there a potential role for honey, green tea, and vitamin C? Complement Ther Clin Pract. 2014;**20**:11–15. doi:10.1016/j.ctcp.2013.11.003

[47] Baumann LS. Less-known botanical cosmeceuticals. Dermatol Ther. 2007;**20**:330–342. doi:10.1111/j.1529-8019.2007.00147.x

[48] Kwon OS, Han JH, Yoo HG, Chung JH, Cho KH, Eun HC et al. Human hair growth enhancement in vitro by green tea epigallocatechin-3-gallate (EGCG). Phytomedicine. 2007;**14**:551–555. doi:10.1016/j.phymed.2006.09.009

[49] Esfandiari A, Kelly AP. The effects of tea polyphenolic compounds on hair loss among rodents. J Natl Med Assoc. 2005;**97**:1165–1169.

[50] Sinn BT, Kelly LM, Freudenstein JV. Phylogenetic relationships in Asarum: effect of data partitioning and a revised classification. Am J Bot. 2015;**102**:765–779. doi:10.3732/ajb.1400316

[51] Oh SM, Kim J, Lee J, Yi JM, Oh DS, Bang OS et al. Anticancer potential of an ethanol extract of Asiasari radix against HCT-116 human colon cancer cells in vitro. Oncol Lett. 2013;**5**:305–310. doi:10.3892/ol.2012.1012

[52] Rho SS, Park SJ, Hwang SL, Lee MH, Kim CD, Lee IH, Chang SY, Rang MJ. The hair growth promoting effect of Asiasari radix extract and its molecular regulation. J Dermatol Sci. 2005;**38**:89–97. doi:10.1016/j.jdermsci.2004.12.025

[53] Sharquie KE, Al-Obaidi HK. Onion juice (Allium cepa L.), a new topical treatment for alopecia areata. J Dermatol. 2002;29:343–346.

[54] Sengupta A, Ghosh S, Bhattacharjee S. Allium vegetables in cancer prevention: an overview. Asian Pac J Cancer Prev. 2004;**5**:237–245.

[55] Park HJ, Zhang N, Park DK. Topical application of Polygonum multiflorum extract induces hair growth of resting hair follicles through upregulating Shh and β-catenin expression in C57BL/6 mice. J Ethnopharmacol. 2011;**135**:369–375. doi:10.1016/j.jep.2011.03.028

[56] Lin L, Ni B, Lin H, Zhang M, Li X, Yin X et al. Traditional usages, botany, phytochemistry, pharmacology and toxicology of Polygonum multiflorum Thunb.: a review. J Ethnopharmacol. 2015;**159**:158–183. doi:10.1016/j.jep.2014.11.009

[57] Sun YN, Cui L, Li W, Yan XT, Yang SY, Kang JI et al. Promotion effect of constituents from the root of Polygonum multiflorum on hair growth. Bioorg Med Chem Lett. 2013;**23**:4801–4805. doi:10.1016/j.bmcl.2013.06.098

[58] Li Y, Han M, Lin P, He Y, Yu J, Zhao R. Hair growth promotion activity and its mechanism of polygonum multiflorum. Evid Based Complement Alternat Med. 2015;**2015**:517901. doi:10.1155/2015/517901

[59] Park KM, Kim DW, Lee SH. Extract of Allium tuberosum Rottler ex Spreng promoted the hair growth through regulating the expression of IGF-1. Evid Based Complement Alternat Med. 2015;**2015**:413538. doi:10.1155/2015/413538

[60] Cho YH, Lee SY, Jeong DW, Choi EJ, Kim YJ, Lee JG et al. Effect of pumpkin seed oil on hair growth in men with androgenetic alopecia: a randomized, double-blind, placebo-controlled trial. Evid Based Complement Alternat Med. 2014;**2014**:549721. doi:10.1155/2014/549721

[61] Khalaf EM, Raizada MN. Taxonomic and functional diversity of cultured seed associated microbes of the cucurbit family. BMC Microbiol. 2016;**16**:131. doi:10.1186/s12866-016-0743-2

[62] Rossi A, Mari E, Scarno M, Garelli V, Maxia C, Scali E et al. Comparitive effectiveness of finasteride vs Serenoa repens in male androgenetic alopecia: a two-year study. Int J Immunopathol Pharmacol. 2012;**25**:1167–1173.

[63] Murugusundram S. Serenoa Repens: Does it have any role in the management of androgenetic alopecia? J Cutan Aesthet Surg. 2009;**2**:31–32. doi:10.4103/0974-2077.53097

[64] Chittur S, Parr B, Marcovici G. Inhibition of inflammatory gene expression in keratinocytes using a composition containing carnitine, thioctic acid and saw palmetto extract. Evid Based Complement Alternat Med. 2011;**2011**:985345. doi:10.1093/ecam/nep102

[65] Wessagowit V, Tangjaturonrusamee C, Kootiratrakarn T, Bunnag T, Pimonrat T, Muangdang N et al. Treatment of male androgenetic alopecia with topical products containing Serenoa repens extract. Australas J Dermatol. 2016;**57**:76–82. doi:10.1111/ajd.12352

[66] Sinclair RD, Mallari RS, Tate B. Sensitization to saw palmetto and minoxidil in separate topical extemporaneous treatments for androgenetic alopecia. Australas J Dermatol. 2002;**43**:311–312.

[67] Shin BK, Kwon SW, Park JH. Chemical diversity of ginseng saponins from Panax ginseng. J Ginseng Res. 2015;**39**:287–298. doi:10.1016/j.jgr.2014.12.005

[68] Ru W, Wang D, Xu Y, He X, Sun YE, Qian L et al. Chemical constituents and bioactivities of Panax ginseng (C. A. Mey.). Drug Discov Ther. 2015;**9**:23–32. doi:10.5582/ddt.2015.01004

[69] Park GH, Park KY, Cho HI, Lee SM, Han JS, Won CH et al. Red ginseng extract promotes the hair growth in cultured human hair follicles. J Med Food. 2015;**18**:354–362. doi:10.1089/jmf.2013.3031

[70] Ryu HJ, Yoo MG, Son SW. The efficacy of 3% minoxidil vs. combined 3% minoxidil and Korean red ginseng in treating female pattern alopecia. Int J Dermatol. 2014;**53**:340–342. doi:10.1111/ijd.12359

[71] Oh GN, Son SW. Efficacy of korean red ginseng in the treatment of alopecia areata. J Ginseng Res. 2012;**36**:391–395. doi:10.5142/jgr.2012.36.4.391

[72] Shin DH, Cha YJ, Yang KE, Jang IS, Son CG, Kim BH et al. Ginsenoside Rg3 up-regulates the expression of vascular endothelial growth factor in human dermal papilla cells and mouse hair follicles. Phytother Res. 2014;**28**:1088–1095. doi:10.1002/ptr.5101

[73] Park S, Shin WS, Ho J. Fructus panax ginseng extract promotes hair regeneration in C57BL/6 mice. J Ethnopharmacol. 2011;**138**:340–344. doi:10.1016/j.jep.2011.08.013

[74] Jahan R, Al-Nahain A, Majumder S, Rahmatullah M. Ethnopharmacological significance of Eclipta alba (L.) Hassk. (Asteraceae). Int Sch Res Notices. 2014;**2014**:385969. doi:10.1155/2014/385969

[75] Datta K, Singh AT, Mukherjee A, Bhat B, Ramesh B, Burman AC. Eclipta alba extract with potential for hair growth promoting activity. J Ethnopharmacol. 2009;**124**:450–456. doi:10.1016/j.jep.2009.05.023

[76] Begum S, Lee MR, Gu LJ, Hossain J, Sung CK. Exogenous stimulation with Eclipta alba promotes hair matrix keratinocyte proliferation and downregulates TGF-β1 expression in nude mice. Int J Mol Med. 2015;**35**:496–502. doi:10.3892/ijmm.2014.2022

[77] Roy RK, Thakur M, Dixit VK. Hair growth promoting activity of Eclipta alba in male albino rats. Arch Dermatol Res. 2008;**300**:357–364. doi:10.1007/s00403-008-0860-3

[78] Tahergorabi Z, Abedini MR, Mitra M, Fard MH, Beydokhti H. "Ziziphus jujuba": a red fruit with promising anticancer activities. Pharmacogn Rev. 2015;**9**:99–106. doi:10.4103/0973-7847.162108

[79] Yoon JI, Al-Reza SM, Kang SC. Hair growth promoting effect of Zizyphus jujuba essential oil. Food Chem Toxicol. 2010;**48**:1350–1354. doi:10.1016/j.fct.2010.02.036

[80] Pazyar N, Feily A. Garlic in dermatology. Dermatol Rep. 2011;**3**:e4. doi:10.4081/dr.2011.e4

[81] Hajheydari Z, Jamshidi M, Akbari J, Mohammadpour R. Combination of topical garlic gel and betamethasone valerate cream in the treatment of localized alopecia areata: a double-blind randomized controlled study. Indian J Dermatol Venereol Leprol. 2007;**73**:29–32.

[82] Jain R, Monthakantirat O, Tengamnuay P, De-Eknamkul W. Avicequinone C isolated from Avicennia marina exhibits 5α-reductase-type 1 inhibitory activity using an androgenic alopecia relevant cell-based assay system. Molecules. 2014;**19**:6809–6821. doi:10.3390/molecules19056809

[83] Jain R, Monthakantirat O, Tengamnuay P, De-Eknamkul W. Identification of a new plant extract for androgenic alopecia treatment using a non-radioactive human hair dermal papilla cell-based assay. BMC Complement Altern Med. 2016;**16**:18. doi:10.1186/s12906-016-1004-5

[84] Mao X, Wu LF, Guo HL, Chen WJ, Cui YP, Qi Q et al. The genus Phyllanthus: an ethnopharmacological, phytochemical, and pharmacological review. Evid Based Complement Alternat Med. 2016;**2016**:7584952. doi:10.1155/2016/7584952

[85] Patel S, Sharma V, S Chauhan N, Thakur M, Dixit VK. Evaluation of hair growth promoting activity of Phyllanthus niruri. Avicenna J Phytomed. 2015;**5**:512–519.

[86] Choi JS, Jeon MH, Moon WS, Moon JN, Cheon EJ, Kim JW et al. In vivo hair growth-promoting effect of rice bran extract prepared by supercritical carbon dioxide fluid. Biol Pharm Bull. 2014;**37**:44–53.

[87] Goufo P, Trindade H. Rice antioxidants: phenolic acids, flavonoids, anthocyanins, proanthocyanidins, tocopherols, tocotrienols, γ-oryzanol, and phytic acid. Food Sci Nutr. 2014;**2**:75–104. doi:10.1002/fsn3.86

[88] Choi JS, Park JB, Moon WS, Moon JN, Son SW, Kim MR. Safety and efficacy of rice bran supercritical CO_2 extract for hair growth in androgenic alopecia: a 16-week double-blind randomized controlled trial. Biol Pharm Bull. 2015;**38**:1856–1863. doi:10.1248/bpb.b15-00387

[89] Takahashi T, Ishino A, Arai T, Hamada C, Nakazawa Y, Iwabuchi T et al. Improvement of androgenetic alopecia with topical Sophora flavescens Aiton extract, and identification of the two active compounds in the extract that stimulate proliferation of human hair keratinocytes. Clin Exp Dermatol. 2016;**41**:302–307. doi:10.1111/ced.12753

[90] Zheng K, Li C, Shan X, Liu H, Fan W, Wang Z. A study on isolation of chemical constituents from Sophora flavescens Ait. and their anti-glioma effects. Afr J Tradit Complement Altern Med. 2013;**11**:156–160.

[91] Wang L, Li F, Lu J, Li G, Li D, Zhong XB et al. The Chinese herbal medicine Sophora flavescens activates pregnane X receptor. Drug Metab Dispos. 2010;**38**:2226–2231. doi:10.1124/dmd.110.035253

[92] Park MJ, Han JS. Protective effects of the fermented Laminaria japonica extract on oxidative damage in LLC-PK1 cells. Prev Nutr Food Sci. 2013;**18**:227–233. doi:10.3746/pnf.2013.18.4.227

[93] Park SK, Park SJ, Park SM, Cho IJ, Park CI, Kim YW et al. Inhibition of acute phase inflammation by Laminaria japonica through regulation of iNOS-NF- κ B pathway. Evid Based Complement Alternat Med. 2013;**2013**:439498. doi:10.1155/2013/439498

[94] Shin K, Kim TS, Kyung J, Kim D, Park D, Choi EK et al. Effectiveness of the combinational treatment of Laminaria japonica and Cistanche tubulosa extracts in hair growth. Lab Anim Res. 2015;**31**:24–32. doi:10.5625/lar.2015.31.1.24

[95] Begum S, Gu LJ, Lee MR, Li Z, Li JJ, Hossain MJ et al. In vivo hair growth-stimulating effect of medicinal plant extract on BALB/c nude mice. Pharm Biol. 2015;**53**:1098–1103. doi:10.3109/13880209.2014.959614

[96] Chang KM, Kim GH. Volatiles of Chrysanthemum zawadskii var. latilobum K. Prev Nutr Food Sci. 2012;**17**:234–238. doi:10.3746/pnf.2012.17.3.234

[97] Guo X, Wang X, Su W, Zhang G, Zhou R. DNA barcodes for discriminating the medicinal plant Scutellaria baicalensis (Lamiaceae) and its adulterants. Biol Pharm Bull. 2011;**34**:1198–203.

[98] Kim AR, Kim SN, Jung IK, Kim HH, Park YH, Park WS. The inhibitory effect of Scutellaria baicalensis extract and its active compound, baicalin, on the translocation of the androgen receptor with implications for preventing androgenetic alopecia. Planta Med. 2014;**80**:153–158. doi:10.1055/s-0033-1360300

[99] Patel S, Sharma V, Chauhan NS, Dixit VK. A study on the extracts of Cuscuta reflexa Roxb. in treatment of cyclophosphamide induced alopecia. Daru. 2014;**22**:7. doi:10.1186/2008-2231-22-7

[100] Patel S, Sharma V, Chauhan NS, Dixit VK. An updated review on the parasitic herb of Cuscuta reflexa Roxb. Zhong Xi Yi Jie He Xue Bao. 2012;**10**:249–255.

[101] Pandit S, Chauhan NS, Dixit VK. Effect of Cuscuta reflexa Roxb on androgen-induced alopecia. J Cosmet Dermatol. 2008;**7**:199–204. doi:10.1111/j.1473-2165.2008.00389.x

[102] Kang JI, Kim EJ, Kim MK, Jeon YJ, Kang SM, Koh YS et al. The promoting effect of Ishige sinicola on hair growth. Mar Drugs. 2013;**11**:1783–1799. doi:10.3390/md11061783

[103] Cho M, Park GM, Kim SN, Amna T, Lee S, Shin WS. Glioblastoma-specific anticancer activity of pheophorbide a from the edible red seaweed Grateloupia elliptica. J Microbiol Biotechnol. 2014;**24**:346–353.

[104] Kang JI, Kim SC, Han SC, Hong HJ, Jeon YJ, Kim B et al. Hair-loss preventing effect of Grateloupia elliptica. Biomol Ther (Seoul). 2012;**20**:118–124. doi:10.4062/biomolther.2012.20.1.118

[105] Murata K, Noguchi K, Kondo M, Onishi M, Watanabe N, Okamura K et al. Inhibitory activities of Puerariae Flos against testosterone 5α-reductase and its hair growth promotion activities. J Nat Med. 2012;**66**:158–165. doi:10.1007/s11418-011-0570-6

[106] Shin JE, Bae EA, Lee YC, Ma JY, Kim DH. Estrogenic effect of main components kakkalide and tectoridin of Puerariae Flos and their metabolites. Biol Pharm Bull. 2006;**29**:1202–1206.

[107] Pumthong G, Asawanonda P, Varothai S, Jariyasethavong V, Triwongwaranat D, Suthipinittharm P et al. Curcuma aeruginosa, a novel botanically derived 5α-reductase inhibitor in the treatment of male-pattern baldness: a multicenter, randomized, double-blind, placebo-controlled study. J Dermatolog Treat. 2012;**23**:385–392. doi:10.3109/09546634.2011.568470

[108] Hossain CF, Al-Amin M, Sayem AS, Siragee IH, Tunan AM, Hassan F et al. Antinociceptive principle from Curcuma aeruginosa. BMC Complement Altern Med. 2015;**15**:191. doi:10.1186/s12906-015-0720-6

[109] Uchiyama C, Ishida K, Tsutsui T, Naito A, Kurita K, Hanihara H et al. Effects of Hura crepitans and its active ingredient, daphne factor F3, on dihydrotestosterone-induced neurotrophin-4 activation and hair retardation. Biol Pharm Bull. 2012;**35**:42–47.

[110] Barbieri L, Falasca A, Franceschi C, Licastro F, Rossi CA, Stirpe F. Purification and properties of two lectins from the latex of the euphorbiaceous plants Hura crepitans L. (sand-box tree) and Euphorbia characias L. (Mediterranean spurge). Biochem J. 1983;**215**:433–439.

[111] Murkute AV, Sahu MS, Mali PY, Rangari VD. Development and evaluation of formulations of microbial biotransformed extract of tobacco leaves for hair growth potential. Pharmacognosy Res. 2010;**2**:300–303. doi:10.4103/0974-8490.72328

[112] Talianova M, Janousek B. What can we learn from tobacco and other Solanaceae about horizontal DNA transfer? Am J Bot. 2011;**98**:1231–1242. doi:10.3732/ajb.1000370

[113] Jaybhaye D, Varma S, Gagne N, Bonde V, Gite A, Bhosle D. Effect of Tectona grandis Linn. seeds on hair growth activity of albino mice. Int J Ayurveda Res. 2010;**1**:211–215. doi:10.4103/0974-7788.76783

[114] Nayeem N, Karvekar M. Anti microbial and anti-oxidant properties of the isolated compounds from the methanolic extract from the leaves of Tectona grandis. J Basic Clin Pharm. 2011;**2**:163–165.

[115] Shimizu K, Kondo R, Sakai K, Shoyama Y, Sato H, Ueno T. Steroid 5alpha-reductase inhibitory activity and hair regrowth effects of an extract from Boehmeria nipononivea. Biosci Biotechnol Biochem. 2000;**64**:875–877.

[116] Tan EK, Millington GW, Levell NJ. Acupuncture in dermatology: an historical perspective. Int J Dermatol. 2009;**48**:648–652. doi:10.1111/j.1365-4632.2009.03899.x

[117] Lee HW, Jun JH, Lee JA, Lim HJ, Lim HS, Lee MS. Acupuncture for treating alopecia areata: a protocol of systematic review of randomised clinical trials. BMJ Open. 2015;**5**:e008841. doi:10.1136/bmjopen-2015-008841

[118] Maeda T, Taniguchi M, Matsuzaki S, Shingaki K, Kanazawa S, Miyata S. Anti-inflammatory effect of electroacupuncture in the C3H/HeJ mouse model of alopecia areata. Acupunct Med. 2013;**31**:117–119. doi:10.1136/acupmed-2012-010240

[119] Shenefelt PD. Hypnosis in dermatology. Arch Dermatol. 2000;**136**:393–399.

[120] Häuser W, Hagl M, Schmierer A, Hansen E. The efficacy, safety and applications of medical hypnosis. Dtsch Arztebl Int. 2016;**113**:289–296. doi:10.3238/arztebl.2016.0289

[121] Willemsen R, Vanderlinden J, Deconinck A, Roseeuw D. Hypnotherapeutic management of alopecia areata. J Am Acad Dermatol. 2006;**55**:233–237. doi:10.16/j.jaad.2005.09.025

[122] Willemsen R, Haentjens P, Roseeuw D, Vanderlinden J. Hypnosis in refractory alopecia areata significantly improves depression, anxiety, and life quality but not hair regrowth. J Am Acad Dermatol. 2010;**62**:517–518. doi:10.1016/j.jaad.2009.06.029

[123] Cohen HA, Barzilai A, Lahat E. Hypnotherapy: an effective treatment modality for trichotillomania. Acta Paediatr. 1999;**88**:407–410.

[124] Iglesias A. Hypnosis as a vehicle for choice and self-agency in the treatment of children with Trichotillomania. Am J Clin Hypn. 2003;**46**:129–137. doi:10.1080/00029157.2003.10403583

[125] Zalsman G, Hermesh H, Sever J. Hypnotherapy in adolescents with trichotillomania: three cases. Am J Clin Hypn. 2001;**44**:63–68. doi:10.1080/00029157.2001.10403457

[126] Almazan TH, Jung JY. Prurigo nodularis after acupuncture. JAAD Case Rep. 2015;**1**:345–347. doi:10.1016/j.jdcr.2015.08.004